TEXTBOOK of PSYCHIATRIC NURSING

Volume – II

Dr. Bimla Kapoor (RN, RM)

Ph.D., M.Phil., M.Sc.(Nursing) PGDDE, M.A. in Sociology
Professor, School of Health Sciences, IGNOU, New Delhi
Formerly Sr. Faculty, R.A.K. College of Nursing,
University of Delhi

KUMAR PUBLISHING HOUSE

Publishers of :
Medical and Nursing Books
PD/11-12B, Vishakha Enclave, Near N.D. Market,
Pitampura, Delhi - 110034 (India)
Tel.: 47074056, 47507880, 32411029, 32911047 | Mob. 9810124056, 9311111029
E-Mail: kphnursingbooks@gmail.com | kumar_bookdepot@yahoo.co.in
Website: www.kphnursingbooks.com

First Edition	:	1994
Reprint	:	1998
Reprint	:	1999
Reprint	:	2000
Reprint	:	2001
Reprint	:	2002
Reprint	:	2003
Reprint	:	2004
Reprint	:	2005
Reprint	:	2006
Reprint	:	2007
IInd Reprint	:	2007
Reprint	:	2008
IInd Reprint	:	2008
Reprint	:	2009
IInd Reprint	:	2009
Reprint	:	2010
IInd Reprint	:	2010
Reprint	:	2011
Reprint	:	2012
Reprint	:	2013
Reprint	:	2014
Reprint	:	2015
Reprint	:	**2016**

Price : ₹400.00

ISBN: 978-81-924060-2-2

Typesetting by Satendra Singh

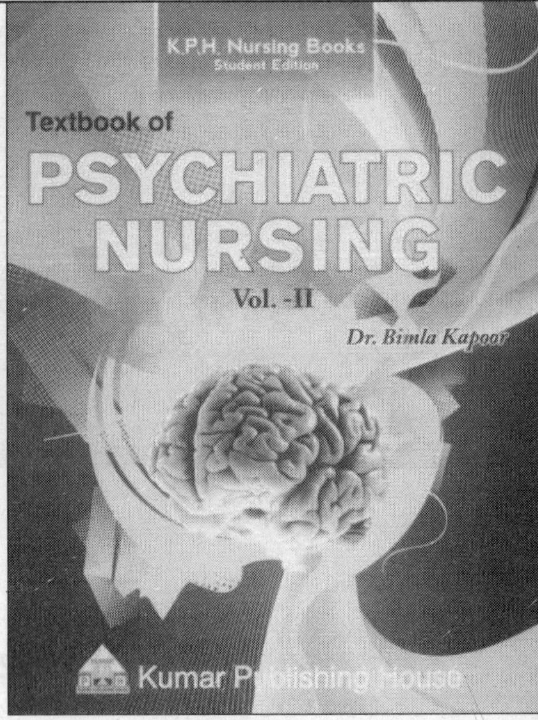

Dr. Bimla Kapoor (RN, RM)

Ph.D., M.Phil., M.Sc.(Nursing) PGDDE. M.A. in Sociology
Professor, School of Health Sciences, IGNOU, New Delhi
Formerly Sr. Faculty, R.A.K. College of Nursing, University of Delhi.

Published by :

Neelam Kumar

Kumar Publishing House

PD/11-12B, Vishakha Enclave, Near N.D. Market, Pitampura, Delhi - 110034 (India)

E-Mail: kphnursingbooks@gmail.com | **Website:** www.kphnursingbooks.com

FOREWORD

I am very happy to write a foreword for the much, expected second volume of the book "A Text Book of Psychiatric Nursing" written by Mrs. Bimla Kapoor, teaching psychiatric nursing at Rajkumari Amrit Kaur College of Nursing, New Delhi.

It is a well known fact that there is a dirth of books in nursing written by Indian authors in Indian context. The present book has tried to make up this difficiency in the field of Psychiatric Nursing.

It is important that text books for nurses must be written in a way that it enables both students and practitioners to improve and enlarge their current knowledge. Since nursing is essentially a profession of practice, the textbooks should also be able to enrich their practice. The present book has taken this point very seriously and one can see the component of theory and practices going side-by-side. The author has vast experience in the field of psychiatric nursing and as such has also taken valuable suggestions from nursing tutors and colleagues to make the book interesting, comprehensive as well as updated with current knowledge in the field of psychiatry and psychiatric nursing.

The teachers teaching the subject and the postgraduate students of nursing will find this book useful for ready reference. I may go one step further to suggest that the medical students will also find this book useful to clear their concepts.

Another area in nursing which must receive active attention of nurse teachers, students and nurse practitioners is in legal aspects of nursing practice. The author has to certain extent dealt with this where she has written on legal aspects of psychiatric nursing.

The teachers, students and the author felt the need to have a comprehensive book on psychiatric nursing which will deal with the content, problems, management emerging trends and current issues. The attempt of the author to write a book of this nature is laudable.

I am confident that the students, teachers and practitioners of psychiatry nursing will make good use of this book to develop better understanding and insight into the problems associated with mental health. This will help them to deal with the various challenges of mental health psychiatric nursing leading ultimately to improve client care.

Bandana Bhattacharya

PREFACE

"Textbook of Psychiatric Nursing Vol.—II" is a continuation of "Textbook of Psychiatric Nursing Vol.—I"

The content of Textbook of Psychiatric Nursing Vol.—II is prepared keeping in mind the need for learning the psychiatric courses in General Nursing and Midwifery, B.Sc. Nursing, Graduate Nurses who have undergone the old nursing curriculum and nurses registered with Open Universities for Post-basic B.Sc. The book can be used as a ready reference by M.Sc. Nursing students.

Textbook of Psychiatric Nursing Vol.—I has four chapters with 11 units. In sequal Volume II contains V to IX chapters with units from 12 to 26 instead of Units from 12 to 22 as mentioned in Preface Vol. I. It is due to the facts that while writing the Vol. II of the book, I felt that it is essential to add four more units to make the book more comprehensive.

The text book of Psychiatric Nursing Volume—II contains accepted contemporary practices in mental health—psychiatric nursing. It includes theoretical approaches to psychiatric nursing, therapeutic modalities, mental and behaviour disorders and their management. The book deals in detail the nursing management aspects using nursing process and has prepared nursing care plans for guidance in practice, to enable the nurses give better client oriented care. It has also focussed on other aspects of psychiatric nursing which includes community & psychiatric mental health nursing the mental health team and the scope of the psychiatric mental health nurse.

The ICD-10 Classification of Mental and Behavioural Disorders, Clinical Description and Diagnostic Guidelines, Geneva, World Health Organization, 1992 (pp. 22-40) is also included.

The last page of the book is a form which is attached to get reader's feedback. Readers can send the suggestions, corrections and reactions for further improvement.

I am thankful to Mrs. Bandana Bhattacharya, Principal "Rajkumari Amrit Kaur College of Nursing", Dr. (Miss) Aparna Bhaduri, Ex. Professor "Rajkumari Amrit Kaur College of Nursing", and Miss Krishna Kumari Gulani, Senior Lecturer, "Rajkumari Amrit Kaur College of Nursing", for constantly encouraging and motivating me to complete this book.

I am indeed thankful to all the Nurse Educators and Readers of Textbook of Psychiatric Nursing Vol—I who had been really a true motivating force behind the completion of book.

My thanks are due to Dr. R.C. Jiloha, Professor, Maulana Azad Medical College, Department of Psychiatry, G.B. Pant Hospital, for going through the content of the book and providing invaluable suggestions and guidance. I am also thankful to the clinical teachers of Rajkumari Amrit Kaur College of Nursing" (Department of Psychiatry Nursing) of endorsing clinical incorporation in the content.

My thanks are also due to World Health Organization for granting the permission to much useful pp. 22-40 from ICD-10 Classification of Mental and Behavioural Disorders, Clinical Description and Diagnostic Guidelines, Geneva, World Health Organization, 1992.

I am also thankful to Mr. Jagan Nath and Mr. S.B. Thapa for editing of this book.

All suggestions are welcome and will be duly acknowledged.

Bimla Kapoor

Contents

CHAPTER V

THERAPEUTIC RELATIONSHIP

CHAPTER VI

THERAPEUTIC MODALITIES

CHAPTER VII

MENTAL AND BEHAVIOUR DISORDERS

CHAPTER VIII

NURSING INTERVENTIONS OF MENTAL AND BEHAVIOUR-DISORDERED PATIENTS

CHAPTER IX

OTHER ASPECTS OF PSYCHIATRIC NURSING

CHAPTER V

THERAUPEUTIC RELATIONSHIP

UNIT-XII

THEORETICAL APPROACHES TO PSYCHIATRIC NURSING CARE

UNIT OUTLINE

Definition of theory.

Types of Theories used by Psychiatric Mental Health Nurse:

- Psycho-analytic Theory.
- Interpersonal Theory.
- Behavioural Theory.
- Humanistic Theory.
- Stress Theory.
- Eclectic Approach.
- Application to Nursing.

- Better Study Section.

INTENDED LEARNING BEHAVIOUR

After reading this unit you will be able to:

a) Explain the concept of theory.
b) List the types of theories used by Psychiatric Nurse.
c) Describe psycho-analytic approach & its uses in psychiatric nursing.
d) Discuss and apply the interpersonal approach.
e) Use the behavioural theory in therapeutic intervention.
f) Identify the stressors.
g) Apply the eclectic approach in caring of patients.

CONTENTS

INTRODUCTION

Nursing practice is based on theoretical concepts. Theory guides the nurse to understand human behaviour and implement the nursing care plan effectively on patients with maladaptive behaviour.

DEFINITION OF THEORY

Theory is a belief, policy or procedure followed as the basis of action. (Webster New Collegiate Dictionary). In selecting a theoretical approach, the psychiatric nurse uses other considerations also such as the client's behaviour, values, belief, resources available, the treatment setting i.e. hospital or community, societal and political influences. One theory may not include all these complex factors. A nurse selects the best from various theories and gives comprehensive care to the patient. In other words, she uses the Eclectic Approach (Selecting what appears to be the best in various methods).

Theories of human behaviour discussed in this unit are used for understanding human behaviour from different perspectives. The theories used by psychiatric/mental health nurses fall into six categories:

* Psychoanalytic Theory.
* Interpersonal Theory.

* Behavioural Theory.
* Humanistic Theory.
* Stress Theory.
* Biological Theory.
* Eclectic Approach.

TO RECALL

* **Theory is a belief, policy or procedure followed as the basis of action.**
* **Eclectic approach is used in nursing i.e. selecting what appears to be the best in all theories.**

PSYCHOANALYTIC THEORY

The psychoanalytic theory is derived from the work of Sigmaund Freud and his followers (Carl Jung and Erik Erikson). The Psychoanalytic theory is based on the following aspects according to Freud :

1. Psychic Energy.
2. Instinct.
3. The Distribution and Disposal of Psychic Energy - ID, Ego and Superego.
4. Cathexis and Anti-Cathexis.
5. Consciousness and Unconsciousness.
6. Anxiety.

PSYCHIC ENERGY

The human organism is a complicated energy system, deriving its energy from the food it eats and expending it for such purposes as circulation, respiration, digestion, nervous conduction, muscular activity, perceiving, remembering, and thinking. Energy takes many forms - mechanical, thermal, electrical, and chemical. It is capable of being transformed from one form to another. The form of energy which operates the three systems of personality is called psychic energy. Psychic energy performs psychological work — e.g. thinking, perceiving, and remembering — just as mechanical energy performs mechanical work.

INSTINCT

All the energy used for performing the work of the personality is obtained from instincts. An instinct is a sum of psychic energy which imparts direction to psychological processes. How many different instincts are there ? There are as many as there are bodily needs, since an instinct is the mental representative of a bodily need. Freud said that the question as to the number of instincts is a matter to be determined by biological investigation.

The form of energy is used by *life instincts* is called *libido*, but no special name was ever given by Freud to the form of energy employed by *death instincts*. In his earlier writings, Freud used the term "libido" to denote sexual energy; but when he revised his theory of motivation, *libido* was defined as the energy of all the life instincts. The final aim of an instinct is the removal of a bodily need. The aim of the instinct of hunger, for example, is to remove the physical condition of hunger. When this is done, no more bodily energy is released, the hunger instinct disappears, and the individual returns to a state of physiological and psychological satisfaction. Stated in another way, the aim of an instinct is to eliminate the source of that instinct.

DISTRIBUTION AND DISPOSAL OF PSYCHIC ENERGY

The distribution & disposal of Psychic Energy are of three types. They are — ID, Ego & Superego.

ID - The energy of the ID is used for instinctual gratification by means of reflex action and wish-fulfilment. In reflex action as examplified by the eating of food, the emptying of the bladder, and the sexual organism, energy is automatically discharged in motor action. In wish-fulfilment, energy is used to produce an image of the instinctual object. The aim of both processes i.e. reflex action and wish-fulfilment is to utilize the instinctual energy in ways that will eliminate the need and bring response to the individual. When ID is blocked by ego or superego processes, it tries to break through the resistances of ego and superego and discharge itself in phantasy or action. When the breakthrough is successful, the rational processes of the ego are undermined, destroyed/damaged. The person makes mistakes in speaking, writing, talking, perceiving, and remembering, and he has accidents because he becomes confused and loses contact with reality. His ability to solve problems and to discover reality is diminished.

EGO - The failure of the ID to obtain relief from tension brings about the emergence of a new line of development which lays a foundation for the formation of the ego. Instead of an image and the real object being regarded as identities, a separation between the two takes place. What happens as a result of this differentiation is the purely subjective, inner world (the mind) and an objective, outer world (the environment). If he is to be properly adjusted, the person is now confronted with the task of bringing these two worlds into harmony with one another.

The separation between mind and the physical world of reality takes place as a result of frustration and learning. As we have said before, the ID cannot satisfy the vital needs of life by reflex action or wish-fulfilment alone. Consequently, the person just has to learn the difference between images and reality if he is going to survive and that is described as Ego.

SUPEREGO - Fear of punishment and a desire for approval cause the child to identify himself with the moral precepts of his parents. This identification with the parents results in the formation of the superego. The parents are equipped with great powers of punishing or rewarding the child. Consequently, the superego is also furnished with the power to reward or to punish. The former is done by the ego-ideal, the latter by the conscience.

CATHEXIS AND ANTI-CATHEXIS

The utilization of energy in the image of an object, or in discharge action upon an object that will satisfy an instinct, is called object-choice or object-cathexis. All of the energy of the ID is utilized in object-cathexis.

The urging forces are to satisfy instinct cathexis and the checking forces are anti-cathexis. As we have seen, the ID has only cathexis while the ego and superego also possess anti-cathexis. In fact, the ego and superego come into existence because it is necessary to check the actions of the ID. However, while the processes which constitute the ego and the superego act as breaks upon the ID, the ego and superego also have their own driving forces.

CONSCIOUSNESS AND UNCONSCIOUSNESS

In the early years of psychoanalysis the central concept of Freud's theory was the unconscious. In Freud's later formulations, beginning about 1920, the unconscious was denoted from its status (as the largest and most important region of the mind to the lesser status of being a quality of mental phenomena.) Much of what had formerly been assigned to the unconscious became the ID, and the structural distinction between consciousness and unconsciousness was replaced by the three-part organization of ID, ego, and superego.

ANXIETY

Anxiety is one of the most important concepts in psychoanalytic theory. It plays an important role in the development of personality as well as in the dynamics of personality functioning. Moreover, it is of central significance in Freud's theory of the neuroses and psychoses and in the treatment of these pathological conditions.

Anxiety differs from other painful states such as tension, pain, and melancholy by some specific quality of consciousness.

Freud recognized that one could be afraid of internal dangers as well as external ones. He differentiated three types of anxiety : reality or objective anxiety, neurotic anxiety, and moral anxiety.

Psychoanalytic approach helps the psychiatric nurse to understand that human behaviour is dominated by instinctual drives, unconscious desires and motives. Though ego helps the individual to make a socially acceptable decision by overcoming conflict and by using various defence mechanisms the conflict may not resolve. As a result, the individual may lean towards maladaptive behaviour.

TO RECALL

- **Psychoanalytic theory is based on an idea that a person's overt behaviour cannot be understood completely. Human behaviour is affected by the subsystem of personality and developmental stages.**
- **Psychodynamic means the pattern of Psychic energy, instincts, the distribution and disposal of Psychic energy i.e. ID, Ego and Superego, Cathexis and Anticathexis, Consciousness and Unconsciousness and anxiety affecting the individual.**

INTER-PERSONAL THEORY

Man is a social being. His behaviour grows out of his attempts to establish a meaningful relationship with others. Significant contributions to the inter-personal theory are made by Harry Stack Sullivan, Adolf Meyer and Eric Berne.

Sullivan believed that the essence of being human is the capacity to live effectively in relationship with others. He also believed that the individual is a social being and personality development depends on the inter-action one person has with another. Inter-action means a relationship between two or more persons that results in a mutual or reciprocal action or influence (Webster New Collegiate Dictionary). Sullivan described the basic principles of the inter-personal theory as

(i) inter-personal relationship and personality development. He believed, like Freud, that development proceeds through various stages. But he described how in each stage there is involvement of different patterns of relationship.

For instance, *infancy* brings interaction with parents and there is need for contact. In *childhood*, more interaction with adults by participation in activities is required. In the stages of *Pre-adolescence* and *adolescence*, there is a gradual withdrawal of the child from parents; peer relationship becomes important. In *late adolescence* or *early adulthood*, intimate relationships with hetrosexual groups are established, resulting in a marital setting.

Failure to make progress satisfactorily through various stages may turn into a maladaptive behaviour.

(ii) The other aspect of Sullivan's theory is anxiety which has relationship in the formation of personality. Since the infant is completely dependent on "significant others" such as mother or father, mother figure like aunt for meeting his physical and psychosocial needs, lack of any of these needs will lead him/her to an insecure and anxious human being. In early childhood, if he/she perceives himself/herself being rejected he/she will have a negative self-concept which will lead him/her to maladjustment.

(iii) Socialization causes a lot of pressure on children. Appreciation and praise by others will enable the child to label him/her as "Good me" and criticism may lead to the label of "Bad me". Over a period an individual develops a "self-system" by using defence mechanisms to reduce anxiety of socialization pressures.

(iv) The other important aspects of the interpersonal theory are social exchange, social role and interpersonal accommodation.

SOCIAL EXCHANGE

Relationship is formed with each other for meeting mutual needs. It can be explained that each person in the relationship wants something from the other.

SOCIAL ROLES

Are those roles which society prescribes i.e. for teachers for priests, role of husband or wife, mother or daughter.

INTERPERSONAL ACCOMMODATION

Is the process where by two persons communicate and interact with each other to achieve their common goals and build a satisfying relationship.

Interpersonal approach will enable the nurse to understand the significance of relationship from infancy till old age. It also helps her in understanding the role expectation of people from various categories. Any problem during the interpersonal relationship with "significant people" may lead to a maladaptive behaviour.

TO RECALL

Inter-personal theory describes the significance of inter-action of an individual from infancy till old age and its effect on the mental health of the person.

BEHAVIOURAL THEORY

Behavioural theory is based on the concept that all behaviour, adaptive or maladaptive, is a product of learning. The contributors to this theory are Ivon Pavlov, John Watson and B. F. Skinner. The basic assumptions of this theory are:

* Skinner describes that behaviour is a response to stimuli from the environment. He also describes that reinforcement is essential to get the response. *Positive reinforcement* is a reward for selected behaviour. Every time a child draws a good picture, the mother's pat on his/her back is a positive reinforcement. In *negative reinforcement* one would like to avoid a response from a child. Every time after drinking milk or water the child throws the glass. As a punishment, the mother takes away the toy from the child till he/she is able to give up the bad habit. So undesirable behaviour is extinguished gradually.

* Human personality is a combination of stimulus - response habits. Neurotic symptoms are viewed as learned habits or responses that are repeatedly reinforced.

* Maladaptive behaviour can be unlearned and replaced by adaptive behaviour if the person receives an appropriate stimulus to eliminate the maladaptive learning. For example, a child can miss the school at will by complaining of headache and vomiting (maladaptive behaviour). She could be corrected by making sure that her school assignments are complete. She could be sent to school by explaining that headache and vomiting will be reduced once she attends her class. (The organic causes should be excluded).

Behavioural approach is used frequently by the psychiatric nurse to control the undesired behaviour of a mentally ill patient specially in one-to-one relationship which will be discussed in this chapter.

TO RECALL

Behavioural theory describes that all behaviour adaptive or maladaptive is a product of learning. Appropriate reinforcement helps in correcting maladaptive learning.

HUMANISTIC THEORY

Humanistic theory is based on the concept that human being has the most reliable source of knowledge about his capabilities, resources and characteristics. An individual is viewed from holistic perspective, physical, emotional, intellectual, social and spiritual. Theorists like William James, Gordon Allport, Abraham Maslow, Carl Rogers and Fritz Perls have contributed towards the humanistic theory. Self is considered as an important aspect in this theory. Carl Rogers summarized the following aspects of this theory:

* Each individual has his own private world where he is able to know about himself. His, I, Me & Myself are clear to him.

* The basic needs of an individual are towards maintenance, enhancement and self-actualization. Maslow devised the hierarchy of needs. The basic needs such as hunger, thirst, security and physical safety must be met. Then the higher needs to belong to a group,to be loved, to be looked on with esteem and to have respect of others are to be met.

The humanistic model will help the nurse to analyse that human beings lead to a friendly, cooperative and constructive behaviour. The maladaptive behaviour is selfishness, aggression and cruelty. The patient can be helped to know about himself and adapt the acceptable behaviour.

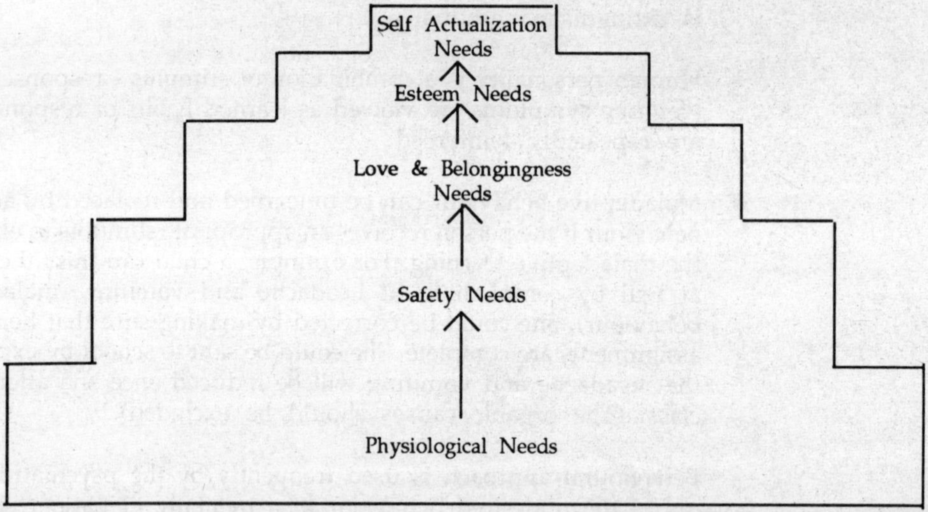

Fig. 1 : Maslow's Hierachy of Need

TO RECALL

In the humanistic theory, human being is viewed from holistic perspective which includes physical, emotional, social, intellectual and spiritual needs for which he has capabilities, resources and characteristics.

STRESS THEORY

The stress theory has contributed towards in understanding the nature and causes of diseases. The work of Walter Canon, Harold Wolff, Hans Selye and R.S. Lazarus is significant in this theory. It describes that certain stimuli perceived as threatening cause reactions which have adverse emotional, behavioural and physiological reactions. The stress theory can be summarized as:

* Stressor may cause physical or emotional disturbances in an individual. Few examples of the stressors are sickness, discomfort, emotional tension etc.

* Canon describes that an individual has a homeostasis mechanism. Homeostasis is defined as the maintenance of a normal steady state in the body. fluid and electrolyte balance, body temperature control and nervous system control are examples of homeostatic mechanisms that help to maintain equilibrium.

* Canon explained Flight-Fight alert of the body to stress. Disease is viewed as a fight to maintain the homeostatic balance of the body tissues.

* Stressor occurs throughout life.

* The process by which people adapt to stress is described as General Adaptation Syndrome (GAS) by Selye. GAS is the process that enables an individual to manage threatening situations through three stages of adaptation: (i) The Alarm Reaction (AR). This is characterized by generalised changes in the body's defence system. (ii) The Stage of Resistance (SR). In this stage the body's homeostasis system plays a role to fight against disease or emotional stress. (iii) The Stage of Exhaustion (SE). This results due to prolonged experience of stress.

* People learn to adapt to the demands of their environment through repeated experience.

From the stress theory the nurse will understand that stressor affects human beings throughout life. When the homeostasis mechanism fails the individual shows symptoms of sickness.

TO RECALL

* **The stress theory emphasizes that there are various types of stressors which may cause emotional and physical disturbances in an individual.**
* **Homeostasis maintains equilibrium.**
* **People learn to adapt to the demands of their environment through repeated experience.**
* **Biological factors are significant in causing maladaptive behaviour/mental illness.**

BIOLOGICAL THEORY

Biological factors predominate the maladaptive behaviour of an individual. Genetics and organic factors significantly influence the development of a person and his psychiatric illness. Biological factors are discussed in detail in *Chapter III Unit-VIII.*

ECLECTIC APPROACH

In the electic approach the psychiatric nurse selects the best from all the approaches and helps her patient.

Case Example:

In a group therapy session Surinder, 28, was quietly observing everyone. He listened carefully but showed inattentiveness to the surrounding. On a comment of Shiela Devi, a female patient, that Surinder was too quiet, he got up and went to his cubicle. After the group therapy was over the psychiatric nurse inquired from Surinder the reason for leaving the session. He said, "I did not want to reply that lady, so I got up and came out."

The nurse has to use a multi-theoretical approach to care for this patient. *Psychoanalytical approach* if the patient has negative transference towards Shiela Devi; Interpersonal approach so that the patient develops confidence in the nurse as well as in the group; *Behaviour approach* of limiting his action of coming away from the group. So the nurse is using an eclectic approach to help Surinder to give up his maladaptive behaviour.

TO RECALL

- **Nursing practice is based on theoretical concepts.**
- **Types of theories used by the Psychiatric/Mental Health Nurse are:**
  - **Psychoanalytic theory**
  - **Interpersonal theory**
  - **Behavioural theory**
  - **Humanistic theory**
  - **Stress theory**
  - **Biological theory**
  - **Eclectic Approach**

APPLICATION TO NURSING

Study of this unit will help the student nurse to comprehend various theories and the aspects which each theory emphasized. This will enable her to apply the knowledge of various theories in caring for the patient.

BETTER STUDY SECTION

1. VOCABULARY (USE DICTIONARY)

Adaptive	Criticism	Significant
Adverse	Driven	Threatening
Analyse	Dominated	
Attainment	Essence	
Attitude	Flight	
Belief	Implement	
Channalize	Inhibit	
Comprehend	Insecure	
Concept	Perspective	
Conflict	Reliable	

2. ASSIGNMENT

* Review Chapter II and III of Volume I. Bimla Kapoor, *A Text Book of Psychiatric Nursing, 1992.*
* Make reading notes of the approaches of theories not described in this unit.

3. EXERCISE

Discuss with your teacher and peer group the various approaches you are able to use in a psychiatric setting.

4. READING REFERENCES

* Beck, Rawlins and Williams. *Mental Health Psychiatric Nursing. A Holistic Life Cycle Approach* (Second edition) The C.V. Mosby Company, Toronto (1988).

* Bimla Kapoor. *A Textbook of Psychiatric Nursing,* Vol-I, Kumar Publishing House, Delhi, 1992.

* Coleman James C. *Abnormal Psychology and Modern Life* (Fifth edition) Scott, Foresman and Company, Glenview, Illinois, U.S.A, (1976).

* Johnson Barbara Schoen. Adaptation and Growth : *Psychiatric Mental Health Nursing.* J.B. Lippincott Company, Philadelphia U.S.A. (1989).

* Calvin S. Hall. *A Primer of Freudian Psychology.* New American Library, New York and Scarborough, Ontario, Canada (1979).

UNIT XIII
THERAPEUTIC NURSE-PATIENT RELATIONSHIP

UNIT OUTLINE

Introduction to therapeutic nurse-patient relationship.

Definition of interpersonal relationship.

Difference between professional and social relationships.

Factors determining effective nurse-patient relationship.

Goals of one-to-one relationship.

Phases of nurse-patient relationship
- * Preinteraction phase
- * Orientation phase
- * Developmental phase
- * Termination phase

Tasks which nurse has to accomplish in each phase.

Barriers in nurse-patient relationship and how to overcome them.

Application to nursing.

Better Study Section.

INTENDED LEARNING OUTCOME

After reading this unit you will be able to:

a Define therapeutic relationship.

b Explain the meaning of Nurse-Patient relationship.

c Differentiate between professional and social relationships.

d Describe the factor determining effective Nurse-Patient relationship.

e Identify the goals of nurse-patient relationship.

f Explain the phases of nurse-patient relationship
- Preinteraction phase
- Orientation phase
- Developmental phase
- Termination phase

g Identify the tasks and barriers of each phase.

h Develop skill in establishing a therapeutic relationship

i Help the patient and terminate the relationship

CONTENT

INTRODUCTION Nurse-patient relationship is a basic requirement of nursing practices. A nurse who is efficient and skillful uses the holistic approach in caring for a patient with any type of problem.

Acceptance of the community health nurse in a community also depends upon how she has developed interpersonal relationship with the people in the community.

DEFINITION OF PSYCHIATRIC NURSING

Nurse-patient relationship is significant in psychiatric nursing too. The objective of psychiatric nursing is the promotion for mental health, prevention of mental illness and care and rehabilitation of the patient with mental illness.

Travelbee Joyce, in ***Interpersonal Aspects of Nursing,*** says about Psychiatric Nursing: "Psychiatric Nursing is defined as an interpersonal process whereby the professional nurse practitioner assists an individual, family or community to promote mental health, to prevent or cope with the experience of mental illness and suffering and, if necessary, to find meaning in these experiences."

During interaction with the patient, the nurse develops a therapeutic relationship. Webster New Collegiate Dictionary (2nd edition) defines "Relationship as a character of being related or interrelated". In the nurse-patient relationship, the patient describes the nurse as "my nurse or care-giver" and the nurse refers to the patients "as patients who have entered in health care system and to be looked after by her".

TYPES OF RELATIONSHIP

The types of relationship can be *social* and *therapeutic* or *professional.* Difference between social relationship and therapeutic relationship are given in the following table:

	THERAPEUTIC RELATIONSHIP	SOCIAL RELATIONSHIP
Technique	It is a planned therapeutic relationship.	It just happens with mutual interests.
Objective	Helping the patient.	Having fun together or satisfying needs of each other.
Interaction time	Interactions are planned for specific time and place.	It may be planned, unplanned and by chance two people meet.
Duration	The length of relationship will depend on the goals. Time is limited.	This varies and may last for years.
Accountability	The nurse focuses on goals during her relationship.	It is shared, both are responsible or accountable in this relationship.
Acceptance	The nurse accepts the patient as "here and now", without attaching judgement and interest.	Acceptance of relationship is based on shared values and beliefs.
Termination	It is considered as an important part of relationship. It is planned and discussed with the patient.	The relationship may exist life long. May terminate gradually. There may be environmental factors like shifting away to another place.

Fig 2 : Table describing characteristics of therapeutic and social relationship.

TO RECALL

> *** Therapeutic relationship is developed during nurse-patient relationship.**
>
> *** Types of relationship are:**
> **- Therapeutic relationship &**
> **- Social relationship.**

DEFINITION OF NURSE-PATIENT RELATIONSHIP

Nurse-patient relationship is an interaction process in which the nurse fulfils her role by using her professional knowledge and skill in such a way that she is able to help the patient physically, socially and emotionally.

ONE-TO-ONE RELATIONSHIP

It is an interaction process between two persons in which the nurse offers a series of purposeful activities and practices that are useful to a particular patient. This therapeutic nurse-patient relationship is also termed as one-to-one relationship.

Travelbee Joyce, in her book *Intervention in Psychiatric Nursing*, defines one-to-one relationship as follows:

"One-to-one relationship is the end result of a series of planned purposeful interaction between two human beings, a nurse and a patient". In this chapter and throughout the text of the book, Nurse-Patient Relationship (NPR), therapeutic relations, one-to-one relations, Interpersonal relationship (IPR) will be used interchangeably.

FACTORS DETERMINING EFFECTIVE NURSE-PATIENT RELATIONSHIP

In the nurse-patient relationship each interaction or encounter is unique because the patient and the nurse are having their own beliefs, values, attitudes and behaviours. But some of the factors which can help her to develop an effective relationship are:

(i) Self-awareness,
(ii) Attitude towards the patient,
(iii) Ability of developing rapport including warmth and genuineness in her approach and empathizing ability.

SELF-AWARENESS

It is an important aspect which a nurse must identify in herself. Self-awareness includes ***self-concept, beliefs and values and life experiences.*** If a nurse has a positive ***self-concept*** about herself, she will be confident of caring for her patients. But if she has developed a negative *self-concept*, she will not be able to help the patient skilfully because she will be prone to criticise self and others. ***Beliefs and Values*** with which a nurse comes will affect the way she takes care of her patient or develops interpersonal relationship. If she values the human life and believes in respecting the person as a human being she will give individualized care to the patient.

Similarly, interpersonal relationship will be affected according to the *life experiences* of a nurse. If she has suffered an emotional trauma of losing mother at a very young age and of having a bad behaviour from her step-mother, then, Probably she will not be able to accept a lady who is a patient and has two step children. A student-nurse who develops self-awareness will be able to assist a patient in an effective way.

ATTITUDE TOWARDS THE PATIENT

The attitude of accetance of the patient with whatever symptoms he or she has, is important for a nurse. The patient develops a feeling that there is a nurse who is prepared to help him. Each patient has a status as an individual in his or her family and environment. The nurse must respect his or her status as an individual. She must develop an attitude of acceptance of the patient, tolerance of his or her disturbed behaviour and helping the patient. She should avoid passing judgment on the patient e.g. "It is bad you smoke so much." She also puts limits on the patient's behaviour i.e. if the patient insists on watching TV at midnight she would say that it is hospital and other patients will be disturbed.

RAPPORT

It is defined as a "relationship of mutual sympathy and understanding especially between patient and therapist". (Medical Dictionary). Some people are good at developing relationship where the patient feels the need to come for help again. This type of relationship describes that rapport has been established. The essential qualities for developing rapport are *warmth, genuineness* and *empathy.*

Warmth means acceptance of the patient with his symptoms, willingness of the nurse to care for the patient, joining the patient's happiness of joy and similing or touching the patient if required.

Genuineness is actual interest or feelings with which the nurse cares for the patient.

Empathy is the capacity for participation in another's feelings or ideas or putting oneself in the same position as other person is going through and feeling for it; and projecting the feelings in how an individual has interpreted it.

Empathetic Ability - People in everyday life tend to show empathy. A woman while watching T.V. cries when the actress is crying because she is going through a stressful life situation of bringing up her children.

In other words, she is emphthizing with the actress on the screen. Empathy is different from sympathy. Empathy allows people to have the feelings of another and respond to, and understand the other person's experience according to his or her experience. But in sympathy a person is having a common feeling or an affinity, association or relationship between persons or things wherein whatever affects one similarly affects the others. In a nursing situation the use of empathy is therapeutic.

TO RECALL

Psychiatric Nursing is defined as an interpersonal process whereby the professional nurse assists an individual, family or community to promote mental health, prevent and cope with mental illness and to find a meaning in life experience.

- **Relationship can be therapeutic or social.**
- **One-to-one relationship is the end result of a series of planned purposeful interactions between a nurse and a patient.**
  Factors determining effective nurse-patient relationship:
  The Nurse's Self-awareness
  The Nurse's Attitude towards patient
  The Nurse's Ability in developing rapport
- **Rapport includes warmth, genuineness and empathetic ability of the nurse.**

GOALS OF NURSE-PATIENT RELATIONSHIP

Travelbee Joyce, in *Intervention in Psychiatric Nursing,* has discussed nine goals in one-to-one relationship.

(I) THE NURSE HELPS THE PATIENT TO COPE WITH THE PRESENT PROBLEMS.

The nurse accepts the patient as "here and now." That is, what are the patient's problems which have hospitalized him/her. How does the patient perceive the problems ? The nurse does not go back to the past history from secondary sources. These sources are collecting information from the patient's relatives and past records. She tries to collect the information from the patient. If the patient talks about his or her past the nurse tries to use this knowledge in helping him/her.

(II) THE NURSE HELPS THE PATIENT TO UNDERSTAND HIS PROBLEM.

The nurse develops this goal throughout her care of the patient. She helps the patient to identify his or her problem. Many a time the patient may say that he is admitted here for a check-up or investigation and refuses the psychiatric care he or she is getting. As the patient continues on treatment the nurse tries to help him/her to identify why he/she is admitted in this hospital or psychiatric unit. She makes the patient understand the problem he/she is going through.

(III) THE NURSE HELPS THE PATIENT TO UNDERSTAND HIS ACTIVE PARTICIPATION IN AN EXPERIENCE.

For example, a patient who gets violent, throws things here and there may be helped to find out the reason for his behaviour. What he thinks can control him ? The moment the patient suggests a remedy, he can be made to realize that he is active in making a decision for his care. This helps him to regain sufficient courage and realise that he is still a worthy person capable of taking decisions.

(IV) THE NURSE ASSISTS THE PATIENT TO IDENTIFY EMERGING PROBLEMS REALISTICALLY.

During the relationship a patient may identify his actual problem as different. For example, the patient who gets violent finds out that his violence is due to loss of money in business which is leading him to insecurity or due to the fear that his children's education in a good school may be affected. So he identifies the problem which he needs to handle.

(V) THE NURSE HELPS THE PATIENT TO FIND OUT A NEW ALTERNATIVE FOR HIS OR HER PROBLEM.

If the patient has any problem, he must have tried all the usual methods to solve it. But when he failed to do so, probably he started feeling helpless, worthless and depressed. The nurse therapist cannot find a solution for the patient's problem, but she can help him with an alternative solution. She can ask the patient, what else can you do to solve this problem ? Who can help you ? The nurse is trying to make the patient understand that there are many alternate solutions to his problem and he has to choose the best which suits him.

(VI) THE NURSE HELPS THE PATIENT TO TRY OUT NEW PATTERNS OF BEHAVIOUR.

While interacting with the patient the nurse is able to identify the nursing needs of her patient. If she finds the patient is not able to socialize and is depressed she starts taking him to the daycare room just for observation. She calls other patients in the same unit to talk about their problems. Gradually, she encourages the patient to go to her neighbouring patient and ask for a magazine. The patient picks up courage and goes to the patient, comes back to the nurse and says, "I have done it but I was very nervous."

The nurse gives a positive reinforcement to the patient by saying, "Good, you could do this, it's not that difficult as you think." The patient develops confidence and may gradually start socializing with a few people. Patient adopts this new pattern of behaviour to reduce his worthylessness and depression.

(VII) THE NURSE HELPS THE PATIENT TO COMMUNICATE.

Mentally ill patients have difficulty in communicating with others, because of thought problems. The patient who is also getting treatment needs help to talk clearly and logically with others. For example, help the patient to describe clearly, step by step, his progress in job. The communication process will be discussed in detail in ***Unit XIV of this chapter.***

(VIII) THE NURSE HELPS THE PATIENT TO SOCIALIZE.

It is known that some of the mentally ill patients have difficulty in socialization. The nurse can use the approach as: One-to-one socialization, one-to-two socialization and one-to-many sicialization. That means she helps the patient to socialize with one person to start with, then with two or three other patients or people and gradually in the group. Of course, the nurse must assess that the patient should have an effective socialization to start with. She should also assess when the patient can be initiated for socialization.

(IX) THE NURSE HELPS THE PATIENT TO FIND A MEANING IN HIS ILLNESS.

It is assumed that an ill person wants to find out the reason or meaning of his suffering. The patient may blame his relatives, his fate or 'karma'. Though it is difficult not to blame anyone, once the patient is able to find out "Why he must live", for "whom he must live", probably his acceptance to illness will not be that difficult. The patient may be explained to accept that his suffering can be due to physical, social, mental or spiritual factors. It will also provide him with a learning experience to solve the problem in future.

The achievement of goals of one-to-one relationship by the nurse will depend on her knowledge of the subject, attitude towards the patient i.e. her values and beliefs, her self-concept, her ability to develop rapport with the patient. The other important factor which helps in developing an effective one-to-one relationship is skill in interviewing and communicating with the patient. This will be discussed in ***Unit XIV.*** It is important for nursing students to learn the different phases or stages of nurse-patient relationship which will be discussed in this unit.

TO RECALL

Goals of one-to-one Relationship:

- **i.** **The Nurse helps the patient to cope with the present problem.**
- **ii.** **The Nurse helps the patient to understand his problem.**
- **iii.** **The Nurse helps the patient to understand his participation in a therapeutic experience.**
- **iv.** **The Nurse helps the patient to face problems realistically.**
- **v.** **The Nurse helps the patient to find out alternative solutions to the problems.**
- **vi.** **The Nurse helps the patient to try out new patterns of behaviour.**
- **vii.** **The Nurse helps the patient to communicate.**
- **viii.** **The Nurse helps the patient to socialize.**
- **ix.** **The Nurse helps the patient to find out meaning in his/her illness.**

PHASES OF NURSE-PATIENT RELATIONSHIP

"Nurse-patient relationship is the end result of a series of planned purposeful interactions between a nurse and a patient." (Travelbee). The definition explains that the interactions are planned and there are a series of interactions, that means the therapeutic relationship goes through various stages or phases. It is very difficult to put a demarcation in the beginning and end of each stage because the stages overlap. But for the purpose of understanding, the nurse-patient relationship can be described in four phases:

(i) Preinteraction phase

(ii) Introductory or Orientation phase

(iii) Working phase

(iv) Termination phase.

PRE-INTERACTION PHASE

DEFINITION

Pre-interaction means a phase which a nurse goes through before the actual interaction with the patient. This phase begins when the nurse is assigned a patient to develop therapeutic relationship with him till she goes to him for interaction.

REACTION OF THE NURSE IN PREINTERACTION PHASE

The nurse thinks and feels about the patient before interacting according to her knowledge, fears and misconcepts. She tries to collect information from secondary sources like the patient's record file, a resource person and other nurses working in the ward. Some student nurses do not collect information from secondary sources; they want complete information from the patient (Primary Source).

— The Nurse plans how she is going to interact with the patient, what she is going to achieve from this interaction and how she is going to help the patient. She plans her objectives for the interaction phase.

— The Nurse may experience anxiety. Anxiety may be manifested by standing in the duty room and going through the records, helping the other nurse to prepare the injection trolly, talking with the clinical instructor on the theoretical aspect of psychiatric nursing, waiting for her friends so that two of them can go together to the patient and using all tactics in delaying a visit to him. It is like "stage fright." A student nurse who is able to approach the patient once overcomes the stage fright.

Anxiety in the nurse may be, "will my patient talk to me ? He may not accept me or like me. He may beat me." But once she goes to the patient, anxiety will be reduced. She can go through the patient's record, talk to the clinical supervisor or other nurses about her fear, can set her goals very clearly and plan a brief interaction with the patient. These strategies will help her to reduce her difficulty in going to the patient.

TASKS OF PREINTERACTION PHASE

* The Nurse explores her fears and anxiety.
* Sets objectives for the interaction phase.
* Takes help of the clinical supervisor or co-workers to overcome fears.

TO RECALL

* **Preinteraction phase begins when the nurse is assigned a patient till the time she goes to the him/her for interaction.**
* **Reactions of the nurse in this phase can be fear and anxiety.**
* **Tasks of the preinteraction phase are:**
  - **The nurse explores her fears and anxiety.**
  - **Sets the objectives for the interaction phase.**
  - **Takes the help of the clinical supervisor to overcome her anxiety and fears.**

INTRODUCTORY OR ORIENTATION PHASE

DEFINITION

Introductory or orientation phase begins when the nurse goes to the patient, introduces herself and gets introduction about him. The nurse and the patient who are strangers meet for the first time and become acquaintances. The orientation phase ends when the nurse and the patient begin to accept each other as a unique human being.

TASKS OF INTRODUCTORY OR ORIENTATION PHASE

Significant tasks of the orientation phase are establishment of contact with the patient, making agreement or pact and talking to him.

ESTABLISHMENT OF CONTACT :- The student nurse locates her patient. She makes an observation of who the patient is and how he has dressed up. She introduces herself to the patient and asks him where they can sit and talk.

PACT :- Pact is the initial encounter. The nurse makes an agreement or pact with the patient to help him towards social recovery. She begins by telling her name, her status and the name of the school of nursing or college of nursing, the length and purpose of her stay and where she will be available. The nurse tells the patient her reason of interacting with him or her and also termination of the relationship. She asks the patient his or her name. Whether he would like to be called by his second name or the first name.

During this phase the nurse starts looking at the patient as a unique individual along with his or her environment.

TALKING WITH THE PATIENT :- While talking with the patient the nurse shows trust in her behaviour. The patient may present a prepared 'SPIEL' to the nurse when she asks, "What is your problem ?" The patient gives his history in detail and asks the nurse, "Hope you know about me now."

This type of feeling comes in the patient when he finds that everybody here is to interview him and collect information, but no one is to help him. If a nurse interrupts the patient for clarification and details, the latter may think differently and give the content of what is being asked.

The nurse also discusses ***confidentiality of information*** shared by the patient. She clearly informs the patient that progress in therapy will be reported to team members by maintaining confidentiality of specific information. Information on harm to self or others will be reported to the concerned member. Trusting relationship is also maintained by keeping up to the time. This will also impose limits on the patient about the timings.

BARRIERS TO ORIENTATION PHASE

* *Establishing an agreement or pact* is considered a barrier in the nurse patient relationship by many nursing personnel. They feel that the patient may think that the nurse is here only for a few weeks. What sort of help could be expected from her in a short span of time. The patient may be explained that other nurses are also working in the ward and he is also interacting with them. If the pact is not developed, the patient may feel deceived and think that nobody is trustworthy. There may be initial difficulty but gradually the patient accepts the fact.

* *Social class of the patient* or the nurse may also act as a barrier in developing the nurse-patient relationship. A nurse coming from a rich family may not feel comfortable to relate with a patient from a low socio-economic class. Likewise, the nurse who has a low socio-economic background may feel uncomfortable to approach the patient with a high social class and may categorise by saying, "An idle rich, there is really nothing wrong with him."

* *Status is* another barrier in the interactive process. The nurse may feel hesitant to approach the patient who is a 'doctor'. She thinks he knows everything so how would she help him. She must know that the patient may know about medicines but he needs psychiatric nursing care because he is a sick human being.

* *Anxiety level of the patient and the nurse* is also a barrier in this phase. The nurse who is anxious to collect history may hardly focus on the patient and his needs. The patient who is trying to know the nurse may also have anxiety. He may not discuss everything in the beginning. There may be resistance in his behaviour. This also acts as a barrier in the interaction process.

* When either the patient or the nurse perceives the other participant as a significant individual from the past — for example, the patient perceives the nurse as his daughter and starts behaving with her like a father it is called *transference.* When the therapist or the nurse perceives a male patient like her father and gives him the same care that she would have given to her father, it is called *counter transference.* Transference and counter-transference are also barriers in the interaction process because the nurse must consider the patient as a unique human being.

TO RECALL

* **Introduction or orientation phase is when the nurse and the patient know each other as unique human beings.**
* **Tasks of the orientation phase:**
  - **Establishment of contact**
  - **Development of an agreement or pact**
  - **Talking with the patient**
* **Barriers of the orientation phase:**
  - **Development of pact**
  - **Social class**
  - **Status of the patient**
  - **Anxiety of the nurse or the patient**
  - **Transference**
  - **Counter-transference**

WORKING PHASE/ PHASE OF EMERGING IDENTITES

DEFINITION

Working phase or phase of emerging identities of the nurse-patient relationship starts when the nurse and the patient are able to overcome the barrier of orientation or introductory phase. During this phase the nurse and the patient actively work on meeting the goals which they had established during the orientation phase. The characteristic features of this phase are that the nurse is able to overcome anxiety and the patient's fear of the unknown is also decreased. Reactions like transference and counter-transference are also reduced.

TASKS OF WORKING PHASE

Therapeutic tasks of the working phase of the nurse patient relationship are as follows:

- The Nurse collects the data in detail from primary and secondary sources and identifies the needs of the patient.
- The Nurse assists the patient to identify his or her problems.
- She helps the patient to communicate.
- She encourages the patient to socialize.
- The Nurse helps the patient to find an alternative solution to his or her problem.
- She encourages the patient to use new patterns of behaviour.
- The Nurse helps the patient to understand that he has a significant role in his treatment.
- She prepares the patient for termination of relationship by reminding him during the interviews. (Refer goals of IPR mentioned in the beginning of this unit).

During the working phase of the nurse-patient relationship, the patient is able to get strength to face the difficulties of illness. He is also assisted to identify the effect of his or her behaviour on others, his relatives or people who are coming in his contact daily.

The working phase helps the nurse to develop knowledge and skill in psychiatric nursing. She identifies her strengths and weaknesses as a nurse while interacting with the patient. She learns to take guidance from experts and the supervisor during difficulty. Group discussion about the patient, helps her to share her knowledge with other team members.

The working phase enables the nurse and the patient to achieve the maximum goals which they have planned for this phase. The end result leads the patient to verbalize, socialize and identify and face his problems realistically. This is the phase which leads to the termination of the nurse-patient relationship.

BARRIERS OF WORKING PHASE

TESTING OF NURSE

The patient tests the nurse for her ability and competence. This arises anxiety in the patient which may act as a barrier in therapeutic relationship. The patient tests the nurse in a number of ways. He may check her ability to set limits. For example, he will tell the nurse, "Please continue talking, I am very upset today........." If the nurse gives in to her demand, it indicates manipulation. He may deliberately be aggressive to test whether he is able to arouse anger in the nurse.

The patient may motivate the nurse to talk about herself. For example he would say, "Sister, how do you come to the hospital ? Who all are there in your family ? Whom do you like the most in your family ?" A skilful nurse understands that the patient is testing her. As soon as the patient asks her questions like "Who all are there in your family", the nurse gives a brief answer and directs and question back, "Who all are there in your family ? And what are their age groups ? How do they occupy themselves ?" The nurse is thus trying to focus attention on the patient.

PROGRESS OF THE PATIENT

A mentally ill patient may not show quick progress. He may progress, then regress and remain stagnant before making further progress. In therapeutic relationship the nurse must understand this realistic progress in the patient.

DIFFICULTY IN COLLECTING AND INTERPRETING THE DATA

The nurse is unwilling to engage in tedious tasks of collecting and interpreting the data, applying the knowledge and skill in helping the patient. She finds it too hard to do. This acts as a barrier in completing the tasks of the working phase.

FEAR OF CLOSENESS

The. nurse feels that she is working closely with the patient. She may find it difficult to terminate the relationship. The patient may not like to discontinue the relationship. To avoid closeness she does not communicate freely (professionally) and makes deliberate attempts to avoid going to the patient. The patient is not able to find confidence in his nurse and therapeutic relationship may not establish. Fear of closeness is also discussed in *Chapter II*..

STRATEGIES TO OVERCOME BARRIERS

The nurse can overcome all these barriers by learning the subject in depth, and by talking to her supervisor and experts. The supervisor can identify from the process recording of the student that she is not making progress in her relationship with the patient. Process-recording shows incompleteness and discontinuity.

Discussion with the peer group is also helpful. Sample of process recording is included in *unit XIV*.

TO RECALL

- **Working phase of the nurse-patient relationship starts when the nurse and the patient are able to overcome the barriers of introductory or orientation phase.**
- **Tasks of working phase:**
  - **The nurse collects the data and identifies nursing needs of the patient.**
  - **Sets goals for the relationship.**
  - **Assists the patient to achieve his goals.**
  - **Encourages the patient towards independence and decision-making abilities.**
  - **Prepares the patient for termination.**
  - **Develops competency in her own clinical experience.**
- **Barriers of Working Phase**
  - **The patient tests the nurse in various situations.**
  - **The nurse thinks that the patient's progress is slow.**
  - **She does not want to do tedious jobs like process recording.**
  - **The nurse fears closeness with the patient.**
- **Strategies adopted to help the nurse to overcome these barriers.**

TERMINATION PHASE

DEFINITION

Termination phase is also called a resolution phase or end phase. The termination phase begins during the orientation phase. In the orientation or introductory phase, the nurse develops 'Pact or Contract' with the patient. In the pact, the nurse explains the patient her purpose of interacting with him or her and terminating the relationship. The main objective of the terminating phase is to bring a therapeutic end to the nurse-patient relationship.

CAUSES OF TERMINATION

The termination of relationship may be due to various reasons:
(i) The patient may be discharged without the knowledge of the nurse. So he or she leaves the ward.

(ii) The patient may go on *parole* and does not come back to the hospital. *Parole* is a method in which the patient has not been discharged from the hospital, but is away from the confines of hospital for two to three days or more.

(iii) The Nurse may terminate relationship due to various reasons i.e. a student nurse completes her psychiatric nursing experience; the patient has improved and no longer needs to have one-to-one relationship. In other words, the patient has reached a state of functioning effectively or the patient may die of a natural cause, or the patient is functioning but he or she may not like to leave a secure environment like hospital. These may be the reasons where the nurse terminates relationship with the patient. So termination of the nurse-patient relationship may be:

(i) When the patient is in hospital and the nurse terminates the relationship.

(ii) When the patient is discharged and the therapeutic relationship is terminated.

TERMINATION WHEN PATIENT IS IN HOSPITAL

— It is significant that the patient should be told about termination. He has a right to know about it.

— The patient should be allowed to express his thoughts and feelings regarding termination.

— Unless the patient communicates, the nurse may not know what he feels about termination.

— The patient who has felt trust, support and caring may be reluctant to terminate the relationship.

— The patient may consider termination as desertion. He feels as if all members of his family and friends have deserted him and now this nurse is also leaving him. Rather than feeling sad about parting, the patient may show anger (acting. out....) and fails to appear for conference or meetings. In other words, he wants the nurse to know that he is leaving her. He may not talk to the nurse during interaction and feels that he is punishing her because she is terminating the relationship.

— The patient may talk about everything except termination. (Non-acceptance).
— The patient may become depressed.

TERMINATION-WHEN PATIENT LEAVES HOSPITAL

— In a situation where the patient is leaving hospital after discharge, he or she does not feel deserted by the nurse.

— Hospital environment is non-threatening and helpful. But once the patient goes home, he has to live in the community and take up social roles as father or mother. All patients don't feel 'Glad to be going home.' The patient may have some doubt about his ability to cope with demands from the family, society and the community.

— The patient may have the doubt that going home does not mean that he or she is not going to come back. His fears get confirmed when another patient in his cubicle comes back in a more violent stage after one week of stay at home.

— The nurse should assist the patient in a frank discussion of his fears. He may be encouraged to talk about problems or persons arousing anxiety in him. Some examples of patient's fears are:

* "I don't know if I will be able to face my friends and relatives."
* "I don't know if I will be able to take care of my children."
* "What will my office people say ?"

PREPARATION OF PATIENT

Though there are no standard methods of helping the patient, still the nurse can try the following strategies:

* The basic method she can adopt is to explain that whatever goals of therapeutic relationship were planned have been met.
* The nurse should allow the patient to talk about his or her fear and an individualistic approach has to be used.
* A psychiatric social worker can be contacted to visit the office and family of the patient.
* The patient may be sent on *'Parole'* before discharge, so that he gradually goes through the weaning-off phase.
* The patient may be sent to a half-way house. Half-way house is a transition facility, such as a group residence, for mental patients who no longer need the full services of a hospital but are not yet ready for a completely independent living.

* The patient may be asked to attend a day-care centre for a few days.

When the patient is getting discharged or leaving hospital, the nurse also has to prepare herself to accept termination of relationship.

PRE-PARATION OF NURSE

* Termination is a period of crisis for the nurse also. If the patient leaves the ward without the knowledge of the nurse because he or she was discharged in her absence, this unanticipated termination may arise anger in her. Probably, she planned a different way of discharging the patient from hospital.
* She may experience depression or anxiety. For, she has now to start looking after another patient.
* She may feel happy subconsciously that the patient has gone. This is probably because of some fears or lack of discussion with teachers about her own inadequancies in helping the patient.
* The termination process for the nurse is *evaluative* and *educative*. *Evaluative* because how far she could help the patient and with more depth of knowledge what better she could do. *Educative* because the nurse gradually develops skill in taking care of a patient with various mental disorders.

Though there is no specific method of terminating the nurse-patient relationship, termination is effective when both the nurse and patient are psychologically prepared.

PROBLEMS AND BARRIERS OF TERMINATION PHASE & STRATEGIES TO OVERCOME

Termination phase of the nurse-patient relationship is definitely a phase of separation and may be associated with a sense of disappointment and feeling of sadness. There are a number of problems which a nurse, specially a student nurse, may face. Some of the problems and strategies to overcome are:

— The patient may ask the nurse to write to him or come back from duty and see him. A student nurse visits the patient in her off duty hours. This indicates that the nurse also has not accepted the termination. She may say, "Just for the happiness of that patient I thought a visit does not matter." But a student-nurse, after discussion with a senior nurse, will understand that she is making the patient more dependent on one particular person.

— The patient may ask for the address or telephone number of the nurse and permission to visit her in hostel. The nurse gives the address. She may say, "I didn't want the patient to be hurt." But, in fact, it is her inability to say "No". She can discuss in the conference room with a psychiatric team and overcome such inabilities.

— The patient should be explained that every relationship terminates. If the patient comes for intervention he or she should be referred to the second incharge. After the termination phase the intervention should not be done by the particular nurse who was interacting with him.

— Gift giving is another problem faced by the student nurse. The patient likes to give a gift to the nurse, who had been caring for him, as a token of his gratitude and in appreciation of her efficient work. The patient needs to be explained about the professional ethics. If he wants to give a gift he may be encouraged to gift out something for the utilization of other patients. Suppose he wants to give a painting, get his name written and put it up in the corridor of the ward. Explain that his work will be seen by many people. This may provide him with a sense of worthiness and achievement.

— The nurse may withdraw earlier from the patient due to her own anxiety. She may not interact with the patient.

— The nurse may not assist the patient which she could otherwise do. She may feel that patients do not die of mental illness, if neglected. But there is psychological dying of mentally ill patients.

— The nurse needs to explore her own feelings and thoughts about separation from the patient which will help her to accomplish the tasks of the termination phase i.e.

TASKS OF TERMINATION PHASE

* Bring a therapeutic end to the relationship.
* Review feelings about the relationship.
* Evaluate progress towards goals, and
* Establish mechanism for meeting future therapy needs.

TO RECALL

* **Termination phase of the nurse-patient relationship begins during the orientation/introductory phase.**

* **Causes of termination can be:**
  - **The patient may be discharged**
  - **He goes on parole and does not come back**
  - **The nurse may terminate relationship due to her change in the posting of clinical experience, the patient becomes functional, or may die of a natural cause.**

- **Termination of relationship has to be done**
  - **(i) when the patient is discharged, or**
  - **(ii) when the patient is in hospital but the nurse no more looks after him.**
- **The nurse needs to prepare herself for the termination.**
- **Tasks of the Termination phase are :**
  - **— Bring therapeutic end to the relationship.**
  - **— Review feelings about the relationship.**
  - **— Evaluate progress towards goals.**
  - **— Establish mechanism for meeting future therapy needs.**
- **Problems and Barriers of the Termination Phase:**
  - **— The patient may ask the nurse to visit him during her off-duty hours.**
  - **— The patient may like to visit or telephone the nurse.**
  - **— Gift giving.**
  - **— The nurse may avoid the patient who is discharged.**
- **Strategies to overcome these barriers.**

APPLICATION TO NURSING

Content presented in this unit on therapeutic relationship is basic in nursing practice and more so in psychiatric nursing practice. The student will be able to differentiate therapeutic relationship from social relationship. The unit provides knowledge about different phases of the nurse-patient relationship, the tasks to be accomplished in each phase, the probable barriers or problems the nurse may encounter and how to overcome them. Content will enable a student nurse to apply this knowledge and develop skill in interpersonal relationship. This skill she can also use in improving her therapeutic relationship in other fields. For example, in community health nursing, medical nursing, surgical nursing.

BETTER STUDY SECTION

I. VOCABULARY (Use Dictionary)

Accountability	Express
Achievement	Holistic
Agreement	Identify
Anxiety	Interchangeably
Arousing	Intervention
Clarification	Participation

Confidentiality	Reaction
Deliberately	Realize
Demarcation	Requirement
Efficient	Standard
Encounter	Tasks
Establishment	Unique
	Worthless

2. ASSIGNEMENT

* List the difficulties you faced during the interaction phase.
* Write the problems you encountered during the termination phase and how you managed to overcome them.

3. EXERCISE

* Define nurse-patient relationship.
* List the goals of one-to-one relationship.
* Enumerate the phases of NPR.
* Describe the significance of NPR for the nurse.

4. READING REFERENCES

(1) Almedia E.M. ***The Interpersonal Basis of Psychiatric Nursing.*** G.P. Putnam's Sons, New York (1972).

(2) Beck, Rawlins and Williams. ***Mental Health Psychiatric Nursing - A Holistic Life Cycle Approach.*** (2nd edition) The C.V. Mosby Company (1988).

(3) Travelbee Joyce. ***Intervention in Psychiatric Nursing Process in the One-to-One Relationship.*** (Ninth edition) F.A. Davis Company, Philadelphia (1976).

(4) Lego Suzanne. ***The American Handbook of Psychiatric Nursing.*** J.B. Lippincott Company, Philadelphia (1984).

(5) Wilson H.S. *Kneis*, C.S. ***Psychiatric Nursing (Second edition)*** Addison-Wesley Publishing Company, Nursing Division, California (1983).

UNIT XIV

COMMUNICATION AND INTERVIEW TECHNIQUES USED IN THERAPEUTIC RELATIONSHIP

UNIT OUTLINE

PART-A Therapeutic Communication

* Definition of Communication.
* Purposes of Communication.
* Modes of Communication.
* Skill Development in Effective Communication.
* Reasons for Break in Communication.

PART-B Interviewing

* Definition of Interview.
* Purposes of Interview.
* Basic Principles of Interview Process.
* Techniques of Interview.
* Attitude of Interviewer.
* Sample of Process Recording.
* Application to Nursing.
* Better Study Section.

INTENDED LEARNING OUTCOME

After reading this unit you will be able to:

a) Define therapeutic communication.
b) Describe the purposes of communication.
c) Identify the modes of communication.
d) Explain the techniques of communication.
e) Discuss the skills required for developing effective communication.
f) Study the reasons of break in communication.
g) Define interview technique.
h) List the purposes of interview.
i) Describe principles of interview.
j) Explain the techniques of interview.
k) Analyse the attitude of interviewer.
l) Develop skill in taking interview and recording.

PART-A THEAPEUTIC COMMUNICATION

CONTENTS

INTRODUCTION Communication refers to the reciprocal exchange of information, ideas, beliefs, feelings and attitudes between persons or among a group of persons. It is a goal-directed process in which people use a system of symbols and signs to convey a message. We communicate when we talk (verbal) and also when we don't talk (non-verbal). We communicate when we move and when we are still. We communicate within ourselves and with others. Communication is very significant in nursing. Nursing process *(Refer Chapter II Unit VI p. 44)* itself is a communication process. The nurse's hastiness in movement, dealing gently or carefully, giving health education, counselling the patient are some of the examples which communicate or send messages to the patient. Hence, nurses must be conscious of therapeutically communicating with patients.

DEFINITION OF COMMUNICATION

Webster's New Collegiate Dictionary defines communication as a process by which information is exchanged between individuals through a common system of symbols, signs or behaviour. A person who sends the message is called sender or encoder and the other who receives the message is called receiver or decoder.

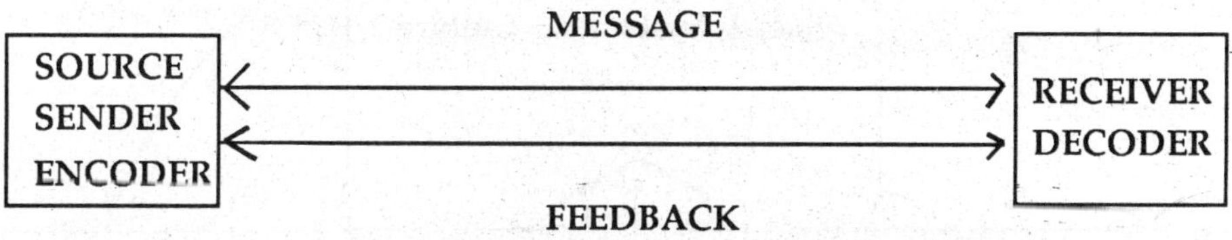

Fig. 3 : Describing Communication is a Two-way Process.

THERAPEUTIC COMMUNICATION

In therapeutic communication the nurse directs the communication towards the patient to identify his current health problems, plan, implement and evaluate the action taken.

Components of communication are described by Berlo in his book *'The Process of Communication'* under four headings, named as the SMCR Model, where 'S' is source, 'M' stands for message, 'C' is channel used for communication and 'R' is receiver.

SOURCE

It is the sender or encoder, the person who initiates the conveying of a message. The message may be verbal or nonverbal. The sender needs to have similiar communication skills, attitude, knowledge, understanding level social system and culture as the receiver or decoder.

MESSAGE

Message should have all the elements properly coded. Content should be clear from the source of the sender to the receiver.

CHANNEL

Various channels are used by the sender/source to communicate a message. For example, as a nurse source, you can use speech for health education to a group of diabetic patients. Listen to complains of the patient. Hence, there are five sensation channels of communication i.e. seeing, hearing, touching, smelling and tasting.

RECEIVER

Receiver or decoder is the person who is receiving the message and interpreting it. To interpret the message correctly the receiver needs to have similar communication skills, attitude, knowledge, social systems and culture, as the source or sender.

To comprehend communication it can be summarized by diagramatic presentation:

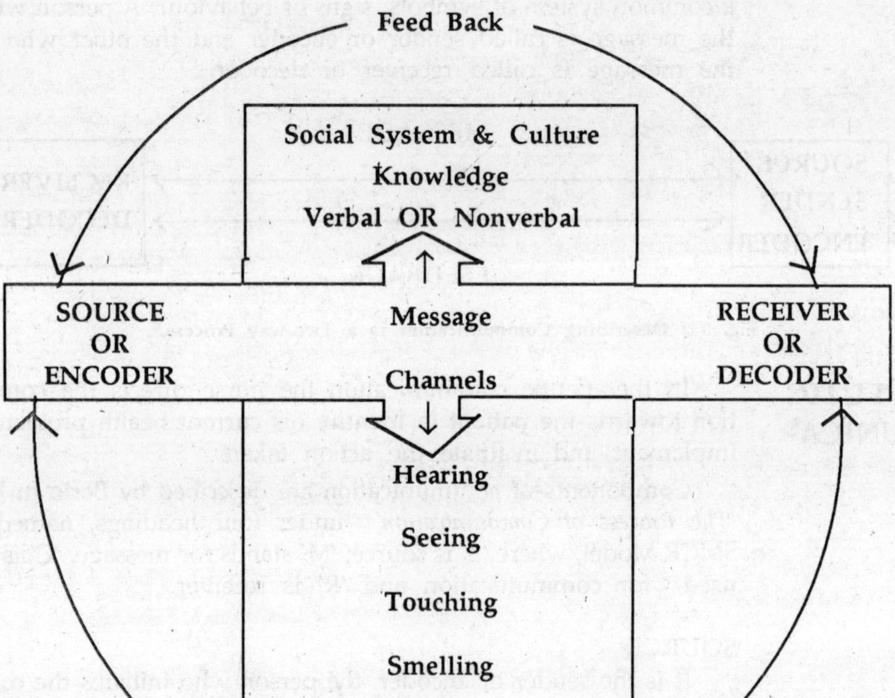

Fig. 4 : Diagram Depicting the Commonness Between Sender and Receiver and Channels Used for Communicating the Message Effectively.

TO RECALL

* Communication is a two-way process.
* In therapeutic communication the nurse directs the communication to work with the patient to identify the current health problems, plan, implement and evaluate the action taken.
* Components of communication are the source/sender/encoder, message may be verbal or non-verbal, channels through which the message is conveyed to receiver or decoder.
* Both sender and receiver need to have commonness for effective communication.

PURPOSE OF THERAPEUTIC COMMUNICATION

In therapeutic communication the purposes are :

a) Understand the meaning of communication.
b) What is to be accomplished during nurse-patient relationship? For example, collecting information from the patient.
c) Why the goals /purposes of nursing are to be achieved? For example to help the patient.
d) How to interact with the patient so as to achieve the goals of IPR? For example, use of various communication techniques.

MODES OF COMMUNICATION

Communication can be verbal and non-verbal.

VERBAL COMMUNICATION

It refers to a written and spoken message exchanged in the form of words. An example of verbal communication is provided by the words, spoken or written like "Sister, I am anxious."

NON-VERBAL COMMUNICATION

It refers to messages that do not involve written or spoken words. The message is conveyed through the behaviour or body language or through any of the five senses. For example, for conveying "I am anxious" the patient's hands may tremble, forehead will have prespiration, lips may be dry and the respiratory rate high. Though these signs may be due to some other reasons, verbal validation should also be sought. Verbal validation is asking the patient if he/she is anxious.

META COMMUNICATION

It refers to how the message should be understood by the receiver. For example, the message "You look fresh and lovely today" is conveyed with wrinkles on the forehead. So the receiver must interpret the sincerity of the sender in giving the compliments.

TO RECALL

* **Purpose of communication can be seeking information and helping the patient.**
* **Modes of communication are verbal, nonverbal and meta communication.**

COMMUNICATION SKILLS OR ABILITIES OF THE NURSE

Skill is the ability of a nurse to use her knowledge effectively and readily. Ability is defined as competency in doing or acquiring proficiency. To communicate effectively, the nurse needs to develop (i) General abilities, and (ii) Special abilities.

GENERAL ABILITIES

Such as :-

— Ability to read.
— Ability to express onself in writing.
— Ability to speak.
— Ability to listen and interpret.

SPECIAL ABILITIES

Such as :-

— Ability to observe and interpret observation.
— Ability to guide the nurse-patient interaction in order to accomplish goals.
— Ability to ascertain if communication is taking place between the nurse and the patient.
— Ability to recognize when to speak and when to be silent - developing a sense of timing.
— Ability to wait - to proceed at the patient's pace/speed.
— Ability to evaluate participation of the patient in the nurse-patient relationship.

TO RECALL

The nurse needs to have an ability to read and write and speak. Listen to the patient and interpret accurately. For effective therapeutic communication special abilities are also required.

TECHNIQUES USED IN COMMUNICATION

To develop skill in effective communication various techniques can be used. During interaction with the patient the psychiatric nurse uses these techniques in combination. No single technique is complete. Some of the techniques used are observing, listening, restating, validating, reflecting, providing information, clarifying, paraphrasing, pinpointing, linking, questioning, structuring, focusing, sharing and summarizing.

THERAPEUTIC COMMUNICATION TECHNIQUE	EXAMPLES
OBSERVING	Observation is made by the nurse of wringing of hands, wiping prespiration, dry lips, speaking in a very low tone. The nurse is making observation of a nonverbal communication
LISTENING	As the patient is talking, the nurse responds by nodding her head, of by saying . "Yes, I follow what you told me". The nurse is actively listening.
RESTATING	The nurse restates or repeats what the patient has been saying. It can be in the form of a question or a statement. For example— **Patient:** My children are going through a financial problem because I am sick. **Nurse :** Your children are going through a financial problem because you are sick. The nurse is restating the statement to increase the patient's awareness of his children's suffering due to his sickness.
VALIDATING	It is a technique which the nurse uses to confirm the accuracy of data or information given by the patient. **Patient :** I get very upset when my husband beats me if I talk anything against my mother-in-law.

THERAPEUTIC COMMUNICA-TION TECHNIQUE	EXAMPLES
	Nurse : Yes, it makes sense that you get upset when your husband beats you on complaining against your mother-in-law. I wonder if you would like to explain further. The nurse is validating the appropriateness of the feeling of being upset about the patient's husband beating her.
REFLECTING	In reflection, the nurse highlights the affective content of the patient's communication that is the feeling or attitude which is implicitly expressed. **Patient :** I am very angry with my wife. **Nurse :** It sounds that you are really angry with your wife. The nurse's use of reflection helps the patient to make further or additional clarification about the statement.
PROVIDING INFORMATION	Providing personal, social and therapeutic information increases the patient's resources. For example, the nurse informs her patient that a social worker will be here from 10 a.m. to 1 p.m. today. Group therapy will be from 2 p.m. to 3 p.m. tomorrow. The patient may ask for more information and utilize the opportunity to clarify doubts.
CLARIFYING	The nurse's formulation of a patient's statement or expression of feelings in clearer terms without indicating approval or disapproval. **Patient:** I am very sad today. **Nurse :** You say you are feeling very sad today. Would you elaborate what is happening ? Explanation given by the patient will clarify further what is making him feel sad.
PARAPHRA-SING	In paraphrasing the nurse restates whatever she has heard from the patient. **Patient:** Sister, all my friends and relatives point out that I will never be able to look after my family members. That makes me depressed. **Nurse:** I hear you saying that whenever you meet anyone, your

THERAPEUTIC COMMUNICATION TECHNIQUE	EXAMPLES
	friends and relatives they point out that you will always remain sick and will be no good to your family. This makes you more sad. The nurse's paraphrasing gives a feeling to the patient to test whether she has understood what he wanted to communicate.
PINPOINTING	The nurse pays attention to certain consistent statements, made by the patient. She pinpoints the difference in what the patient says and what he does. **Nurse:** So, you and your father don't agree to the girl you want to marry. (Makes observation of the patient's behaviour). The nurse may point out, "You say you are sad, but you are smiling."
LINKING	The nurse tries to link the patient's two events, feelings or persons together. **Nurse :** You fight with your wife because her friends visit her too frequently and you feel neglected.
QUESTIONING	Questioning in coomunication is used when the nurse wants clear information. Too many questions should be avoided. The Nurse can use open-ended or close-ended questions. Close-ended questions are with the answer of 'Yes' or 'No', 'Right' or 'Wrong'. Open-ended questions gives more chance for the patient to speak. **Nurse :** "Do you feel sad when your mother does not come to visit you?" This is an example of a close-ended question.
FOCUSING	Concentrating on one single point. **Nurse :** Since when did you start taking alcohol ? **Patient :**. 20 years. **Nurse :** How did you start taking it ?
SHARING	The Nurse thinks about the patient other than the time she looks after him. She may evaluate whether their interactions are helping the patient. She may say : "I was thinking of you yesterday." This is definitely a gesture of warmth and thinking caring according

THERAPEUTIC COMMUNICA-TION TECHNIQUE	EXAMPLES
	to Indian culture. The patient may also feel that the nurse is caring for him.
SUMMARIZING	In summarizing the nurse highlights the main theme of what has been discussed. Summarizing is useful in focusing the patient's attention on what he has discussed. If he would like to add or delete anything. **Nurse :** Yesterday, we were discussing about the various career lines your son could choose. Today, we have discussed two main points. Some of the other techniques like structuring, confronting, processing, checking perceptions, asking for demonstration and illustration, are also used in communication. Non-therapeutic communication techniques are reassuring, rejecting, giving approval, advising, defending, requesting, belittling the feelings of the patient are some of the examples. These non-therapeutic techniques should be avoided.

Fig. 5 : Table Describing Techniques Used in Communication.

COMMUNICATION FAILURE

In a clinical situation there may be failure in communication between the nurse and the patient. It can be due to the following factors:

* Failure to perceive the patient as a human being. For example, thinking that all female patients are fussy. The patient is not being perceived as an individual female patient.

* Failure to recognize the level of meaning in communication. For example, "pain is pretty bad" may mean two different things to the nurse and the patient. Pretty bad may be very severe from the nurse's point of view and dangerous from the patient's point of view.

* Failure to listen.

* Using a value statement without reflection. "Isn't it wonderful that you are going home ?" It may not be wonderful from the patient's point of view.

* Failure to interpret with knowledge. For example, "Now that you are going home everything will be alright." The patient knows that he has to join duty, pay back the debt and face society.
* Use of close-ended questions only.
* Conflicting verbal and non-verbal messages.
* Giving false reassurance.
* Changing the subject if one becomes uncomfortable.

TO RECALL

* **Therapeutic communication techniques are : observing, listening, restating, validating, reflecting, providing information, clarifying, paraphrasing, pinpointing, linking, questioning, focusing, sharing and summarizing.**
* **Break in communication occur due to various factors.**

PART-B INTERVIEW TECHNIQUES

CONTENT

INTRODUCTION

Every human being is engaged in interview. Sometimes one interviews and sometimes one may be interviewed. It is felt that if there were some rules of interviewing, a beginner could follow them. But the interview takes place between human beings who are too individualized to be reduced to a formula. Thereby the interview is considered to be the most important assessment tool.

DEFINITION

Webster defines, "Interview is a meeting at which information is obtained from a person." Interview is professional goal-directed interaction between two people. Erickson describes the essential elements of interview as "It is a face-to-face meeting and conversation between individuals attempting to arrive at a solution of the same problem. A conversation with a specific purpose."

PURPOSES OF INTERVIEW

The purpose of interview varies according to need or situation. In a psychiatric nursing interview, the purpose can be :

INTRODUCTORY

The nurse and the patient are getting acquainted with each other. Rapport or relationship is being established.

INFORMATION GETTING

The nurse interacts with the patient to collect data on his sickness. This helps her to make a nursing diagnosis and plan the care.

INFORMATION GIVING

The patient may require information on the treatment he is getting, progress of his disease and rehabilitation facilities. This information can be given during interview or interaction.

THERAPEUTIC PURPOSE

During the process of interview the patient talks, talks and talks about his problem. This process, called verbal catharsis, reduces his tension. During interaction the nurse can encourage the patient towards constructive planning i.e. expressing his emotions, through paint and brush.

EVALUATIVE PURPOSE

The nurse and the patient may sit and discuss how far the latter has made progress in socializing, in communication and in decision-making. She can also restate to the patient the coping mechanisms used by him to overcome his anxiety.

TO RECALL

- **Interview is a face-to-face interaction between two persons. It is goal-directed.**
- **Purposes of interview are :**
  - **Introduction**
  - **Information getting and giving are :**
  - **Therapeutic**
  - **Evaluative**

BASIC PRINCIPLE OF UNDERSTAD-ING HUMAN NATURE

Annette Garrett in her book on *Interviewing, its Principles and Methods,* explains that understanding of facts of a human being is very essential for interacting. The patient may have motives different from what he is projecting.

UNDERSTANDING FACTS ABOUT HUMAN MOTIVATION

The nurse needs to be patient, tolerant, less condemning and better helpful. Many a time the patient disguises himself, pretands to be bold. This may be the source of his anxiety. It is common that a person apparently likes someone but deeply dislikes him. She may forget the lunch invitation because internally she dislikes the person. Human motivation needs to be interpreted the way the patient projects during interaction.

OBJECTIVE AND SUBJECTIVE FACTS

Death of a wife is an objective fact. But the subjective facts are loss of money as the wife was working, loss of a mother figure for children at home and loss of a compatible partner.

MORAL PIGEON-HOLING

Moral pigeon-holing is putting a person in a right and wrong category. The nurse should recognize the danger involved in passing judgement on the patient's attitude. She must avoid imposing her own moral judgement on the patient. "I feel cigarette smoking is bad." The nurse is trying to impose her own judgement that those who smoke are not good. It should be avoided.

CONFLICTING PULLS

During interaction, a patient talks about his marital life and suddenly stops or changes the topic. He is in a conflict whether to talk to the nurse or not. This situation makes the patient uncomfortable during interview. The patient may develop an ambivalence feeling towards the nurse because he has talked everything about himself to her. The patient may develop a positive transference or a negative transference.

TECHNIQUES OF INTERVIEW

Techniques of interview are discussed in Part-A of this unit. These are : Observing, listening, restating, validating, reflecting, providing information, clarifying, paraphrasing, pinpointing, linking, focusing, sharing, summarizing and questioning. The technique may be elaborated with illustrations.

Questioning - An effective method of interviewing is the art of question.

* In questioning the patient, friendliness should be used.

* Questions asked should be in small sentences and in a simple language.

* Avoid putting questions accusingly or suspiciously.

Nurse : You think you are sick because your father did not care for you. (Accusingly)

Nurse : Are you looking for something ? (may sound suspicious).

* The manner and tone are more important than the words.

Nurse : "Radha, you thought you could avoid group therapy ? Isn't that so ?" It can also be said as, "Radha, today you were not able to come for group therapy. Were you busy in something else ?"

* Avoid showing pleasure of seeing through the patient.

Nurse - Sham Lal, did you go for your bath ?

Patient - Yes, sister, at 6.00 a.m. I finished my bath.

Nurse - Did you change your clothes ?

Patient - Yes.

Nurse - You were wearing the same clothes yesterday also. That means you have not taken your bath as yet (The nurse smiles and walks towards the duty room as if saying, "Mr. Sham Lal, I caught you red-handed").

* Avoid being interested in mysterious data about the patient unless he wants to talk and the nurse uses it for therapeutic purposes.

Patient - Sister, when I was 16 years old, I fell in love with a girl. Now I am happily married and have two children.

Nurse - What happened, you could not get married to that girl ?........

* Avoid in built answer questions. It shows values of the nurse.

Nurse - I am sure you don't smoke, Neeraj.
Isn't it bad to smoke ?

* Answering a personal question, the nurse should be truthful, brief and frank in answering a personal question and then she should redirect the question to the patient.

TO RECALL

- **The basic principle of interviewing is understanding human nature in terms of:**
  - **What is the patient's motivation ?**
  - **Discrepancy between objective and subjective facts.**
  - **Moral pigeonholing by the nurse therapist.**
  - **The patient's conflicting pulls.**
  - **Feelings towards the nurse interviewer.**
- **Techniques of interview (discussed in Part-A of this unit under Techniques of Communication).**

ATTITUDE OF INTERVIEWER

Interview skills are developed gradually. The nurse needs to develop the following attitudes as an interviewer:

— She must guard against herself. If she discovers that she is prejudiced towards drug abusers, she needs to interact with her team members to overcome it.

— Acceptance of patient. "Here and now" with his problem. By accepting the patient the nurse tries to understand the psychodynamics of his behaviour.

— Control rather than absence of feelings. Otherwise the interviewer becomes artificial.

— Avoid offering a false reassurance. To a chronic schizophrenic patient the nurse says, "You will be completely all right. Don't worry." It is not a right approach.

— Build on strengths of the patient. For example, in a day-care centre, the patient is able to play at the carrom board very well. Reinforce his success so that he develops a sense of achievement.

— Avoid passing judgement of right and wrong.

— Avoid saying, "Yes, I understand you." The patient thinks, "If the nurse understands, what's the need for me to talk."

— Look for attainable goals. Goals which can be achieved. The Goal of helping the patient financially may be achieved through the occupational department but it may not be achieved all the time.

— Allow the patient freedom of expression during the interview.

— Win the patient's confidence, by stressing his strength.

— Try to make the interview helpful. Help the patient to identify his problem and use coping mechanisms to overcome it.

— Close the interview carefully. Stop at the fixed time.

THINGS TO LOOK FOR INTERVIEW

In an interview, the nurse must look for salient features, i.e.

(i) ***Association of ideas :*** Give time to the patient for free association, allow him to talk as and whatever he wants to talk.

(ii) ***Note for shifts of conversation:*** Maybe, the patient does not want to reveal something which is too painful or personal to him. Strained relationship between father and mother may be painful for the patient.

(iii) ***Note for recurrent reference :*** The patient may during conversation, refer many a time to the difficulty he is facing with his boss.

(iv) ***Note for inconsistencies:*** The patient's report is not consistent. There are gaps in his conversation, Indicating confusion and guilt.

(v) ***Look for a concealed meaning :*** An unmarried mother may say, "I don't want to see the father of the child." In fact, now she wants to meet him to share her joy of having a child.

(vi) ***Note for the opening and closing sentences:*** "Sister, so many people have come. I am just the same, so what would you do ?" This indicates a feeling of remorse and helplessness and rejecting the nurse.

In the closing sentence, "Sister, I think after talking to you today I am feeling a little light or comfortable. Thank you, Sister. "This indicates that the rapport is being established.

ESSENTIAL CONDITIONS OF INTERVIEWING

The essential conditions for a good interview are :

PHYSICAL SETTING

Some degree of privacy should be maintained, a comfortable and relaxed atmosphere will enable the patient to develop confidence. Interruption like even phone calls must be avoided. The length and place of the interview should be prefixed. Avoid waiting and don't let the patient wait either.

RECORDING

Explain the purpose of recording to the patient. With his permission a tape-recorder can be used. Otherwise, scribbling of a few points. Complete the record immediately as the patient leaves. It should be recorded VERBATIM (word for word). As the patient speaks recording should be done in the same form.

CONFIDENTIALITY

It is very significant to allow the patient to feel free. However, the patient should be explained that if there is need to inform members of the team about any information, he will be told about it. For example, if the patient has suicidal ideas the members need to be informed for his safety.

TO RECALL

Things to look for in an interview are:

- Association of ideas.
- Shifts of conversation.
- Recurrent reference made by the patient.
- Inconsistencies while talking.
- Concealed meaning.
- Opening and closing sentences.

Essential Conditions of a Good Interview are:

- Physical setting.
- Recording.
- Confidentiality.

PROCESS RECORDING

The interaction or interview is recorded by the nurse by using various communication techniques. During conversation she draws inference. Recording of the interview is called a process recording, which includes participants, conversation and inference.

(i) Participants are the therapist and the patient

(ii) Conversation is an aspect where recording is verbatim, i.e. word for word.

(iii) Inference is drawing a conclusion from the facts. The nurse draws her conclusion from the conversation based on psychopathology behaviour in psychiatric illness. *Sample of outline for process- recording* is as follows:

I. IDENTIFICATION DATA:

Name:	Marital Status:
Age:	Occupation:
Sex:	Language:
Literacy:	Date of Admission:
Ward No.:	Address:
Bed No.:	
ORD No.:	
Religion:	
Income:	
Reliability:	

II. PRESENTING COMPLAINTS:

a) According to the patient

b) According to the relatives

III. HISTORY OF PRESENTING COMPLAINTS:

IV. AIMS AND OBJECTIVES OF INTERVIEW:

— Patient's point of view

— Student's point of view

First Interview

Date:

Time and Duration:

Specific Objectives:

Participants	Conversation	Inference

Summary

1. Summary list of reference
2. Introspective observation
3. Interview techniques used

Total Summary

(Summarized after severel interviews)

1. Phases of one-to-one relationship relating to the patient's behaviour in the ward: psychological, social and emotional.

2. Evaluation of goals.

3. Interview tactics used with illustrations and outcome.

4. Areas to be improved.

5. Evaluation of the patient's condition at the time of termination of relationship and his response to various therapies received.

APPLICATION TO NURSING

Reading of this unit on communication and interview provides the basic concepts to nursing personnel for interacting with psychiatric patients. This unit will help the student-nurse to use various communication techniques in developing effective therapeutic N.P.R. The unit also provides the methods by which the nurse can interview the patient skilfully. The sample form in the unit will provide her with a guideline to apply the knowledge in a clinical setting while interacting with psychiatric patients.

BETTER STUDY SECTION

1. VOCABULARY (USE DICTIONARY)

Accomplished	Encoder	Tremble
Appropriateness	Engages	Wringing
Attainable	Element	
Attitude	Fussy	
Awareness	Implicit	
Belittling	Indicating	
Catharsis	Interpret	
Concentrating	Motives	
Consistent	Mysterious	
Decoder	Nodding	
Disguises	Reciprocal	

2. ASSIGNMENT

a) Make a list of communication techniques used while interacting with the psychiatric patient.

b) Explain the special abilities required by the psychiatric nurse in communicating effectively.

c) Describe how the attitude of a nurse affects in the interview process.

3. EXERCISE

Select a patient during your clinical posting in a psychiatric ward, interact and do the process-recording according to an outline of the sample form.
(Refer to the Sample of Process Recording).

4. READING REFERENCES

Berlo, D.K. ***The Process of Communication.*** Holt, Rinehart & Winston, New York (1963).

Taylor C.M. ***Essentials of Psychiatric Nursing.*** (Eleventh edition) The C.V. Mosby Company, London (1982).

Shives L.R. ***Basic Concepts of Psychiatric-Mental Health Nursing.*** (Second edition), J.B. Lippincott Company, Philadelphia (1990).

Wilson H.S. & Kneisl C.R. ***Psychiatric Nursing.*** (Second edition) Addison-Wesley Publishing Company, California (1983).

Williams, Beck & Rawlins. ***Mental Health Psychiatric Nursing - A HolisticLife Cycle Approach.*** (Second edition) The C.V. Mosby Company, Toronto (1988).

SAMPLE OF PROCESS RECORDING

I. History

Identification Data :

Name	: Mr. K.L.	Address	:	9/144, Arya Nagar, Sonepat,
Age	: 29 years			
Sex	: Male	Language	:	Hindi
Ward No. 10, Bed No. 2		Informant	:	Brother-in-law
Education	: 7th pass	Reliability	:	Poor
Occupation	: Carpenter	- He is not staying with the patient.		
Religion	: Hindu	- Knows the patient only for 3 years.		
Marital Status	: Married.			

II. Presenting Complaints

A. According to the Patient :

1. He has been seeing faces of people - mother-in-law, a Muslim man resembling his father showing an angry face for two months.
2. He can hears a razor talking to him and he can call its voice whenever he wants.
3. Breathlessness.
4. Lack of interest in talking to others.
5. Getting violent and beating parents.
6. Lack of interest in having sexual relationship with wife.

B. According to the Relatives :

Abnormal behaviour consists of :

- Irrelevant talking, for example talking about jharna (spring) and children and saying they have strong relationship amongst each other.
- Incoherent speech at times which they cannot understand.
- Abusive, aggressive, violent-beating parents.
- Laughing and crying on his own.
- Drug abuse - sulffa, a product of the bhang plant-since 1976.
- Selling household things like the gold ring, utensils etc. for buying the drug.
- Tearing of clothes.
- Poor personal hygiene.
- Lack of interest in work.

According to the relatives, these symptoms are present since the time they know him, i.e. Since his marriage in May 1986. These symptoms are gradually increasing.

III. History of Presenting Complaints

Mr. Krishan Lal had been taking drugs since 1976 when he was working in the "Atlas Cycle Co". Four or five years ago, he started beating his parents and once even threatened them with a knife. According to the informant, since marriage itself the patient had been talking irrelevantly and at times incoherently. He was abusive, aggressive and violent. He used to beat his parents but never had beaten his wife. Many a time he used to sit alone and talk to himself and sometimes he will start crying or laughing on his own. On several occasions he used to tear off his clothes and never took care of his personal hygiene. The tools for carpentary were bought for him but he never worked with them. He used to say that he could hear some voices calling him and also he could see the faces of his mother-in-law and a man resembling his father. He was never interested in socializing. He loves his children. He believes that Panditji had heard a voice during their marriage ceremony because of which they had just five "Pheras" (circles round the holy fire) in place of seven, so he feels his marriage is incomplete. He also has a feeling of impotency. He also says that the kids are not his own because he never had sexual relationship with his wife.

His sleep is not disturbed and appetite is normal. He has regular bowel and bladder habits.

For the above symptoms he has been taken to various doctors and hospitals. Since January 5, 1992 he has been under treatment in one of the hospitals in Delhi.

IV. Aims and Objectives of Interview

1. Patient's Point of View

i. To help the patient to come out of his problems.
ii. To help the patient to conceptualize his problems.
iii. To help the patient choose alternatives and try them out.
iv. To help the patient to communicate.
v. To help the patient to socialize.
vi. To help the patient to change his attitude towards family members and life.
vii. To provide the patient with corrective interpersonal experience.
viii. To help the patient develop insight.

2. Student's Point of View:

i. To gain the patient's confidence and get his cooperation.
ii. To establish rapport with the patient.

iii. To know about the patient's illness and understand the psychodynamics of illness.

iv. To identify the role of the socio-cultural background on the patient's behaviour.

v. To help the patient help himself.

vi. To gain skill in taking interview.

vii. To practise various communication/interview techniques to get information from the patient and to help him.

I. Interview

Date : January 27, 1994.
Time : 10.00 AM to 10.30 AM
Duration : 30 Minutes

Specific Objectives :

1. To gain the confidence of the patient.
2. To assess the condition of the patient.
3. To collect the psychiatric history of the patient.
4. To identify the patient's problems.

Before this interview the therapist had one interaction with the patient on January 1, 1994, to assess his mental status.

INTERVIEWING THE PATIENT AND DRAWING INFERENCE

Participant	Conversation	Inference
P	Namaste, Sister (he folds his hands to wish)	Gait normal.
N	Namaste, Krishan Lal, come and sit (the patient sits) Did you have your breakfast ?	Immediate memory intact.
P	No.	
N	Today, you are looking more fresh.	
P	Yes, Sister, I am better now. I want to get discharged.	
N	APKA MAN KAISA HAI (How is your mood today ?)	
P	MAN KHUSH HAI (I am happy) (the patient looks apathetic)	Affect is inadequate and inappropriate.
P	AB MUJHE KAL SE KOI AWAZEN NAHIN SUNAI DE RAHI HEIN. SHAKLEN BHI DIKHAI NAHI DE RAHI HEI. PAHELE MUJHE MERI SAS DIKHAI DETI THEE. AUR EK MUSLIM ADMI JO GUSSE MEIN THA, AUR MERE PJIA JI JAISA DEKHAI DETA THA.	No auditary and visual hallucination. The patient perceives father as an angry man.
N	Yes, hmm.	
N	Was your father very strict with you ?	He didn't like father being strict.
P	Yes, he was very strict and used to beat us.	
N	Is he strict now also ?	
P	No, now during illness I had beaten my parents.	
N	You were beating your parents ? Do you think this is right ?	Realises his mistake by analysing his behaviour.
P	No	
N	What are you doing these days ?	
P	I am a carpenter. In 1976 I worked in the Atlas Cycle Co for four years and then stopped working there.	Remote memory intact.
N	Why did you leave that job ?	
P	The owner told me to leave the job. Then I worked as a conductor in a truck and after learning driving I became a driver. After marriage I stopped that.	The patient had changes the job.
N	Why did you stop that work ?	
P	It was long-route driving.	
N	When did you get married ?	Remote memory intact. Paranoid delusion present.
P	Three years back but my marriage is not real, it was incomplete. I had just 5 pheras instead of seven.	
N	Why just five ?	
	Panditji got some order and he stopped. I just stayed with my wife for a day.	Delusion of control present.
N	Do you have children ?	
P	Yes, I've got a two-year-old son and three-month-old daughter.	
N	If you've stayed with your wife just for a day, how do you have two children.	
P	My wife had illicit relations with someone else.	Paranoid delusion.

N	Do you love your children and wife ?	
P	I like my children but I don't want to have any relationship with my wife.	The patient is attached with his children. Libido creased decreased.
N	Why ?	
P	Because our marriage was incomplete	
N	Is your wife staying with you now ?	
P	No	
N	What is your plan after discharge ?	
P	I will work as a carpenter, I've a machine at home.	Willing to work after discharge.
N	Are you taking medicines regularly ?	
P	Yes.	
N	Once you get discharged you must come for regular follow-up and continue taking the medicines till the doctor says.	Concentration good.
P	O.K. Sister.	
N	Do you want to ask any question.	
P	No.	
N	O.K. then we will stop our interview here. Thank you for being with us.	

SUMMARY

1. Summary List of Inferences

Mr. K.L. was cooperative, communicating well. His gait was normal. Immediate, recent and remote memory intact. Affect inadequate - apathetic. No auditory and visual hallucinations present. Paranoid delusion present, he has decreased libido.

He has got his negative feeling i.e. of anger towards father because of the old man's strictness. He was beating his parents but now he realises his mistake. He plans to work as a carpenter after discharge. He likes his children but does not want to have any relationship with his wife because of his delusion of an incomplete marriage.

2. Introspection

The nurse was able to assess the condition of the patient while interacting and gain confidence. The problems which she could identify were: the patient had a paranoid delusion towards his wife, and marriage. Gradually, with subsequent interactions she will be able to help Mr. K.L.

3. Interview Techniques Used

i. Listening
ii. Direct questioning
iii. Reflection - feeling
  - content
iv. Pinpointing
v. Non-verbal communication of nodding of the head.

COMPREHENSIVE TEST ON CHAPTER V

1. List the types of theories used by the psychiatric nurse:-

(i)
(ii)
(iii)
(iv)
(v)
(vi)

2. Define the following terms:

(i) Therapeutic relationship/one-to-one relationship/nurse-patient relationship is defined as ....
(ii) Communication process is defined as ....
(iii) Interview is defined ....
(iv) SPIEL is defined ....

3. List the factors determining effective nurse-patient relationship:

(i)
(ii)
(iii)

4. Tasks of the preinteraction phase are :

(i)
(ii)
(iii)

5. Barriers of the interaction phase are :

(i)
(ii)
(iii)
(iv)
(v)
(vi)

6. Problem/Barriers of termination are :

(i)
(ii)
(iii)
(iv)

7. Match the following:

COLUMN A	COLUMN B
_ (1) It is also known as a body language.	A. Verbatim
_ (2) It is one of the effective methods of interviewing.	B. SMCR
_ (3) Placing the patient in the right and wrong category is called	C. Verbal communication
_ (4) It is an essential feature of interviewing	D. Observation
_ (5) "I am feeling sad" is an example of	E. Confidentiality
_ (6) Recording of interaction done 'word for word' is also called as	F. Moral Pigeonholing
_ (7) When the patient is restless, pacing up and down, the technique used by the nurse is	G. Clarifying
_ (8) When he patient says that he is very happy today and the nurse ask's him to elaborate, the technique used by the nurse is	H. Non-verbal communication
_ (9) Concentrating on one single point is a technique called	I. Focusing
_ (10) These are the major components of communication.	J. Pinpointing
	K. Questioning.

COMPREHENSIVE KEY TEST OF CHAPTER V

I. (i) Psychoanalytic theory (ii) Interpersonal theory
(iii) Behavioural theory (iv) Humanistic theory
(v) Stress theory (vi) Eclectic approach

2. (i) The end result of a series of planned purposeful interaction between two human beings, a nurse and a patient.

(ii) Communication process is defined as exchange of information between individuals through a common system of symbols, signs or behaviour.

(iii) Interview is a face-to-face interaction between two persons.

(iv) SPIEL is defined as narration by the patient of total history of his sickness as part of routine.

3. (i) **Self-Awareness** of the nurse including her self-concept, beliefs and values, and life experiences.

(ii) **Attitude** of acceptance of the patient.

(iii) **Developing rapport.** The essential qualities for developing rapport are warmth, genuineness and empathetic ability of the nurse.

4. Tasks of the preinteraction phase are :
(i) The nurse explores her fears and anxiety.
(ii) Sets the objectives for the interaction phase.
(iii) Takes help of the clinical supervisor/teacher to overcome her anxiety and fears.

5. (i) Development of pact or contract.
(ii) Social class of the patient.
(iii) Status of the patient.
(iv) Anxiety of the nurse or the patient.
(v) Transference.
(vi) Counter-transference.

6. (i) The patient may ask the nurse to visit him during the latter's off-duty hours.
(ii) The patient may like to visit or telephone the nurse.
(iii) Gift giving by the patient.
(iv) The nurse may avoid the patient who is discharged.

7. Match the following:
(1) H (2) K (3) F (4) E (5) C (6) A (7) D
(8) G (9) I (10) B.

CHAPTER VI
THERAPEUTIC MODALITIES

UNIT XV

PSYCHOPHARMACOLOGY AND ROLE OF PSYCHIATRIC NURSE

UNIT OUTLINE

- Definition of Psychotropic drugs.
- Classification of Psychotropic drugs.
  * Antipsychotic agents.
  * Antiparkinson/Anticholinergic agents.
  * Antidepressant agents.
  * Antimanic agents.
  * Antianxiety agents.
    Sedatives and Hypnotics
- Description of drugs
  * Sub-classification of drugs.
  * Indication or use of drugs.
  * Contraindication.
  * Side-effects of drugs.
  * Nurse's role in giving drugs.
- Application to Nursing
- Better Study Section

INTENDED LEARNING BEHAVIOUR

After reading this unit you will be ableto:

- define psychotropic drugs
- classify the psychotropic drugs i.e.
  * Antipsychotic drugs,
  * Antiparkinson/anticholinergic agents.
  * Antidepressant agents.
  * Antimanic agents.
  * Antianxiety agents.
    Sedatives and Hypnotics
- describe each major drug in terms of:-
  * Types of drugs.
  * Indication and use.
  * Contraindication.
  * Dose, action and side-effects.
  * Nurse's role.
- Apply knowledge while administering drugs.
- Make early diagnosis and prevent complication due to toxicity.

CONTENT

INTRODUCTION

Over a span of several decades the psychotropic drugs are proving effective in controlling a broad range of mental and emotional disorders. These various chemical agents have revolutionised the treatment of mental illness. With increased use of these drugs, their action and side-effects have also increased.

DEFINITION OF PSYCHOTROPIC DRUGS

Pshychotropic drug is any drug that has a primary effect on behaviour, experience, or other psychological functions (Logman Dictionary of Psychology and Psychiatry). Psychotropic or psychoactive drugs can also be defined as chemicals that affect the brain and nervous system, alter feelings and emotions. These drugs also affect the consciousness in various ways. A Broad range of these drugs is used in emotional and mental illnesses.

CLASSIFICATION OF PSYCHOTROPIC DRUGS

Psychotropic drugs can be classified under five major groups:

A. Antipsychotic Agents
B. Antiparkinson Agents
C. Antidepressant Agents
D. Antimanic Agents
E. Antianxiety Agents, Sedatives & Hypnotics.

A. ANTIPSYCHOTIC AGENTS

DESCRIPTION

Antipsychotic agents are also known as neuroleptics, major tranquillizers, or phenothaiazines. This group of drugs has a major clinical use in the treatment of psychosis. Psychosis is a state in which a person's ability to recognize reality, to communicate and to relate to others is severely impaired (Wilson H.A. Kneisel).

INDICATIONS OR USE

Antipsychotic agents are commonly used in the followings conditions:

* Schizophrenic disorders
* Paranoid disorders
* Mania
* Organic dementia
* Acute brain syndrome

Symptoms for which antipsychotic or neuroleptic drugs are used include impaired communication, inability to relate to others, delusion, hallucinations and inability to identify reality, disordered thinking and emotional withdrawal.

MODE OF ACTION

Antipsychotic agents are thought to block the dopamine receptors. Dopamine is a chemical which is released in the brain and causes psychotic thinking. Increased production of dopamine transmits the nerve impulses to the brainstem faster than normal. This results in strange thoughts, hallucinations and bizarre behaviour. Antipsychotics help in blocking or reducing the activity of dopamine. Antiemetic is another property of antipsychotic agents. They are also used in hiccoughs.

CONTRA-INDICATIONS

Antipsychotics are contraindicated in children under three years of age, comatose patients, patients with drug hypersensitivity, severe depression, and bone marrow depression.

Antipsychotic agents should be used cautiously in patients with a history of epilepsy, pregnancy, Parkinson's disease, peptic ulcer etc.

CLASSIFICATION OF ANTIPSYCHOTIC AGENTS

Types of antipsychotic or neuroleptic or phenothiazine agents, with chemical name, trade name, oral dose, effects, and side-effects are given in the form of a Table.

CLASSIFICATION OF ANTIPSYCHOTIC AGENTS

CHEMICAL GROUP & GENERIC NAME	TRADE NAME	RANGE OF DAILY DOSAGE IN mgm	FORM OF AVAILABILITY Tab.	liquid	Injection	ACTION
I PHENO-THIAZINES ALIPHATIC						
i. Chlorpromazine	Largectile	50-1200 mgm/day	√	√	√	Higher sedation, hypotension, lower extrapyramidal symptom (EPS) I/M form has low potency, thereby more injections with large doses are required. May lead to injection abcesses or sciatic nerve complications.
	Thorazine		√	√	x	
	Promapar		√	√	-	
	Sonazine		√	√	-	
ii. Triflupromazine	Siquil	30-150 mgm/day	√	√	√	More potent than chlorpromazine so EPS are more.
iii. Promazine	Sparine	100-400 mgm/day	√	√	√	
PIPERAZINE						
i. Trifluoperazine	Eskazine	5-40 mgm/day	√	√	√	Lower sedation, hypotension, higher EPS
* ii. Perphenazine	Trilafon	6-64 mgm/day	√	√	√	-do-
* iii. Acetophenazine	Tindal	40-120 mgm/day	√	x	x	
iv. Carphenazine	Proketazine	25-400mgm/day	√	√	x	Lower sedation, hypotension, higher EP
v. Procholoperzine	Stemetil	15-150 mgm/day	√	√	x	
vi. Fluphenazine	Prolixin Permitil Anatensol Deconoate	1-20 mgm/day	√	√	√	short acting can be used for testing the tolerance. Prolimitin Enanthate can be used as long acting for mintenance dose.
PIPERADINES						
i. Thioridazine	Mellaril	50-800 mgm/day	√	√	x	These drugs have lowest extra pyramidal symptoms (EPS) of the phenothiazines.

CLASSIFICATION OF ANTIPSYCHOTIC AGENTS

CHEMICAL GROUP & GENERIC NAME	TRADE NAME	RANGE OF DAILY DOSAGE IN mgm	FORM OF AVAILABILITY			ACTION
			Tab.	Liqure	Injection	
ii. Mesoridazine		150-400 mgm/day	√	√	√	The other effects are orthostatic hypotension, cardiac effect, ejaculatory inhibition. Should be used carefully for elderly and suicidal patients.
iii. Piperacetazine	Serentil Quide	40-160 mgm/day	√	x	√	
II. BUTYRO-PHENONES						
i. Haloparidol	Haldol	2-100 mgm/day	√	√	√	EPS more common than phenothiazianes.
ii. Triperidol			x	x	√	
III. THIOXAN-THENES						
i. Thiothixene	Navane	5-60 mgm/day	√	√	√	More potent than chlorporthixene Potency and side-effects similar to phenothiazine
ii. Chlorprothixene	Taractan	75-600 mgm/day	√	√	√	
iii. Fluphenthixol	Fluanxol	3-10 mgm/day	√	√	√	
IV. OXINODLES						
i. Molindone	Moban, Endo Lidone	15-225 mgm/day	√	x	x	Similar to phenothiazine.
V. DIBENZO-XAZIPINES						
i. Loxapine	Daxolin Loxapac	15-100 mgm/day	√	x	x	Same as phenothiazine.

* Drugs are not available in India Pesently.

Fig. 6 : Table Describing Classification of Antipsychatic agents.

SIDE-EFFECTS OF ANTI PSYCHOTICS/ NEUROLOPTIC AGENTS

Side-effects are described according to the effect on various systems.

1. CENTRAL NERVOUS SYSTEM CHANGES

Extrapyramidal symptoms such as motor restlessness, Parkinsonism, dystonia, tardive dyskinesia and neuroleptic malignant syndrome.

Parkinsonism: Occurs in 40% of the patients presenting extrapyramidal symptoms. There are two varieties of Parkinsonia Symptoms:

(i) Akinetic Form - Appears in the first week of administration of antipsychotic drugs. The characterstics of akinetic form are:

Difficulty in masticating movements, weakness and muscle fatigue.

(ii) Agitating Form of Parkinsonian Symptoms include: Tremors at rest, rigidity and mask-like face. Most characterstic features of Parkinsonism are:

(i) Rigidity of muscles
(ii) Motor retardation
(iii) Salivation
(iv) Slurred speech
(v) Mask-like face
(vi) Shuffling gait

Anticholinergic drugs are given as treatments.

Akathisia : Akathisia occurs in 50% of all the patients presenting extrapyramedal symptoms. The common characterstics are: Restless "walking in place." Difficulty in sitting still, or strong urge to move about - referred to as "Walkies and Talkies" by Haris (De Gennaro, A.J.N. 1981,P. 1326). Generally occurs after two weeks of treatment. Before administering anti-Parkinsonian medication anxiety should be ruled out.

Dystonia : Dystonia occurs in 6% of total number of patients presenting EPS. The characteristic features are: rapidly developing contraction of muscles of the tongue, jaw, neck (producing torticollis) and extraocular muscles. Combined torticolis and extraocular spasm results in an ***OCULOGYRIC CRISIS*** in which eyes look upward, head is turned to one side. Dystonia is painful and gives a frightening experience to the patient. Constant observation of the patient should be made. Dystonia occurs within a few minutes of giving medicine or after several hours.

Tardive Dyskinesia : This occurs due to abrupt termination or reduction of the antipsychotic drug after long-term-high-dose therapy. Tardive dyskinesia is characterized by involuntary rhythmic, stereotyped movements, protrusion of the tongue, puffing of cheeks, chewing movements, involuntary movements of extremities and trunk. These symptoms occur in 3% of patients. Antipsychotics shoula be stopped immediately. There is no treatment, symptoms may appear for years. It is irreversible.

Neuroleptic Malignant Syndrome (NMS) : This is a rare complication of antipsychotic agents and is usually fatal. May develop within hours or after years of continued drug use. Symptoms include hyperpyrexia, severe muscle rigidity, altered consciousness, blood pressure changes, increased count of W.B.C. Symptoms appear suddenly when medication is started and can persist for 10-14 days or longer. Symptomatic treatment is given to patients.

2. AUTONOMIC NERVOUS SYSTEM

Dry mouth, blurred vision, constipation, urinary hesitance or retention and under rarer circumstances paralytic ileus.

3. CARDIO-VASCULAR

Tachycardia, orthostatic hypotension and reversible arrhythmias.

4. BLOOD OR HEMATOPOIETIC

Agranulocytosis (marked decrease in leukocytes system especially with chlorpramozine) leukopenia, leukocytosis.

5. ENDOCRINE DISRUPTIONS

Menstural irregularities, including amenorrhea and false positive pregnancy tests, breast enlargement, lactation, weight gain, changes in libido, impotence, glycosuria, hyperglycemia.

6. GASTRO-INTESTINAL

Anorexia, constipation, diarrhoea, hypersalivation, nausea, vomiting, obstructive jaundice.

7. ALLERGIC EFFECTS

Dermatitis, photosensitization, pigment deposits.

8. OCCULAR EFFECTS

Blurring of vision, Pigmentation of cornea and lens and Rationpathy.

9. HEPATIC SIDE-EFFECTS

Liver toxicity occurs in 0.5% of cases presenting EPS. It is a hypersensitivity reaction and not dose dependent. Onset of symptoms is within the first one month of treatment. Symptoms may be fever, chills, nausea, malaise, prurites and jaundice

NURSE'S ROLE

On reading side-effects of the antipsychotic drugs, it is evident that the role of the nurse is very significant in the thserapeutic effect of the drug, early observation and prevention of complications, limiting the complications if already occurred.

* *Close Observation,* specially when the antipsychotics are just started. The expected results are reduction in aggressive hyperactive behaviour and disorganized thoughts. Look for the possible side-effects.

* *Extrapyramidal reaction,* i.e. Parkinsonism, akinesia, akathisia, dystonia, and tardive dyskinesia. These symptoms are reduced/ treated with early observation, reporting and use of anti-Parkinsonion or anticholinergic medication (Refer antiparkinsonian drugs described in this unit).

* *Observe drowsiness.* Medicine should be administered at bed time. Report if the drowsiness persists for a very long time. The patient should be advised not to drive and handle hazardous machinery while taking antipsychotic drugs. Observe for sore throat, fever due to agranulocytosis.

* *Record blood pressure* of the patient on antipsychotic drugs. If the blood pressure drops by 20 to 30 mm of Hg in the patient, immediate reporting and intervention should be done. The patient should be made aware of the possibility of dizziness and injuries after receiving medication and injection due to orthostatic hypotension.

* *Accurate route of medication* - Antipsychotic drugs are not given subcutaneously unless specially prescribed as they cause tissue irritation. These drugs should be given deep 1/M.

* *Dry mouth* may be reduced by encouraging the patient to rinse his or her mouth frequently. Give a piece of lemon or chewing gum. Good oral hygiene should also be maintained.

* *Blurred or impaired vision* in the patient causes anxiety and annoyance to him. The patient should be encouraged to inform these symptoms immediately. Blurred vision or brown coloured vision, night blindness can be permanent due to pigmentary retinopathy.

* The patient on antipsychotic drugs may have *weight gain.* Weight record should be maintained. The patient may be encouraged on a low salt and planned caloric diet.

* The patient may complain of *gastric irritation.* He should be discouraged to take antacids as there will be decreased absorption of antipsychotic drugs.

* An *intake output chart* should be maintained specially for male patients who are confined to bed and have an enlarged prostate gland. Encourage at least 2,500 ml of liquid intake.

* The patient snould be advised to *protect his skin,* by not going in the sun and to wear protective clothing and sunglasses.

* The patient should be explained not to *increase or decrease or stop taking drugs* without discussing with his doctor. The drugs should be withdrawn slowly to avoid nausea or seizures.

* The nurse should find out the *menstrual changes* from the female patient. Sometimes the patient may complain of fever, upper abdominal pain, nausea, jaundic and diarrhoea. These symptoms can be due to cholestatic jaundice. The nurse should stop the medicine immediately and inform the doctor.

* *Reasurance to relatives* - The patient and his relatives should be explained that desired effects will be achieved after weeks of medication, so the relatives need to wait for the effects of the drugs.

TO RECALL

— Antipsychotic/Neuroleptic/Major Tranquillizers/Phenothiazenas are the drugs used in psychosis

— Indications/Uses:
* Schizophrenic disorders
* Paranoid disorders
* Mania
* Organic Dementia
* Acute brain syndrome

— Mode of Action
Antipsychotic agents are thought to block the dopamine receptors.

— Contraindications
Comatose patients, drug hypersensitivity, severe depression, bone marrow depression.

— Classification
* Phenothiazine
* Butyrophenones
* Thioxanthenes
* Oxinodles
* Dibenzoxazipines

— Side-Effects on
* Central nervous system - Extra pyramidal symptoms (EPS); parkinsonism; akathesia, dystonia, tardive dyskinesia, neuroleptic malignant syndrome (NMS).
* Autonomic Nervous System - dry mouth, blurred vision, constipation
* Cardivascular system
* Blood or hematopoietic system
* Endocrine
* Gastro-intestinal system
* Allergic Effects

— Nurse's Role.

B ANTIPARKINSONIAN AGENTS

DESCRIPTION

Antiparkinsonian agents are the specific drugs to treat the extrapyramidal side-effects of antipsychotic agents. Side-effects are parkinsonism, akathisia, acute dystonia and tardive dyskinesia. (Refer side-effects of antipsychotic agents).

Anticholinergics, antihistamines and amantidne are used to treat these side-effects.

INDICATIONS OR USE

Antiparkinsonian drugs are used to treat the extrapyramidal symptoms. (EPS)

MODE OF ACTION

Anticholinergic drugs block the secretion, thereby reducing the symptoms of akathesia and acute dystonia. It is not effective against tardive dyskinesia.

Antihistamines have effects like anticholinergic drugs. Amantadines are dopamine-releasing agents from central neurones. Studies show that this drug may affect some clients with tardive dyskinesia.

CONTRAINDICATION

Patients with a history of closed angle glaucoma, urinary or intestinal obstruction, hypersensitivity, prostatic hypertrophy, tachycardia are not given these drugs. The drugs are given with caution to patients with myasthenia gravis, artherosclerosis and chronic respiratory problems. Anticholinergic drugs: Amantadine is given with caution to patients with renal impairment as most of the medication is excreted through the kidneys.

CLASSIFICATION OF ANTIPARKINSONIAN DRUGS

Chemical and Generic Name	Trade Name	Dose Range per day mgm/day	Form of availability
I. ANTICHOLINERGIC			
i. Benztropine	Cogentin	0.5-6.0	Tab, Injection
ii. Biperiden HCl Hydrochiride	Akinetone Dyskinon	2.0-8.0	-do-
iii. Trihexyphenidyl Hydrochiride	Pacitane Parbenz	2.0-12.0	Tab.
iv. Procyclidine Hydrochiride	Kemadrin	5.0-20mg	Tab.

Contd.

Chemical and Generic Name		Trade Name	Dose Range per day mgm/day	Form of availability
II.	ANTIHISTAMINE			
i.	Diphenhydramine	Benadryl	75-100	Capsule & Syrup
III.	DOPAMINE DRUGS			
i.	L. Dopa	Larodopa	2.gms-3gms.	Tab.
ii.	Amantadine Hydrochiride	Symmetrel	100-200mgm	Tab.
iii.	Selegline	Deprenyl	5mg-10mg	Tab.
iv.	Carbidopa & L. Dopa.	Sinemet	10mg-100mg	Tab.

Fig. 7 : Table Describing Classification of Antiparkinsonian Drugs.

SIDE-EFFECTS OF ANTIPARKINSONIAN DRUGS

Anticholinergic : Side-effects are dry mouth, flushed, dry skin, blurred vision, photophobia, increased heart rate, constipation, urinary retention, mental confusion and excitement.

Antihistamine : Side-effects are drowsiness, dizziness, anorexia, nausea, vomiting, euphoria, orthostatic hypotension, weight gain, weakness and tingling of hands.

Amantadine : Side-effects are mood changes, slurred speech, insomnia, inability to concentrate, dry mouth, livedo reticularis that is a red-blue netlike discolouration of the skin which becomes worse in winter.

NURSE'S ROLE

* Observation - Observation of the patient for side-effects of anti-parkinsonian drugs such as tachycardia, palpitation, sedation, drowsiness and blurred vision.
* Maintain an intake output chart in case the patient has urinary retention or constipation.
* Encourage adequate intake of fluids and roughage in the diet.
* Record vital signs such as B.P., pulse and respiration every four hours.
* Advise the patient not to get up quickly from a lying -down position

to sitting because of orthostatic hypotension.

* Educate the patient not to use hazardous machinery or driving when he is on anticholinergic drugs.

* Encourage the patient to get his routine eye check-up done for early detection of blurred vision or glaucoma.

* Record the medicine and side-effects accurately.
* Report and record any side-effects observed to the physician.

TO RECALL

*** Antiparkinsonian agents are used to prevent and treat the extrapyramidal side-effects of antipsychotic agents.**

*** Antiparkinsonian drugs are classified as :**
— Anticholinergic
— Antihistamine
— Amantadine

*** Nursing implications are significant in terms of :**
— Observation
— Recording
— Educating the patient

C. ANTIDEPRESSANT AGENTS

DESCRIPTION

Antidepressant agents are used in affective disorders or disturbances mainly to treat depressive disorders caused by emotional or environmental stressors. Several groups of affective disturbances are treatable by antidepressants.

INDICATIONS OR USE

Antidepressants are used in the following depressive states:

* *Grief reaction* which may follow due to loss of money or a significant person. It may lead to shock, denial, sadness, excessive crying, irritability and anger, usually between two months.

* *Pathological Grief* - Grief reaction continues. A person withdraws socially, presents somatic symptoms.

* *Depression* due to adjustment disorders, loss of self-esteem, discontent,

feeling of worthlessness, lack of initiative and increased sleep.

* *Endogenous Depression* - It does not have relationship with events. There is a slowing of thought, speech, severely depressed mind, agitation, vegitative signs; early morning insomnia. (Refer Chapter VII).

* *Agitated Involutional Depressive Syndromes* - Patient over 45 years of age suffering from depression. It is a subgroup of endogenous depression; including agitation, delusion and guilt.

MODE OF ACTION

Antidepressant drugs are classified as Tricyclics, Tetracyclics and MAO inhibitors. Research studies have shown reduced levels of norepinephrine (NE) and serotinin (5-HT) (neurotransmitters) in the space between nerve endings carrying message from one nerve cell to another cause depression. Tricyclic antidepressants and MAO inhibitors increase these neurotransmitters i.e. norepinephrine and sertinin to the synaptic receptors in the central nervous system *(Refer Unit IX Fig. 13, Page No 71)*. Tricyclic inhibitors block the reuptake of NE and 5-HT and MAO inhibitors block the action of Monoamine oxidise in breaking down excess of NE and 5-HT at the presynaptic neuron.

CONTRAIN-DICATIONS

Antidepressants are given with caution to patients with cardiovascular disorders because they cause arrhythmias. They increase symptoms of psychosis and mania in cases of manic-depressive psychosis. Drugs are given with caution to patients with liver disorders.

CLASSIFICATION OF ANTIDEPRESSANT AGENTS

CHEMICAL GROUP & GENERIC NAME	TRADE NAME	RANGE OF DAILY DOSAGE IN mgm	AVAIL-ABLE FORM	ACTION
I. TRICYCLIC ANTIDEPRES-SANTS				
i. Impramime	Tofranil Depsanil Imavate Janimine Presamine	50-200 mgm/day 75-300 mg/day	Tab.	Tricyclic and tetracyclic antidepressants are used to treat symptoms of depression. For example, insomnia, decreased appietite, decreased libido, fatigue, indecisiveness, difficulty in thinking and concentration.

Contd.

CLASSIFICATION OF ANTIDEPRESSANT AGENTS

CHEMICAL GROUP & GENERIC NAME		TRADE NAME	RANGE OF DAILY DOSAGE IN mgm	AVAIL-ABLE FORM	ACTION
ii. Trimipramine		Surmontil	50-300 mgm/day	Tab.	Somatic symptoms and feelings of worthlessness.
Amitriptyline		Tryptanol	75-300 mgm/day	Tab.	
		Quietal	50-200 mgm/day	Tab.	
		Amiline			
Desipramine	*	Petrofrane	75-300 mgm/day	Tab.	
	*	Norpramine			
Nortriptyline		Aventyl	40-100 mgm/day	Tab.	These drugs are effective in 85 per cent of those people who exhibit symptoms of depression.
		Pamelor			
Protriptyline	*	Vivactil	30-60 mgm/day		
Doxepin		Spectra			
		Doxepin	25-150 mgm/day	Cap/	
	*	Exipeaca		Tab.	
II. TETRACYCLIC ANTIDEPRESSANTS					
i. Maprotilene		Lidiomil	75-300mgm/day	Tab.	
ii. Mianseril		Tetradep	60-150 mgm/day	Tab.	
III. MONOAMINE OXIDASE INHIBITORS					
i. Isocarboxazid	*	Marplan	10-60 mgm/day		MAO inhibitors are used in severe endogenous depression when patients do not respond to Tricyclic and Tetracyclic antidepressants.
ii. Phenelzine sulphate	*	Nardil	15-90 mgm/day		
iii. Tranylcypromine sulphate		Parnate	10-60 mgm/day		

* These dugs are not available presently.

Fig. 8 : Table Describing Classification of Antidepressant Agents.

SIDE EFFCTS OF ANTIDEPRESSANT DRUGS

Side-effects of antidepressants can be described under the following systems:

* **Central Nervous System** - Drowsiness, sedation, delusion, hallucination, extrapyramidal symptoms. Taradive dyskinesia with amoxapine (Ascendin).

* **Autonomic Nervous System** - dry mouth, urinary retention, constipation, dilated pupils.

* **Cardio-Vascular** - Postural hypotension, Tachycardia, cardiac arrythmias, agranulocytosis.

* **Gastro-intestinal** - Nausea, vomiting, loss of appetite, jaundice.

* **Endocrine** - Galactorrhea (formation of milk even mother though is not a nursing mother), gynecomastia (large mammary glands in male may sometimes secrete milk), hyperglycemia and hypoglycemia.

* Allergic rash to drugs in some patients.

NURSE'S ROLE

* Observation of the side-effects and monitoring the changes noted are very significant to prevent complications due to antidepressant agents.

* Encourage the patient to take medicine at bed time due to a sedative effect. Dryness of mouth to decrease.

* Give plenty of fluids orally. Lemonade or chewing gum should be given. A few sips of water also help the patient.

* Do not give medicine empty stomach as the patient complains of nausea and vomiting.

* Accurate recording of intake and output of the patient should be maintained to check if he has retention of urine.

* To relieve constipation plenty of fluids and roughage should be encouraged in the diet.

* If the patient complains of dizziness or light headedness he/she should be encouraged to get up slowly and sit in the bed before standing. These symptoms may be due to orthostatic hypotension. The patient should be reassured that these symptoms are for a short period only. Some patients may present hypertension.

* Accurate recording of vital signs like B.P. and Pulse.

* The nurse should be able to interpret the blood reports specially blood sugar level and W.B.C. count. If the patient complains of sore throat, fever, malaise, it should be reported to the physician on duty. These symptoms may be due to agranulocytosis or hyperglycomia.

* If the patient complains of sexual disfunction inform the physician immediately and stop the drug.

* If the patient is presenting symptoms of pressure of speech, increased motor activity and elated mood, the physician should be informed and the drug should be stopped immediately.

* Antidepressant tricyclic drugs begin therapeutic effects within four to eight weeks.

* Accurate recording of the observation made.

TO RECALL

* **Antidepressant agents are used to treat depressive disorders caused by emotional or environmental stressors.**

* **Indication or use of antidepressants is in grief reaction, endogenous depression and agitated involutional depressive syndrome.**

* **Mode of Action : Tricyclics and MAO inhibitors increase the level of neurotransmitters i.e. norepinephrine and Serotonin and reduce depressive symptoms.**

* **Contraindications - Arrhythmias, mania and patients with liver disorders.**

* **Classification - Antidepressant agents are classified as :**
  - **Tricyclic antidepressants**
  - **Tetracyclic antidepressants, and**
  - **Monoamine oxidase inhibitors (MAO inhibitors)**

* **Side-Effects are on various systems such as central nervous system, autonamic nervous system, cardio-vascular system, gastro-intestinal, endocrine and skin.**

* **The nurse's role is significant to protect the patient from drug-induced complications.**

D. ANTIMANIC AGENTS

DESCRIPTION

Antimanic agents are also called mood stabilizers. Lithium is considered a treatment of choice for the manic phase of the bipolar disorders, more commonly understood as mania or manic depression. It has also been tried in the treatment of depressive and schizoaffective disorers.

INDICATION OR USE

The major use of an antimanic agent is for treatment of mania and recurrent manic episodes.

MODE OF ACTION

The specific biochemical mechanism of action of antimanic agents is unclear. Anatimanic agents produce many neurochemical changes in the area of brain. These changes may affect norepinephrine and serotonin in the part of CNS involved in emotion. It may decrease the activity of the nerve impulse, resulting in depression or increase in the nerve impulse, causing mania. Lithium also helps in maintaining the sodium concentration in the brain, thereby regulating the mood swings as well as impulse along the nerve cells.

CONTRA-INDICATIONS

* Patients's with renal impairment are not given the drug as 80 per cent of a lithium dose is reabsorbed in the proximal renal tubules and excreted by the kidneys.
* Patients with sodium depletion or receiving diuretics (diuretics are the drugs which increase urine output.)
* Patients with cardio-vascular problems.
* Pregnant woman can have foetal anomalies.
* Patients with hypothyrodism would require monitoring of their dose for hypothyrodism also.

CLASSIFICATION OF ANTIMANIC AGENTS.

Chemical Group or Generic Name	Trade Name	Daily Dosage Range in mgn	Form Caps & Tablets	Action
I. LITHIUM CARBONATE	Licab Eskalith	600-1200mg (divided dosage) serum level range 0.5-1.5m Eq/L,	Caps & Tab.	Reduces symptoms of mania.
	Lithane Lithonate Lithobid Lithonafe-s(Syrup) Lithocarb	900-1800 (divided dose)		
II. CARBAMAZEPINE	Tegretol Mezetol	400-1600mgs (dose range and serum level to be maintained between 8-12 mgm/ml.	-do-	Given to patients when lithium is not very effective.

Fig. 9: Table describing Classification of Antimanic Agents, Trade name, Dosage and Action.

SIDE-EFFECTS Side-effects can be summarized under various systems as well as according to the serum lithium level in the blood.

A. **According to Various Systems:**

* *Central nervous and autonomic nervous system* : Tremors, muscle irritability, tinnitus (Ringing or tinkling sound in the ears that is purely subjective), confusion, slurred speech and convulsions, blurred vision.

* *Cardiovascular System* - Arrhythmias, hypotension, bradycardia, generalized odema.

* *Gastro-intestinal:* Euthyroid goiter, myxedema.

* *Urinary:* Albuminuria, oliguria, polyuria.

* *Allergic:* Drying and thinning of hair, alopecia, itching.

B. ACCORDING TO SERUM LITHIUM LEVEL

SERUM LITHIUM LEVEL	Symptoms
Below lm Eq/L	Nausea, diarrhoea, fine hand tremors and malaise
1 - 2 m Eq./L	Drowsiness, vomiting, abdominal pain, lethargy, dizziness, confusion, ataxia.
2 - 2.5m Eq/L	Anorexia, persistent nausea and vomiting, blurred vision, seizure, acute circulatory failure, stupor, coma.
Above 2.5 m Eq/L	Generalized convulsion, oliguria, death.

Fig. 10 : Table describing Serum Lithium Level and Side-Effect.

NURSE'S ROLE

* Give medicine during or after meal to decrease gastric irritability. It will also reduce the metallic taste in the mouth.
* Make observation of the side-effects. Record and report immediately.
* Make note of the serum lithium level, and observe the side-effects and plan the nursing intervention (Refer Fig. on Page 79)
* Weight should be recorded before lithium therapy. Excessive weight gain or swelling of ankles and wrists should be noted. Weekly weight record should be maintained.
* Intake/output chart is to be maintained to note the kidney functioning.
* Fluid intake is to be balanced because retention of fluid will increase weight.
* Any change in the diet should be reported immediately. Less intake of diet will affect the lithium level in the blood.
* Salt should not be restricted in the diet unless instructed by the physician.

✻ Advise the patient not to increase or decrease medicine unless advised.

TO RECALL

✻ Antimanic agents are also called mood stabilizers.

✻ Indication or use of these agents is specifically for treatment of mania and recurrent manic episodes.

— Mode of action:- Antimanic agents produce many neurochemical changes in the brain.

— Contraindications:- Patients with renal impairment, sodium depletion or receiving diuretics, and cardiovascular problems. Pregnant women can have foetal anomalies.

— Classification of Antimanic Agents, Lithium Carbonate and Carbamazepine.

— Side-Effects,:- Side-effects occur due to imbalance in the serum lithium level.

— Nurse's role.

E. ANTIANXIETY AGENTS, INCLUDING SEDATIVES AND HYPONOTICS

DESCRIPTION OF ANTIANXIETY AGENTS

Anxiety is a state which occurs in all human beings at sometime or the other. It is also a cardinal symptom of many psychiatric conditions. The drugs used to relieve anxiety are called *ANTIANXIETY OR ANXIOLYTIC AGENTS.* Antianxiety drugs relieve moderate-to-severe anxiety and tension.

INDICATION OR USE

— Antianxiety agents are used to relieve mild, moderate and severe anxiety associated with: emotional disorders physical disorders excessive environmental stress neuroses and mild depressive states without causing excessive sedation or drowsiness.

— For control of alcohol withdrawal symptoms.

— To control convulsions.

— To produce skeletal muscle relaxation

— To provide short-term sleep preoperatively, prior to diagnosis and insomnia.

Antianxiety agents should always be used in time-limited regimen.

MODE OF ACTION

These non-barbiturate benzodiazepines act as CNS depressants. It is believed that these drugs increase or help the inhibitory neurotransmitter action of gama-aminobutyric acid (GABA). This GABA mediates both presynaptic and postsynaptic inhibition in all areas of CNS. So, there is inhibition or control on the cortical and limbic system of the brain, which is responsible for emotions such as rage and anxiety.

CONTRAINDICATIONS

Patients with renal or liver and respiratory impairment are given antianxiety drugs with caution.

PART-A. CLASSIFICATION OF ANTIANXIETY AGENTS

	CHEMICAL GROUP & GENERIC NAME	TRADE NAME	RANGE OF DAILY DOSAGE IN mgm	ACTION
I.	NON-BARBITURATES			
A.	BENZODIAZEPINES			
i.	Chlordiazepoxide	Librium; Equibrome	15-100mgm	These are non-barbiturate Benzodiazepines.
ii.	Diazepam	Valium; Calmpose	6-50 mgm	They produce a tranquillizing effect without
iii.	Oxazepam	Serepax	30-120 mgm	much sedation.
*iv.	Prazepam	Verstran	20-60 mgm	These drugs are potential for abuse.
*v.	Chlorazapate	Tranzene Azene	11.25-60 mgm	
vi.	Flurazepam	Dalmane, Nitravet	15-60 mgm	
vii.	Nitrazepam	Mogadon	10-30 mgm	
viii.	Lorazepam	Ativan	2-6 mgm	
B.	NON-BENZODIAZEPINES PROPANEDIOLS			
i.	Meprobamate	Equanil	1.2-1.6 gms	These drugs have sedative action and present a
		Miltown	1.2-1.6 gms	high risk of abuse and physical dependence.
		* Tybamate	1.2-1.6 gms	
II	ANTIHISTAMINES	* Atarax	30-200 mgm.	* These drugs are not available in India presently.
		* Vistaril	30-200 mgm.	
i.	Hydroxyzine			

Fig. 11 : Table Describing Classification of Antianxiety Agents.

PART-B. CLASSIFICATION OF SEDATIVES AND HYPNOTICS

	CHEMICAL GROUP & GENERIC NAME	TRADE NAME	HYPNOTIC DOSE RANGE - DAILY	SEDATIVE DOSE - DAILY	ACTION
III.	**BARBITURATES**				
i.	Amobarbidtal SA	Amytal	100-200 mgm	60-150 mgm	These drugs cause drowsiness lethargy, decreased alertness and sleep. Tolerance to drugs can occur within seven to fourteen days, resulting in physical dependence.
ii.	Butabarbital SA	Butisol	100-200 mgm	20-200 mgm	
iii.	Pentobarbital LA	Nembutal	100-200 mgm	60-150 mgm	
iv.	Phenobarbital LA	Luminal	100-200 mgm	30-90 mgm	
v.	Thiopental USA	Pentothal	Used for anasthesia		
IV.	**NONBARBITURATES** Refer classification of antianxiety agents.				
V.	**QUINAZOLINES**				
i.	Methaquualone	* Quaalude * Parest * Optimil Mandrax	150-300 mgm	250-300 mgm	
VI.	**ACETYLINIC ALCOHOLS**				
i.	Ethchlorvynol	Placidyl	0.5gm-1 gms	200-600 mgm	
VII.	**CHLORAL DERIVATIVES**				
	Chloral hydrate	Noctaec	0.5gm-2 gms		
	Chloral betaine	Beta-chlor	870mg-1 gm.		
VIII.	**MONOUREIDES**				
	Paraldehyde	Paral	3gm-8 gms.		

* Drugs not available in India presently.

Fig. 12 : Table Descrbing Classification of Sedatives and Hypnotics.

SIDE-EFFECTS OF ANTIANXIETY SEDATIVES-HYPNOTICS

Side-effects of antianxiety and sedativehypnotics can be described acording to systems.

* Central nervous system: drowsiness, ataxia, confusion, depression, blurred vision.
* Cardiovascular system: Hypotension, palpitations, syncope (fainting or form of unconsciousness)
* Endocrine - changes in libido.
* Allergic - Skin rash
* Physical/Psychological dependence non-benzodiazepines and barbiturate group of drugs has a high risk of abuse and physical dependence.
* Acute toxicity of barbiturates that can be fatal when taken in excessive dosage usually for suicide attempts. Overdose can cause tachycardia, hypotension, shock, respiratory depression, coma and death.

NURSE'S ROLE

* Assessment of the patient, prior to the use of antianxiety, sedative-hypnotic agents. If the patient complains of sleep disturbance the causative factor should be identified.
* Appropriate nursing measures to induce sleep should be taken such as a calm and quiet environment, a cup of hot milk, good back care, allowing the patient to read magazines, sitting with the patient for sometime for reassurance purpose.
* While administering the drugs daily dose should be given at bed time to promote a normal sleep pattern, so that day-time activities are not affected.
* Give I/M injection deep into muscles to prevent irritation.
* Look for side-effects, record and report immediately.
* If the patient complains of drowsiness tell him to avoid using knife or any other dangerous equipment. He should be instructed not to drive.
* Instruct the patient not to take any stimulants like coffee, alocohol as they alter the effect of drugs.

* Avoid excessive use of these drugs to prevent the onset of substance abuse or addiction.

* Drug should be reduced gradually, Sudden stoppage of the drug may cuse REM (Rapid Eye Movements), insomnia, dreams or nightmare, hyperexcitability, agitation or convulsions.

TO RECALL

* **Antianxiety or Anxiolytic agents are used to treat overt anxiety and somatic complaints.**

* **Sedatives and hypnotics are used to induce sedation.**

INDICATIONS - To reduce anxiety, to control convulsions, to control alcohol withdrawl symptoms, to reduce muscle spasm, to induce sleep.

MODE OF ACTION - Nonbarbiturates benzodiazepines work selectively on the limbic system of the brain which is responsible for emotions such as rage and anxity. Sedatives - hypnotics induce sleep.

CONTRAINDICATION - Patient with renal, respiratory and liver impairment.

CLASSIFICATION OF ANTIANXIETY SEDATIVE HYPNOTICS

I. Non-barbiturates
Benzodizepin
Non-benzodiazepines
II. Anthistamins
III. Barbiturates
IV. Quinazolines
V. Acetylinic Alcohols
VI. Choloral derivatives
VII. Monoureides

SIDE-EFFECTS are according to each system significant in drug abuse or physical dependency.

NURSE'S ROLE is very significant to prevent complications and physical dependence on the drug.

APPLICATION TO NURSING

Reading of this unit will help the nursing personnel to understand the types of psychotropic drugs. Classification of psychotropic drugs will enable her to understand the implication of using a particular drug and how it helps the patient. Reading of this unit will also enble the nurse to identify side-effects, plan the nursing intervention and save the patient from complication. The list of drugs may not be exhaustive but nursing personnel will be able to identify the effect of a particular classified drug on change in the behaviour of the patient. Knowledge of this unit will enable her to assist the physician to reduce, increase or stop a particular drug.

BETTER STUDY SECTION

1. VOCABULARY (USE DICTIONARY)

Abuse	Inhibitory	Rage
Assessment	Intervention	Retention
Dizziness	Monitoring	Rigiding
Drowsiness	Odema	Slurred
Euthyroid	Physical dependence	Syndrome
Gradually	Presynaptic	Termination.
Hesitance		
Impaired		
Impulse		

2. ASSIGNMENT

Make a tabular chart of antipsychotic antidepressant drugs under the following headings.

Generic Name	Trade Name	Dose	Action	Side-Effect	Nurse's Role

3. EXERCISE

a) Define the following terms:
   i. Psychotropic agents
   ii. Antianxiety agents
   iii. Physical dependence
   iv. Syncope

v. Tardive dyskinesia

b) Describe the role of the nurse while administering antipsychotic drugs.
c) List the E P S (Extrapyramidal symptoms).

4. READING REFERENCES

Shives L.R. *Basiç Concepts of Psychiatric-Mental Health Nursing* (2nd edition) J.B. Lippincott Company, Philadelhia (1990)

Lego S. *The American Handbook of Psychiatric Nursing.* J.B. Lippinoott Company, Philadelphia (1984).

Tripati K.D. *Essentials of Medical Pharmacology* Jaypee Brothers R.P. & Williams S.R.

Mental Health Psychiatric Nursing - A Holistic Life Cycle Approach. The C.V. Mosby Company, Washington, Dec. (1988).

Johnson, B.Sc. *Adaptation and Growth Psychiatric - Mental Health Nursing* (2nd edition) J.B. Lippincott Company, Philadelphia (1989).

Kapoor, Bimla - *A Text Book of Psychiatri c Nursing.* Kumar Publishing House, (1992).

UNIT XVI

PSYCHOSOCIAL THERAPIES AND ROLE OF NURSE

UNIT OUTLINE

- Definition of psychotherapies
- Goals of Psychosocial therapies
- Types/Techniques of Psychosocial therapies
- Individual Psychotherapy:
  * Psychoanalyses
  * Hypnosis
  * Abreaction
  * Reality therapy
  * Uncovering
  * Supporting therapy
- Behaviour modification
  * Systematic desensatization
  * Aversion therapy
  * Assertiveness training
  * Cognitive behaviour therapy
  * Implosive therapy/flooding
  * Positive reinforcement
- Interpersonal Therapy
  * Marital therapy
  * Family therapy
  * Transactional therapy
- Group Psychotherapy
- Other psychosocial therapies
  * Therapeutic Community/ Milleu Therapy
  * Attitude Therapy
  * Application to Nursing
  * Better Study Section.

INTENDED LEARNING BEHAVIOUR

After reading this unit, you will be able to:

- Define psychotherapy
- Classify the types/techniques of psychosocial therapy
- Describe the individual psychotherapies
- Apply the knowledge of individual psychotherapy in therapeutic nurse-patient rela tion-ship
- Explain behaviour therapy and its types
- Utilize the knowledge in the clinical field and community.
- Discuss the interpersonal therapy
- Develop skill in using types of interpersonal therapies in hospital and community
- Develop skill in conducting group therapy
- Participate in Millieu therapy
- Develop skill in using appropriate attitude-therapy

CONTENT

INTRODUCTION

In treatment modalities for psychiatric patients the approaches used are: Psychopharmacology *(Unit XV)*, Psychotherapies or Psychological treatments and somatic therapy or physical treatment. In this unit the emphasis will be on psychological treatment or psychotherapies. Psychotherapy is the treatment used for a patient with emotional and personality problems. It is also used for problems which originate due to psychological factors. The basic principle in psychotherapy is the Therapist-Patient Relationship. *(Refer Chapter V, Unit XHI)*. In all psychotherapies the therapist respects the client, remains non-judgemental and accepts the client as an individual human being. Use of psychotherapy by nursing personnel is an independent role where the nurse uses an appropriate psychotherapy approach to help her patient.

DEFINITION OF PSYCHO-SOCIAL THERAPY

Psychotherapy is the treatment of personality problems, maladjustments and mental disorders by psychological means. Wolberg (in Longman Dictionary of Psychology and Psychiatry) defines psychotherapy as, "A form of treatment for problems of an emotional nature in which a trained person deliberately establishes a professional relationship with the objective of removing, modifying or retarding existing symptoms, of mediating disturbed patterns of behaviour, and of promoting positive personality growth and development."

Lego S. defines psychotherapy as, "A method of treatment based on the development of intimate (therapeutic) relationship between client/patient and therapist for the purpose of exploring and modifying the client/patient's behaviour in a satisfying direction."

A Psychiatric Glossary (1980) defines psychotherapy as, "A process in which a person who wishes to relieve symptoms or resolve problems in living or is seeking personal growth enters in implicit or explicit contract to interact in a prescribed way with a psychotherapist." *(p. 116)*.

All the three definitions emphasize the basic concepts that: (1) in psychotherapy a therapeutic relationship is established between the patient and the therapist; (2) the purpose of psychotherapy is to modify, remove or reduce the factors causing a disturbed behaviour and, (3) to help the patient to grow and develop coping mechanism to face the problems in future, and improve in social functioning.

GOALS OF PSYCHOSOCIAL THERAPY

The goals of psychotherapy are to help the patient in:

(i) Changing maladaptive behaviour patterns.

(ii) Reducing or eliminating environmental conditions that may be causing such a behaviour.

(iii) Improving interpersonal and other competencies, i.e. communication skills.

(iv) Helping the patient to resolve inner conflicts and overcome feelings of handicap (such as the patient feels he can't socialize, or take a decision or communicate effectively).

(v) Modifying an individual's accurate assessement of himself and the world around him.

(vi) Helping him to develop a sense of self-identity.

So, psychotherapy helps in reducing the patient's discomfort, improving his social functioning and ability to perform or act appropriately.

TYPES/TECHNIQUES OF PSYCHO-SOCIAL THERAPIES

Types or techniques of psychotherapies used are many. Types/ techniques of psychotherapy adopted in this text are presented diagramatically.

TYPES/TECHNIQUES OF PSYCHO-SOCIAL THERAPY

INDIVIDUAL PSYCHOTHERAPY

* Psychoanalysis
* Hypnosis
* Abreaction
* Reality Therapy
* Uncovering
* Supportive Therapy
  - Ventilation
  - Environmental Modification
  - Persuasion
  - Reeducation
  - Reassurance

BEHAVIOURAL PSYCHOTHERAPY

* Behaviour modification
* Systematicdesnsatization
* Aversion Theropy
* Assertiveness Training
* Coginitive behaviour therapy
* Implosive Therapy (Flooding)
* Positive Reinforcement
  - Response shaping
  - Modelling
  - Token economy

INTERPERSONAL PSYCHOTHERAPY

* Marital Therapy
* Family Therapy
* Tranactional Therapy

GROUP PSYCHOTHERAPY

OTHER PSYCHO-SOCIAL THERAPIES

* Therapeutic Community/ Millieu Therapy
* Attitude therapy

Fig. 13 : Types/Technique of Psychosocial Therepy.

TO RECALL

— Psychotherapy is a method of treatment based on the development of an intimate (therapeutic) relationship between client /patient and therapist for the purpose of exploring or modifying the patient's behaviour in a satisfying direction.

— Goals Of Psychotherapy Are:

- **Changing maladaptive behaviour**
- **Modifying environment causing maladaptive behaviour**
- **Improving I.P.R. skills**
- **Helping the patient to overcome a feeling of handicap**
- **Helping him to make an accurate assessment of himself and develop self-identify.**

— Types Of Psychotherapies

i. Individual Psychotherapy
ii. Behavioural Psychotherapy
iii. Interpersonal Psychotherapy
iv. Group Psychotherapy
v. Other Psychosocial Theropy

INDIVIDUAL PSYCHO-THERAPY

Psychotherapy conducted on a one-to-one basis. The therapist treats one person at a time. The effectiveness of such a therapy depends on the Patient-Therapist Relationship. Types of individual psychotherapy include:

Psychoanalysis, Hyponsis, Abreaction, Reality Therapy, Uncovering and Supportive Therapy.

TYPES OF INDIVIDUAL PSYCHO-THERAPY

PSYCHOANALYSIS

Psychoanalytical therapy was developed by Freud. The therapeutic technique focuses primarily on the influence of unconscious forces such as repressed impulses and memories, internal conflicts and childhood traumas on the mental life and adjustment of the individual. Its foundation is based on problems in early psychosexual development. The Oedipus Complex; the pleasure and reality principles, the systems of personality, i.e., Id, ego and super ego and the central importance of anxiety and defences against anxiety and neurotic reactions. *(Refer Units II and III of Chapter I).*

Psychoanalysis as a form of therapy is used primarily in psychoneuroses by bringing about basic modification in the personality. This is done by establishing a constructive therapeutic relationship.

The specific methods used to achieve the effect of therapy are: free association, dream interpretation analysis of resistances and defences used by the patient, working through the feelings and experiences revealed by the patient during transference.

Every interaction lasts for 45 minutes, four to five days a week for approximately three to five years. It is an expensive form of therapy in terms of money and time.

HYPNOSIS AND HYPNOTHERAPY

Hypnosis is a superficial or deep trance (a somnolent state/sleep like) resembling sleep. It is induced in a patient by suggestions of relaxation and concentrating attention on a single object. The patient/client becomes highly suggestible, submissive and abandons control and response to therapist's influence. He can be induced to recall forgotten events, becomes insensitive to pain, gains relief from tension, anxiety and other psychological symptoms. It affects behavioural change and control of attitudes.

Hypnosis is considered effective in obesity, hypertension, asthma, smoking, peptic ulcer, overeating and other addictive disorders. A person under hypnosis cannot be forced to perform actions that conflict with his values and belief.

ABREACTION

It is a therapeutic technique in which the patient talks about repressed emotions by reviving and reliving painful experiences that have been buried in the unconscious. When the psychiatrist considers that it could be helpful, he may use an intervenous injection of a drug such as pentothal.

REALITY THERAPY

This is a psychotherapeutic technique which focuses on the present behaviour and development of a patient's ability to cope with the stresses of reality and take a greater responsibility for the fulfilment of his needs.

To achieve these purposes the therapist becomes involved in an active relationship with the patient, rejects his unrealistic behaviour and teaches better ways to meet his needs in the real world. The patient needs to be stressed on, that the past cannot be changed; so he must take responsibility of right or wrong actions of the present.

UNCOVERING OR INSIGHT PSYCHOTHERAPY

This technique is used to break through the patient's repressed conflicts and traumatic experience to the surface. It helps the patient in gaining an insight. The patient explores different methods to cope with the problem, once he gains an insight into his conflict or problem.

SUPPORTIVE PSYCHOTHERAPY

It is a form of "surface therapy". The therapist helps the patient/client to relieve emotional distress and symptoms without probing into the past or attempting to change or alter the basic personality of the individual. The therapist reinforces the existing defences used by the client and utilizes various techniques such as: (i) Ventilation, (ii) Environmental manipulation; (iii) Persuasion. (iv) Reeducation and (v) Reassurance.

(I) VENTILATION

It is a free expression of feelings or emotions. The patient is allowed to talk freely whatever comes to his mind. It is also described as *MENTAL VENTILATION.* The therapist will note that during free talking the patient avoids certain events or mentions them superficially. The client/patient is encouraged to talk about them more freely until they no longer cause emotional disturbance in the client/patient. It helps the client to unburden his feelings by sharing and revealing himself which makes the client/patient less tense. For example, a student feels that her way of talking to the teacher was not appropriate. She feels it and becomes uncomfortable or tense until a day she gets an opportunity to talk to the teacher and ask for apology. The teacher might not have even thought of the harshness in the student's behaviour.

(II) ENVIRONMENTAL MODIFICATION OR MANIPULATION

A method of improving the well-being of mental patients by changing their living conditions. If there is a restless patient in the ward due to whom the other patient is not able to sleep, the former may be transfered to a cubicle where no other patient is allowed for a day or two.

(III) PERSUASION

Persuasion psychotherapy is used in which the therapist attempts to induce the patient to modify his faulty behaviour by using his power of reasoning, will and self-criticism. For example, a mother who is neglecting her girl child may be helped to modify her behaviour.

(IV) REEDUCATION

The patient learns more effective ways of dealing with problems and relationship through therapist-patient relationship or group therapy.

(V) REASSURANCE

It is a supportive approach that encourages the patient to believe that there are possibilities of improvement. It is also used to diminish anxiety e.g. by explaining to the patient that the period of heightened depression is a temporary phase.

TO RECALL

- **Individual Psychotherapy is conducted on a one-to-one basis. The therapist treats one person at a time.**
- **Types of Individual Psychotherapy**
  - **— Psychoanalysis**
  - **— Hypnosis or Hypnotherapy**
  - **— Abreaction**
  - **— Reality Therapy**
  - **— Uncovering or Insight Psychotherapy**
  - **— Supportive Psychotherapy includes:**
    - **Mental Ventilation**
    - **Environmental Modification or Manipulation**
    - **Persuasion**
    - **Reeducation**
    - **Reassurance**

The principles of achieving goals of individual psychotherapy are described by Shives L.R. as follows:

(a) Establishing a therapeutic therapist-patient relationship.

(b) Providing an opportunity for the patient to release tension as problems are discussed.

(c) Assisting the patient in gaining an insight into the problem.

(d) Providing an opportunity to practise new skills.

(e) Reinforcing an appropriate behaviour as it occurs.

(f) Providing consistent emotional support.

BEHAVIOURAL PSYCHOTHERAPY AND ITS TYPES

DEFINITION

It is a form of psychotherapy which focuses on modifying faulty behaviour rather than basic changes in the personality. Insetad of probing the unconscious or exploring the patient's thoughts and feelings, behaviour therapist tries to eliminate the symptoms and modify ineffective or maladaptive patterns by applying basic learning techniques.

Behaviour therapists believe that problem behaviour are learned and therefore can be eliminated or replaced by a desirable behaviour through new learning experiences. Behaviour techniques include behaviour modification systematic desensitization, cognitive behaviour therapy, aversion therapy, assertiveness therapy, implosive therapy, and positive reinfocement therapy.

BEHAVIOUR MODIFICATION

It is also called "Simple Extinction". Learned behaviour pattern becomes a waste or disappears if it is not reinforced. To eliminate a maladaptive behaviour one has to remove the reinforcement for it. It is effective when reinforcement is being used without the knowledge of the affected individual. Every time Sonu, a nine-year-old girl bites her nails, her mother gives her an angry look. Sonu understands the mother's anger and tries not to repeat the bad habit. A maladaptive behaviour is gradaully removed. Mother's anger is a punishment for Sonu. Rewards are also provided to reduce the maladaptive learning. Rishu, 11-year-old boy, is told that if he studies one hour regularly on his own in class VI he would be allowed to buy a cricket set of his choice.

SYSTEMATIC DESENSITIZATION

It is a form of behaviour therapy developed by J. Wolpe and others. The objective of the therapy is to reduce or eliminate fear or anxieties in which (i) the patient is trained in deep muscles relaxation, (ii) he has various anxiety-provoking situations or specific phobia; such as fear of death, fear of animals. These problems are placed from the strongest to the weakest order i.e. the client is anxious about which one is causing anxiety the least. (iii) Each of these situations is presented in imagination or in reality beginning with the weakest. Once the patient relaxes while imagining, that means the anxiety is getting reduced gradually.

For example, a child is having fear of crossing the road. For a few days the mother can take the child to the road and just stand and talk about other things. The child keeps observing people crossing to and fro. Then after two or three days mother and child cross the road while they are talking. This may reduce the anxiety in a child as he is allowed to cross the road in a relaxed manner. Therapy is very useful for patients who have developed certain fears specially to domestic animals like dog.

AVERSION THERAPY

It is a form of behaviour therapy in which the patient is conditioned to avoid an undesirable behaviour or symptom by associating them with painful or unpleasant experiences, such as putting a bitter taste on nails or tongue for nail biting. Giving drugs like apormorphine which cause nausea or vomiting on taking alcohol or an electric shock to treat a child with enuresis.

Aversion therapy has been used for alcoholism and compulsive unacceptable social behaviour like homosexuality.

ASSERTIVENESS TRAINING

It is a behaviour therapy technique in which the patient is given training to bring about change in emotional and other behavioural patterns by asserting himself. In other words, one is encouraged not to be afraid of showing an appropriate response, negative or positive, to an idea or suggestion. Many people hold back their feelings. The assertive behaviour training is given by the therapist first by role playing and then by practice in a real life situation. Attention is focused on more effective interpersonal-skills. For example, a timid patient will become less anxious if he is made to realize that giving voice to his feelings is appropriate such as complaining about poor service.

Assertiveness training teaches one to ask for: what is wanted, take a position on various issues and take action to obtain what one wants; of course, taking care of other persons' rights. This training can be used for mentally healthy and mentally ill persons.

COGNITIVE BEHAVIOUR THERAPY

It is a psychotherapeutic approach based on the idea that emotional problems in an individual arise due to faulty ways of thinking and distorted attitude towards onself and others. The therapist takes the role of a guide who helps the patient to correct and revise his perceptions and thoughts. This helps the patient to change his thoughts, feelings and behaviour about himself. Congnitive Behaviour therapy is considered effective in the treatment of depression and adjustment difficulties.

IMPLOSIVE THERAPY

It is a behaviour therapy technique opposite to systematic desensitization. It is also called FLOODING. In this therapy, an individual is exposed directly to a maximum intensity fear-producing situation either in imagination or in real life. The patient gradually feels no actual danger in the situation. For example, he has developed intense phobia of a lizard. During a psychotherapy session suddenly the therapist puts a rubberized lizard on the table. For a minute the patient may get scared but gradually may start handling a rubberized lizard while talking.

POSITIVE REINFORCEMENT

It is a stimulus or stimulus situation which is given to the patient

or individual after the response. When the stimulus is given after the response it is on the basis that the strength of the response is increased and that the response will appear again. For example, as soon as the infant gets up and walks, the mother claps and gives the infant a piece of chocolate to enjoy.
Positive reinforcement can be done by (i) Response Shaping, (ii) Modelling, and (iii) Token Economy.

(I) RESPONSE SHAPING

Positive reinforcement is used in response shaping or incorporating or establishing a response which is not existing in an individual's behaviour. This technique is used in a behaviour problem or mental retardation.

For example, Shubam, 14, has an intelligence level of a five years old child. He had never done any of his activities such as washing after defecation, wearing shoes and socks. The therapist trained the family member to encourage Shubam to wear his socks and shoes. When he wears them he should be taken for a ride (car) which he enjoys the maximum. In this way he can be encouraged to learn those behaviours which he has never learnt.

(II) MODELLING

Modelling is a behaviour therapy technique in which learning occurs through observation. The client/patient watches someone else perform a particular action such as answering the telephone. Models are often parents or other adults and children. Modelling is a form of social learning and is often called Observational Learning.

(III) TOKEN ECONOMY

It is a behaviour therapy programme usually conducted in a hospital or classroom setting. In token economy the desired behaviour is reinforced by offering tokens that can be exchanged for special foods, games, comics or other rewards.

For example, a patient with schizophrenia does not maintain personal hygiene. The day he maintains he gets a token as reinforcer that he can watch T.V. when he desires. Like this he is able to collect many tokens and adapt s behaviour which is socially acceptable. Like maintaining personal hygine. Sometimes in return of tokens the patient may exchange them by asking for PAROLE.

So the use of tokens as reinforcers for an appropriate behaviour has many advantages: (a) By the number of tokens the patient earns he knows the number of times he has exhibited the desired behaviour, (b) Tokens do not give immediate satisfaction, so the patient learns to use the opportunity appropriately; (c) How the patient uses these tokens will enable him to make a decision.

Gradually, the patient will require no reward in terms of a **token;** he would be able to adapt to a certain behaviour with **guidance and** help

TO RECALL

- **Behaviour psychotherapy is a form of psychotherapy which focuses on modifying a faulty behaviour rather than basic changes in the personality.**
- **Types of Behavioural Psychotherapy:**
  - **Behaviour Modification**
  - **Systematic Desensitization**
  - **Aversion Therapy**
  - **Assertiveness Training Therapy/Assertive training**
  - **Cognitive Behaviour Therapy**
  - **Implosive Therapy (Flooding)**
  - **Positive Reinforcement**
- **Response shaping**
- **Modelling**
- **Token Economy**

INTERPERSONAL PSYCHOTHERAPY AND ITS TYPES

DEFINITION

Interpersonal therapy is the term used by J.L. Morena for a type of psychotherapy in which there is emphasis on the interpersonal relationship of the various persons involved, such as husband, wife, and one or more other parties.

Coleman J.C. included marital and family therapy and transactional analysis in interpersonal psychotherapy.

MARITAL THERAPY

This psychotherapy is directed at improving a disturbed marital relationship. It is centred on efforts to change the psychodynamics and behaviour of the partners. The sessions are usually conjoint. In a conjoint session two partners meet the therapist in joint sessions. Marital therapy may be conducted on a problem solving level in which grievances are aired and clashes worked through or on a more analytic level focusing on dreams, unspoken communication and the sources of defensive or aggressive attitude.

For example, the husband may say during the sessions. "She does not have any complaint against me, but still she is not happy;

that makes me uncomfortable." During the session the wife may start crying and confess, "Often I wanted to reply him back but seeing his anger and children around me I have been withdrawing into silence. But what's the use of talking ?"

In other words, insight is shared by the couple which may help them in a satisfactory marital relationship.

FAMILY THERAPY

It is a form of group psychotherapy in which the family is a therapeutic unit. Family is the matrix out of which all human interactions develop. The objective of family therapy is not merely to improve relationship but to modify home influences that contribute to the disorder of one or more family members. In this process, the therapist helps individual members to become aware of their distorted reactions and defensive patterns used by them. The therapist also encourages the members to communicate more meaningfully and handle their difficulties in a constructive manner.

Most of the psychopathology in an individual occurs due to the way he deals with his intimate relationship with family members. Changes in the individual behaviour can only occur if there is a change in all the members of the family.

TRANSACTIONAL ANALYSIS

It is a form of interpersonal psychotherapy developed by Eric Berne, which focuses on characteristic interactions that reveal internal 'ego states' and the 'Games People Play'. The ego states are - Child, Adult and Parent. Our parent is that part of our behaviour which we have learnt from others or our parents. "Go to sleep now", is an example of our parent talking. These statements as an adult, if used for another adult like wife or husband, create a problem. The child in the individual may obey immediately. Being an adult, the wife may start crying. Or an adult in an individual/wife may reply to her husband, "I will sleep after sometime."

In a transactional analysis the therapist analyses the interaction among the group members (often married) and helps the participants understand the ego state in which they are communicating with each other. 'Games People Play' are not 'for fun' but because they are played according to a set of unspoken rules. Allowing the individual to adopt a sick role and act. A response like "Yes but............" and allow the individual to continue. This provides an opportunity to an individual to reveal how we often unknowingly manipulate and harm other people as well as ourselves.

TO RECALL

* **Interpersonal therapy is a type of psychotherapy in which the emphasis is on the interpersonal relationship of various persons involved, such as husband, wife and one or more parties.**
* **Types of Interpersonal therapy**
  - **Marital Therapy**
  - **Family Therapy**
  - **Transactional Therapy**

GROUP THERAPY

DEFINITION

Group psychotherapy is a treatment of psychological problems in which two or more patients interact with each other on both an emotional and cognitive levels in the presence of one or more psychotherapists who serve as catalysts (the person who can be related to or who can understand the other's point of view), facilitators or interpreters. Three major kinds of groups are: Group Therapy, Therapeutic Groups and Adjunctive Groups. Sadocks (1985) suggests that in **Group Psychotherapy** members gain a personal insight, improve their interpersonal relationship, change destructive behaviour and make a necessary alteration in their behaviour.

Therapeutic Group is a group of patients who meet under the leadership of a therapist to work together to improve mental and emotional health. Example - groups of expectant mothers, people who have just lost their husband or wife. Group of people with a chronic illness. Therapeutic groups are self-help groups like Ashiana, Saheli in Delhi, who conduct these groups for drug addicts.

Adjunctive Groups deal with selected needs of a group. For example, for sensory stimulation allow them to have music therapy, for self-expression art therapy, for expression of feelings and emotions through dance therapy. These are a few examples which can be used for adjunctive groups.

Though group approaches vary, the basic principle is that in a group there is intimate sharing of feelings, ideas and experiences. There is an atmosphere of mutual respect and understanding which improves self-respect and self-understanding due to which the individual is able to live with others.

TYPES OF PSYCHOTHERAPY GROUPS

Psychotherapy groups can be classified in various ways such as:

(i) Traditional Groups.
(ii) Encounter Group or T. Group.
(iii) Homogeneous or heterogeneous groups,
(iv) Open or close groups,
(v) Groups for Psychosis or neurosis.

TRADITIONAL GROUPS

Traditional groups include mainly the patients with mental illness and are from the hospital inpatient department. In the didactic group therapy, lecture is given to the patient along with some filmshow, like in the case of excessive drinking or use of drugs.

Psychodrama is a technique of psychotherapy in which a patient acts out his feelings in front of a group of patients. The therapist guides and directs the patient and interprets the actions of the patient. This type of acting out provides an insight into the patient about his faulty patterns of learning which he can eliminate.

ENCOUNTER GROUP

Encounter group is a form of small group in which an individual learns how his feelings and behaviour affect him and others. This group is not necessarily a group of people with mental illness. The individual may have some coping difficulty which he would like to resolve at the right time. For example, a suspicious feeling gradually being developed about his wife or any other illusions. These groups are based on sensitivity training or T-groups.

HOMOGENEOUS AND HETEROGENEOUS GROUPS

Homogeneous groups are composed of patients of the same age, race, sex, socioeconomic level and similar category of illness. Heterogeneous groups vary on all these aspects.

OPEN GROUPS AND CLOSED GROUPS

In open groups members may join and leave the group at anytime. Closed groups have a specific number of people, specific time to start and close the group sessions; the duration is three to four weeks. Inpatients and outpatients both are included in this group.

Open and closed groups are used extensively in the hospital.

GROUP ACCORDING TO MENTAL ILLNESS

Neurotic group or patients suffering from psychotic illnesses come under this category.

STEPS OF GROUP THERAPY

The steps of group therapy can differ from an individual group therapist to therapist. Some of the common steps are : (i) Selecting the members in a group: (ii) Developing contact in a group, (iii) Selection of group leader (generally the therapist).

SELECTING GROUP MEMBERS

It is a very important function of a group therapist. She has to decide based on the condition of the patient who all can be included in the group. A very depressed patient may lead to withdrawal of other members of the group, whereas too many excited patients included in the group may lead to unsuccessful group therapy.

DEVELOPING CONTACT

It is a very significant factor.

* The purpose should be made clear to all the members in the group.
* Time, length and place of the meeting should be announced.
* Starting and ending time and how frequently the group sessions will be conducted.
* Attendance of members.
* Confidentiality to be maintained within the group.
* Role of the members is : to report punctually, maintain confidentiality and interact freely.

SELECTION OF GROUP LEADERS

* Role of the therapist - the therapist acts as a facilitator and helper. The goals of the nurse therapist as identified by De Mocker (1981) are:

  i) to provide information to the group.
  ii) allow emotional catharsis.
  iii) share members' perception.
  iv) share feelings of fear, loneliness and frustration.
  v) improve communication skills.
  vi) provide a role model.
  vii) help to know what is reality.
  viii) set limits for some patients.
  ix) make observation of all the non-verbal techniques being used by the patient.

TO RECALL

- **Group psychotherapy is a treatment of psychological problems in which two or more patients interact in the presence of a psychotherapist**

- **Types of group psychotherapy**
  - **Group therapy**
  - **Therapeutic group**
  - **Adjunctive group**

- **Types of Psychotherapy groups**
  - **Traditional groups**
  - **Encounter groups or T. groups**
  - **Homogeneous or heterogeneous groups**
  - **Open or closed groups**
  - **Groups for psychosis and neurosis**

- **Steps of Group Therapy**
  - **Selecting the members in a group**
  - **Developing contact in a group**
  - **Selection of a group leader**
  - **Role of a therapist**

OTHER PSYCHOSOCIAL APPROACHES

In other psychosocial therapies two major concepts are also included i.e. **MILLIEU THERAPY OR THERAPEUTIC COMMUNITY AND ATTITUDE THERAPY.**

MILLIEU THERAPY

Milieu is a French word derived from Mi means 'middle', lieu means 'place'. So milieu means environment or setting. Therapeutic milieu means providing a healthy environment which helps in the recovery of a patient. Most of the psychiatric illnesses occur because of an unhealthy environment. So a therapeuic environment helps the patients to become socially productive individuals. **Longman Dictionary** of Psychology and Psychiary describes the term Therpeutic Community as follows, "Therapeutic community is a term applied by the English Psychiatrist Maxwell Jones (1953) to a mental hospial that utilizes Milieu therapy. In this approach the entire environment of a mental hospital or a psychiatric ward is organized in such a way to achieve the aim of promoting recovery in the patient and preventing complications which may occur due to stay in the hospial." In his approach only standard treatment prescribed by the psychiatrist is not included, it also considers:-

(a) the interaction between the patient and all members of the staff.

(b) Social relationship among the patients.

(c) Participation of the patient in a ward meeting and physical set-up

(d) Participation in making a decision regarding occupational and recreational activities for the patient.

(e) Participation in certain policies of the ward.

HISTORICAL OVERVIEW

During World War II to rehabilitate neurotic patients it was discovered that

(i) the programme of treatment was more effective when careful attention was paid to the Milieu in which the casualty was kept;

(ii) The social system i.e. the I.P.R. of an attendent provided emotional support during stress,

(iii) Immediate treatment, if provided where close friends were also available, improved the daily activity of the patient and reduced the length of disability.

(iv) An opportunity to ventilate or talk about frightening or anxiety-provoking experience before or during sickness was helpful to the patients.

This basic approach was used in a psychiatric setting by bringing more interaction between the staff and the patient and was called *THERAPEUTIC COMMUNITY* by Maxwell Jones (1953). Dr. Jones wrote a book on social psychiatry which was published with a changed title, The Therapeutic Community (to start with, it was a report of efforts of the Belmot Hospital in England to rehabilitate neurotic patients through the use of a group method during and after World War II). Dr. Jones dedicated his book to the "Nursing Staff", justifying that it is the nursing staff who have formed a framework around which the therapeutic communities have been built.

DEFINITION OF THERAPEUTIC COMMUNITY/ MILIEU THERAPY

Milieu Therapy or Therapeutic Community approach attempts to make the maximum use of (i) the social system and its constituents (i.e. the patient, his relatives and neighbours), (ii) Personnel and the hospital community (i.e. psychiatrist, nurse, psychologist, social worker, other patients) to modify the patient's behaviour so that he may manage his life and his personal relationship in a more constructive manner.

GOALS OR PURPOSES OF THERAPEUTIC COMMUNITY/ MILIEU THERAPY

The goals can be described as follows:

* To minimize the antitherapeutic environment for the patient in the ward. For example, telling other nurses that he is always sad; let him stay in the bed only. (Example of antitherapeutic environment).

* To minimize prolongation of hospitalization by helping in early recovery.

* To minimize maladaptive behaviour. Creating an environment where maladaptive behaviour is discouraged.

* To provide a free and favourable climate in which the patient can talk and gain awareness of his own feelings, impulses and behaviour.

* To help the patient to improve his self-esteem by helping him understand that he can also make decisions, can take responsibilities, and his activities are appreciated if he performs them well.

PRINCIPLES OF MILIEU THERAPY

The essential principles of Milieu therapy can be described as:

(i) Therapeutic community is an approach used for the care of mentally ill patients through group activity.

(ii) Democracy is observed in a hospital setting. Democracy helps in increasing the self-respect of a patient.

(iii) The patient is involved in his own therapy which helps him in making decisions.

(iv) Decision-making ability improves the self-confidence of patients.

(v) It provides an environment of free communication. Hospital authoritativeness is reduced.

(vi) The patient is also directed to focus his attention not only on his own needs but also on the needs of other patients.

(vii) In a mental hospital or psychiatric ward, patients are away from society. So they feel isolated. Milieu therapy reduces social isolation and dehumanization of a large hospital. In large hospitals it is difficult to maintain one-to-one contact. Patients are considered as Bed No. suffering from types of schizophrenia and not by *name.*

(viii) It attempts to reduce the feeling in the patient about the supreme power of the doctor. The patient feels that he can approach the doctor.

(ix) Though the nurse sets limits and has various roles to play, still the patient considers her part of the milieu in which he is living. The nurse needs to be consistent in setting limits.

(x) Continuous assessment should be made to evaluate the progress of a patient. Modification should be made in nursing interventions.

IMPORTANT ASPECTS OF THERAPEUTIC COMMUNITY

Therapeutic Community or Milieu Therapy is based on several principles discussed in this unit. In this approach certain basic factors are considered which influence the effective Milieu Therapy.

GOVERNING SYSTEM

i. Communication is open and free.

ii. The goals are(a) to improve self-esteem (b) minimize hospital stay and disability, and (c) to minimize antitherapeutic environment.

iii. The patient and the staff get frequent opportunities to participate in hospital administration. For example, if tea is served at 7 o'clock, the patient may discuss and make arrangement that it is served at 8 o'clock as most of the patients are on sedatives and get up late.

iv. Emphasis in a therapeutic community is placed on social and group interaction with an individual patient and staff. Both are important members of the community.

v. A successful therapeutic community requires that both the staff and the patient become fully aware of their roles, limitations and responsibilities.

vi. Though staff members are in a position of final authority, much of the operation of the administration is in the hands of the patient.

vii. The hospital unit remains in close contact with outside agencies so that the patient can be provided with required information. Maybe job opportunities, half-way homes.

ADMINISTRATIVE ORGANIZATION

Therapeutic or antitherapeutic effect of Milieu therapy will depend on the hospital setting. If the hospital organization believes in this type of approach for mentally ill patients, the effect can be achieved. Otherwise, it is difficult for a unit to achieve these goals. In our country it may be difficult initially but once the hospital gets to know the advantages for the patients, such an approach will be practical!

ADVANTAGES FOR PATIENT

i. Milieu Therapy creats a different type of attitude and behaviour in the patient because the environment is like home.

ii. Instead of adopting a sick role, the patient makes decisions in the ward management and cares for other patients. In other words, he becomes less dependent and passive.

iii. The patient learns to adopt a behaviour which is acceptable in the therapeutic environment like learns to control hostility.

iv. The patient learns to make a decision which improves his self-confidence.

TYPES OF STAFF

The types of staff are professional i.e. Psychiatrist, Nurse, Psychologist, Technical Staff, Support Personnel. Each staff member asks repeatedly: "How do I perceive the needs of the patient ?" "How can I help the patient by improving my own knowledge and behaviour according to my capacity ?" For achieving these objectives the PRESCRIBED ATTITUDE approach can be used. In this approach the team leader forms a diagnosis of the patient's behaviour and provides the attitudinal approach to the patient based on the understanding of his behaviour. The attitude approach will be discussed under a separate heading in this unit.

ROLE OF NURSE

In a therapeutic community or Milieu Therapy. The role of the nurse is discussed by Jones as: Tripartite Role

(i) *Authoritarian Role* - when she controls the group and sets a limit.

(ii) *Social Role* - where the nurse encourages support in various ways. Talking to the team member, discussion during conference, encouraging the patient to communicate.

(iii) *Therapeutic Role* - By giving medication, maintaining therapeutic relationship. Making observation and reporting.

TO RECALL

> * Therapeutic Community or Milieu Therapy or Therapeutic Environment are interchangeably used terms.
>
> Definition - Milieu Therapy is an approach in which there is maximum use of a social system, hospital personnel and hospital community to modify the patient's behaviour so that he may manage his life and his personal relationship in a more constructive manner.
>
> * Goals of Milieu Therapy
> * Principles of Milieu Therapy
> * Important aspects of Milieu Therapy
>   — Governing System
>   — Administrative Organization
>   — Advantage of Milieu Therapy to the patient
>   — Types of Staff
>   — Tripartite Role of the Nurse

ATTITUDE THERAPY

In a therapeutic community or milieu therapy the effects can be best achieved if it is managed properly. To achieve the proper therapeutic effects an appropriate attitude is adopted by the nurse and team members.

DEFINITION OF ATTITUDE THERAPY

Attitude therapy is a form of Milieu Therapy in which all staff members assume a consistent, prescribed attitude designed to be therapeutic towards patients.

CRITERIA OF PLANNING OF ATTITUDE THERAPY

Attitude therapy is planned:

i. When the patient is in the hospital for a long time:
   * The patient is interviewed to assess his emotional state and activity level.
   * Family members are interviewedto acquaint them with the attitude therapy which will be used for the patient.

ii. After this, a staff meeting is held in which all the team members are present.

iii. A clinical diagnosis is made by the psychiatrist.

iv. A plan of attitude to be adopted for a particular patient is discussed with purpose.

v. *One Principal Line of Approach at a Time* is used by all the team members.

The attitude therapy is basically meaning to change the attitude of the patient in specific situations. A general attitude which the nurse needs to adopt for psychiatric patients is kept in mind. This has been discussed in earlier chapters.

ADVANTAGES OF ATTITUDE THERAPY FOR PATIENTS

Key and Hoffling have described the advantages of attitude therapy as:

i. The patient starts feeling that an organized approach is being used for his/her treatment.

ii. Guesswork and haphazard plans by individual members of the team are reduced.

iii. The patient's problems or conflicts are solved in less time.

iv. This approach also provides an opportunity for the members to explore, test and change the therapeutic attitude which will bring best results in patients.

v. It brings members of the team together to plan, work and evaluate each other's efforts and to discover new ways of helping the patient.

K.A. Menninger has worked on the concept of prescribed attitude therapy. Based on Menninger's work, the prescribed attitudes, their description and for which types of patients they can be used are given in the form of a table.

TABLE. DESCRIBING ATTITUDES, EXPLANATION OF ATTITUDES AND PATIENTS FOR WHOM THEY CAN BE USED

ATTITUDES	EXPLANATION OF ATTITUDE	TYPES OF PATIENTS
VIGILANT OBSERVATION OR WATCHFULNESS	The staff supervises the patient carefully without his knowledge.	Patient with * suicidal ideas and suicidal attempts * Patient with ideas of running away from the hospital.
INDULGENCE	Staff members accept or grant harmless favours, allow a certain amount of divergence from his routine such as delaying food or activities.	Patient in a withdrawal state.
ACTIVE FRIENDLINESS	Staff play an active role in the therapeutic professional interpersonal relationship.	* For patients who are in convalescent schizophrenia. * Patients who are emerging from severe depression.
PASSIVE FRIENDLINESS	The patient is allowed to take initiative in therapeutic relationship. The nurse gives the message that she is available to him. For example, she sits with the patients quietly and watches T.V. or reads a magazine. If the patient takes initiative, staff members follow quickly.	It is appropriate for patients who are extremely withdrawn, confused, frightened, paranoid schizophrenics, suspicious elderly patients, and patients with organic brain syndromes.
MATTER OF FACTNESS	The nurse uses an approach of casualness in interaction specially in requests, manipulative behaviour. Reassurances and emotional response are avoided.	Hysterical patients, Manic patients.
KIND FIRMNESS	Staff members put firm limitations. Direct, clear and confident rules are calmly imposed on the patient. Directions are specific and coincise with expectations that the patient will follow them.	* Paranoid patient. * Manic patient's jokes * Hysterical patient asking for attention.

Fig. 14 : Table Describing Attitude, Explanation of Attitudes and Patients for whom they can be Used.

ATTITUDE TO BE USED IN ANSWERING A REQUEST OF THE PATIENT

Grant, if feasible. Help the patient to evaluate the question and come to a decision. The patient will be able to perceive the childish nature. If he makes a request at 11 P.M. "Sister, can I sing loudly ?" it is to be restricted.

Direction or Substitute - For example, the patient wants to watch T.V. at 11.30 p.m. Allow him to watch but with a very low volume so that other patients are not disturbed. He may be given in substitute magazines to read.

Attitude to be used with regard to privileges or restrictions. Ignore the misuse. For example, two patients are playing cards in the recreation room till 11.30 p.m. when they should be sleeping. Is an example of misuse of privileges which should be ignored at times. Encourage use of privileges. For example, if a patient is good in painting, encourage him to borrow colours of his choice from a social worker and use the privilege effec-tively.

TO RECALL

- **Attitude therapy is a form of Milieu Therapy in which all staff members assume a consistent, prescribed attitude de-signed to be therapeutic towards patients.**
- **Criteria of planning attitude therapy**
- **Advantages of attitude therapy for patients**
- **Common attitudes used**
  - **— Vigilant observation or watchfulness**
  - **— Attitude of indulgence**
  - **— Attitude of active friendliness**
  - **— Attitude of passive friendliness**
  - **— Attitude of matter of fact**
  - **— Attitude of kind firmness**
- **Attitudes to be used in specific situations.**

APPLICATION TO NURSING

Reading of the unit on psychosocial therapies will enhance the knowledge of nursing personnel about different types of psychosocial therapies used for patients. Reading of this unit will build on the knowledge of readers that these psychosocial therapies can be used in any setting, not necessarily with sick hospitalized persons only. Any child or adult having a maldaptive behaviour can be assisted to overcome his problem with the help of psychosocial therapies. This unit will also enable the students how to conduct various types of therapies and also group therapy. It will provide an insight into the pivotal role of a nurse in facilitating the recovery and rehabilitation of the patient by providing a therapeutic milieu in the ward and use of appropriate attitudes.

BETTER STUDY SECTION

1. VOCABULARY (USE DICTIONARY)

Acceptable	Eliminate	Privileges
Achieve	Emphasis	Reinforced
Appropriate	Harshness	Resolve
Catharsis	Heightened	Reviving
Constituents	Hostility	Stimulus
Casualty	Intimate	Substitute
Competencies	Manipulative	Tripartite
Conflict	Meditating	Unburden
Cogntion	Minimize	
Defensive	Modalities	
Democracy	Modify	
Destructive	Pivotal	

2. EXERCISE

* Define psychotherapy.
* List types of psychosocial therapies.
* Enumerate the goals of psychotherapies.
* Conduct group therapy in a clinical setting under the guidance of your teacher.
* List the common attitudes used by the psychiatric nurse.

3. STUDY QUESTIONS ASSIGNMENT

* Read Chapter I Unit III & VI and XIII by Kapoor, Bimla from the *Text Book of Psychiatric Nursing* (1992).
* Make notes on different types of psychosocial therapies ***(Use reading reference of this unit).***

4. READING REFERENCE

1. Chapman A.H. & Almeida Elza M. *The Interpersonal Basis of Psychiatric Nursing*. G.P. Putnam's Sons, New York (1972).

2. Goldenson R.M. *Longman Dictionary of Psychology and Psychiatry.* New York (1984).

3. Kalkman M.E. & Davis A.J. *New Dimensions in Mental Health Psychiatric Nursing.* (Fourth Edition) McGraw Hill Book Company, New York (1974).

4. Kapoor, Bimla. *Textbook of Psychiatric Nursing.* Kumar Publishing House (1992).

5. Keys J. and Hoffling C.K. *Basic Psychiatric Concepts in Nursing* (Fourth Edition) J.B. Lippincott Company (1980).

6. Lego S. *The American Handbook of Psychiatric Nursing.* J.B. Lippincott Company (1984).

7. Mitchell R.G. *Essential Psychiatric Nursing.* Churchill Living Stone, New York (1986).

8. Taylor C.M. *Essentials of Psychiatric Nursing* (Eleventh Edition) The C.V. Mosby Company, London (1982).

9. Topalis M. and Mathency R. *Psychiatric Nursing* (Fifth Edition) The C.V. Mosby Company (1970).

UNIT XVII

SOMATIC THERAPY AND ROLE OF NURSE

UNIT OUTLINE

- Introduction to Somatic Therapy.
- Description of Electro-Convulsive Therapy.
- Historical Development of ECT.
- Techniques/ methods of giving ECT.
  * Placement of Electrodes.
  * Amount of current and observation of production of seizures.
  * Number and frequency of ECT.
  * Mode of action.
  * Indication of ECT.
  * Contraindication of ECT.
  * Complications or Adverse effect.
  * Role of Nurse in ECT Treatment
  * Preparation of physical set-up
  * Waiting room or resting room.
  * Treatment room or ECT room.
  * Recovery room or after-care room.
- Nursing care to the patient
  * Before ECT treatment.
  * During ECT treatment.
  * After-care of patient.
- Insulin shock treatment.
- Psychosurgery.
- Application to Nursing.
- Better Study Section.

INTENDED LEARNING BEHAVIOUR

After reading this unit you will be able to:

- Define somatic therapy.
- Define ECT treatment.
- Explain the historical development of ECT.
- Discuss the techniques of giving ECT in terms of
  * Direct ECT
  * Modified ECT
  * Placement of Electrodes
  * Amount of current and production of seizure
  * Number and frequency of ECT
- Underline the mode of action
- Recognize the indications and contra-indications of ECT
- List the complications of ECT
- Build skill in preparation of a physical set-up
- Demonstrate skill in giving care to the patient
  * Prior to ECT
  * During ECT
  * After ECT
- Recall the other types of somatic therapies
  * Insulin Shock Treatment.
  * Psychosurgery.

CONTENT

INTRODUCTION In 1900-1930, specific treatments for mentally ill patients were not known much. One of the reasons could be that the causes of psychiatric illness were not clearly identified. However, with technological changes and constant research various treatment modalities have been adopted. These are: **Somatic Therapy,** which includes psychopharmacology, *(Chapter VI, Unit XV),* Electroconvulsive therapy, Insulin coma therapy and Psychosocial therapy. *(Chapter VI, Unit XVI).*

DESCRIPTION OF ECT

It is a painless form of electric therapy, primarily used for patients with depression and schizophrenic disorders. The patient is prepared by administration of barbiturate anesthesia and an injection of a chemical relaxant. An electric current is then applied for a fraction of a second through electrodes placed on the temple region. This immediately produces two-stage seizures or convulsions (Tonic and Clonic Stage).

HISTORICAL DEVELOPMENT OF ECT

In 1934, Dr. Ladislau Von Meduna, a Hungarian psychiatrist, found that producing fits like epilepsy helps schizophrenic patients. He believed that patients from epilepsy did not suffer from schizophrenia. Based on this belief, he found an appropriate epileptogenic substance: camphor oil which produced epilepsy— like fits in patients with psychoses. Later, camphor oil was replaced by a synthetic agent, Pentyleneterazol (Metrazol) which was used to produce major motor seizures. This was called the pharmacoconvulsive technique.

In 1937, Ugo Cerletti and Lucino Bini, the Italian Neuropsychiatrists, discovered during animal experiments that a brief electrical stimulus of sufficient intensity would immediately be followed by a major motor seizure (convulsions). This was effectively used thereafter. In late 1950s and early 1960s with the development of anaesthetic gas the Electro-convulsive Therapy was effectively used. It was initially termed as Electric Shock Therapy (EST) which is now being called Electro—Convulsive Therapy (ECT).

TO RECALL

- **Electro-Convulsive Therapy (ECT) is a physical/somatic therapy in which with the help of two electrodes, current is passed through the temporal region in between the two hemispheres of the brain, to produce a grand mal—type of seizures**
- **Cerleti & Bini are the first neuropsychiatrists who used ECT in 1937.**

TECHNIQUE/ METHOD OF GIVING ECT

ECT can be given by a direct and indirect method. Electroconvulsive Therapy (ECT) has been used **directly** on patients. The patient is administered atropine sulphate subcutaneously 0.6 mgm to 1.0 mgm, half an hour before the treatment or I/V immediately before the treatment. Minor Tranquillizer like *Colmpose* is also used. A grand mal seizure is induced in the patient by passing an electric current through the temporal lobe. Atropine prolongs the period of disorientation after the seizures. It also reduces vomiting. Immediately after the ECT treatment appropriate rescuscitative and other emergency management equipment and supplies are kept ready. A skilled person and nurse to rescuscitate the patient should be available. ECT given by this technique causes a lot of anxiety to the patient.

Electroconvulsive Therapy is **modified** with the use of Anaesthesia, muscle relaxation and oxygenation. The use of anaesthesia is necessary to allay anxiety and achieve the maximum effect. It is used to modify the force of convulsion and to avoid complications like bone fractures. Modified ECT is also used for the patients who are recovering from heart conditions.

A short acting barbiturate, methohexial sodium (Brevital Sodium) or Theopental (Pentothal) 5 ml to 10 ml (1 ml = 10 mgm) and ultra short acting depolarizing agent succinylcholine 0.3 ml to 0.5 ml (1 ml = 20 mgm) are given interavenously.

PLACEMENT OF ELECTRODES

The location of electrodes depends on the unilateral or bilateral electroconvulsive therapy. Bilaterally, ECT involves the placement of electrodes in the bitemporal region. An imaginary line is drawn from the outer canthus of the eye to the targus of the ear. The midpoint of this imaginary line is located and the electrode is placed one inch above the midpoint. Refer Fig.

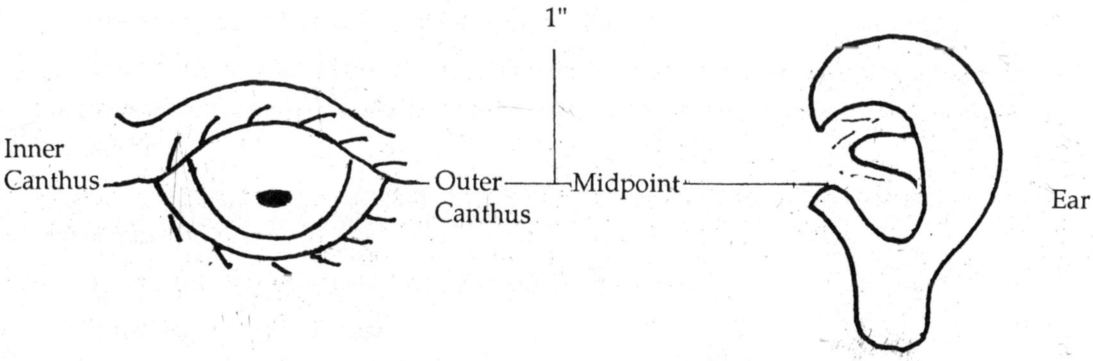

Fig. 15 : Site for Placement of Elctrodes in Bilateral Technique.

To minimize post-convulsive confusion and amnesia, unilateral ECT has been devised in which the electrodes are placed so as to avoid the dominant temporal lobe. One electrode is placed for bitateral ECT (in a right handed person on the left side and left-handed person on the right side in the temporal area). The second electrode is placed on the nondominant. Centroparitel. scalp, just lateral to the midline vertex. Refer Fig.

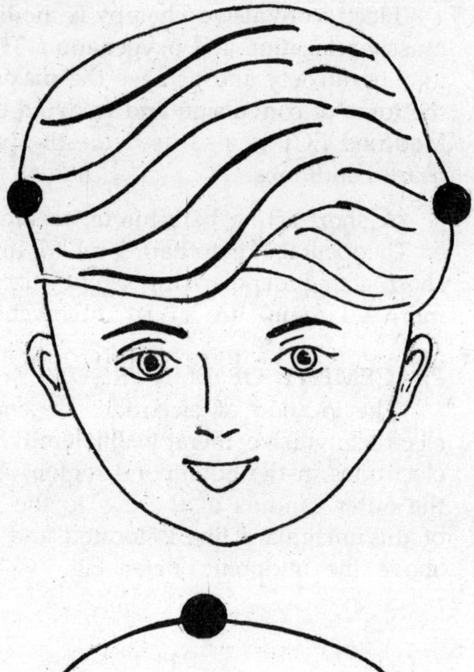

BILATERAL

UNILATERAL

Fig. 16 : Site for Placement of Electrodes in Bilateral and Unilateral Technique.

In both methods sufficient electricity has to be passed to produce grand mal seizures. Properly administered unilateral and bilateral ECT are equally effective. However, the possibility remains that some patients may respond rapidly to bilateral ECT, for example, a patient with hypomanic or manic symptomatology.

AMOUNT OF CURRENT

The nature and range of a stimulus intensity setting varies from device to device: 70 to 130 volts for 1 to 1 second will produce a convulsive effect. The actual amount of the current passed during the treatment was found to rannge from 200 to 1600 milliamphers. Most therapists in their routine apply more than the lowest possible range of current according to the threshold of the patient so that he may go in seizures which, in a way, resemble the seizures of epilepsy where the patient is less prone to fractures. Some therapists approach from a higher range of passing current and then reducing its intensity.

OBSERVATION OF PRODUCTION OF SEIZURE

The production of grand mal seizure is necessary for direct and modified ECT. In direct ECT, the *TONIC PHASE* that is muscle contractions last for 10 seconds approximately. The *CLONIC PHASE* that is movement or convulsion lasts for 25 to 30 seconds approximately. Then the patient goes in to the relaxation phase. The physician can see changes in EEG (Electroencephlograph) also. With the use of anaesthesia in modified ECT, mild grimace or blepharo-spasm, (a tonic spasm of the eyelid muscles) is observed when the current is applied. There is a slow planter flexion (reverse Babinski) during the tonic phase and there are fine movements of the toes during the clonic phase.

NUMBER AND FREQUENCY OF ECT TREATMENT

There is no clinical justification for a fixed number of treatments. However, patients being treated for depression trypically show some signs of improvement after the first few treatments. Peak response is attained between five and ten treatments for patients with bipolar disorders, manic type, schizoaffective disorders, or catatonic schizophrenia. Twenty to 25 treatments may be required for chronically ill schizophrenic patients.

ECT treatment is most often given three times a week. The frequency of treatment can be reduced if the patient shows a severe confusional state. With an extremely agitated, psychotic or suicidal patient it may be useful to give the first few treatments on a daily basis.

ECT does not prevent relapse. So maintenance treatment should be with drugs and psychotherapy.

TO RECALL

- ✻ **Types of ECT — Direct and Modified ECT**
- ✻ **Electrodes can be placed unilaterally or bilaterally.**
- ✻ **Intensity of the current varies between 70 and 130 volts for .1 to 1 second.**
- ✻ **Seizure occurs in Tonic and Clonic phases**
- ✻ **ECT can be given three times a week**
- ✻ **Five to Ten ECT's help in bringing improvement in patients.**

MODE OF ACTION

The mode of action is difficult to be based on one single factor. However, some of the hypotheses concerning mechanism of ECTare discussed in this unit.

Changes in behaviour due to ECT are attributed to an acute amnesic change in the patient. Many patients who are getting ECT, seem to forget what had been bothering them during the depressive episode. Biological mechanism by which a therapeutic effect has been brought about by ECT includes Neurochemical, Neuroendocrine and Neurophysiological.

Catecholamine hypothesis is a theory used to explain affective disorders and the effect of anti-depressent medication, *(Refer antidepressant in Unit XV).* Catecholamines are a group of hormones, including epinephrine, norepinephrine and dopamine produced in adrenal glands and cells of CNS and autonomic nerves. A primary functior is that of neurotransmission. Catecholamines' production usually increases in body tissues as emotional stress goes up.

Neurochemical investigations have shown that the role of catecholaminergic effect is due to presynaptic and postsynaptic receptor effect and may not be due to neurotransmission. This effect is also achieved due to seizures caused by ECT Treatment. Decreased availability of serotonin (5-HT) is considered to be a potential causative factor for depressive illness. Tricyclic agents have been used to reduce depression, whereas ECT-induced seizure has been used in Mania. ECT Convulsions also have an effect on GABA receptors like antimanic agents i.e. Lithium carbonate.

Neurophysiological effect due to ECT seizure is achieved probably due to a cerebral hypometabolic state.

Neuroendocrine changes have effects on depressive illnesses. Polypeptides from the hypothalmus change the neuroendocrine acvtivity which affects thalamocortical pathways.

The axioms or widely accepted theoretical concepts are:

(i) The persistent behavioural or therapheutic effect i.e. changes in the CNS are due to repeated ECT seizures and not changes in the peripharal or visceral component.

(ii) The rate of change in behaviour and improvement direcly depends upon the number and frequency of seizures. Repeated seizures alter many brain functions like in psychotic state, perception recall, concentration, memory and orientation as well. Sometimes these changes may create anxiety in the patient and his relatives.

(iii) The target population for convulsive therapy is endogenous psychotic patients. These patients show many physiological and behavioural characteristics — which reflect the organization of the brain. These characteristics are particularly responsive to repeated seizures.

(iv) Improvement in behaviour (clinical remission) is characterized by a gain in weight, increased appetite, increased duration of sleep, increased libido, increased interest in the environment.

TO RECALL

* **Mode of action is still not very clear.**
* **Biological effects brought about by Neurophysiological, Neuro-endocrine and Neurochemical aspects by ECT, are considered upto some extent. However, it is the catechol-amine hypothesis due to the effect of ECT which gained more popularity.**

INDICATIONS OF ECT

The indication of ECT depends upon the availability or non-availability of psychotropic drugs. The common conditions for ECT treatment are:

* Major depressive episode is a primary indication for ECT; 80 percent patients with major depressive episode respond to ECT treatment.
* Involutional Melancholia: 80 to 90 percent of patients show marked improvement with ECT treatment, better than with drugs.
* Psychotic depression.
* Unipolar-Bipolor depression.
* Depression of old age as long as there is no arteriosclerosis and brain changes.
* Post-partum depression.
* Manic phase if the patient is terribly disturbed and exhausted.
* Catatonia.
* Schizophrenia when they are not responding to other therapies.
* Other responsive groups to ECT treatment are patients with:
    - — Premorbid personality
    - — Stupor (Catatonic)
    - — Previous depressive episode
    - — Paranoid delusion
    - — Anorexia
    - — Early morning insomnia
    - — Weight loss
    - — Lack of concentration
    - — Ideas of guilt and worthlessness.
    - — Suicidal thought and suicidal attempts.

ECT treatment is **not effective** in:

* Reactive depression. (Neurotic)
* Psychoneurosis, hysteria, hypochondrias, and anxiety states.

* Schizophrenia only hebaphrenic and simple.

* Drug dependence.

CONTRAINDICATION OF ECT

There is no absolute contraindication of ECT. The only situations in which there is increased risk i.e. patients with increased intracranial pressure, including tumors, hematomas, and subarachnoid hemorrhage, may undergo neurological deterioration with ECT.

The presence of an acute myocardial infarction raises risk because of increased decompensation of heart due to ECT. Hypertension is also a cause of concern because due to ECT there is an increase in blood pressures and heart rate temporarily. Increase in blood pressure due to ECT in patients with cardiac disease, aneurysm, thrombophelebitis, bleeding disorders or where there is increased risk of embolism should be taken care of before planning to give ECT.

Pregnancy and old age are not contraindicated.

COMPLICATIONS OR ADVERSE EFFECTS

Complications of ECT treatment are much reduced with modified ECT. Some of the risks or complications are explained as:-

* Impairment of memory may vary from mild tendency to forget names to a severe confusion.

* To start with, the patient has a tendency to forget all types of events but gradually it limits to the events just before the ECT treatment.

* This causes disturbance to the patient and his relatives. They should be explained that these changes are temporary.

* The memory returns fully within a few weeks to a month.

* However, the learning capacity of the patient improves, though there is impairment of retention in memory function.

FRACTURES AND DISLOCATIONS

* Most frequently the fracture and dislocation are caused by muscular contraction due to ECT.

* Compression fracture of vertebrae of dorsal area between the second and eighth-usually third, fourth and fifth vertebrae-is common.

* Fracture of femur and humerus occurs in young muscular individuals. There may be complete rupture between head and shaft of femur due to tight restraints applied during the convulsion phase.

* Fracture of acetabulum is very rare. It can be due to sudden contractions of the muscles which pull the head of the femur towards the pelvis.

* Impacted fractures are more frequent in elderly people.

* Dislocation of jaw is the most frequent complication of the tonic phase. It can be totally prevented by supporting the jaw or applying pressure on the chin upward.

COMPLICATIONS IN THE RESPIRATORY SYSTEM

Apnea is a physiological phenomenon in any epileptic seizure. Airway should be kept clear by use of metal airway. Prevent collection of saliva in the mouth by suction. Turn the head to one side. Oxygen therapy for a short duration is used by the therapists prophylactically. However, if apnea is prolonged, artificial respiration should be applied. To reduce the effect of barbiturates, Coramine 1 m.gm to 2.5 gm should be given intravenously.

Neurological and cardiac complications are very rare. Thorough physical examination is required prior to the ECT treatment.

OTHER COMPLAINTS OF PATIENT DUE TO ECT

Headache, backache, painful mastication, injury to mouth and tongue. Fear due to an unpleasant experience on waking up after the treatment. These complications can be prevented by observation and early intervention by nursing care.

STUNS OR SUBSHOCKS occur due to an insufficient current applied to the patient which does not result in a full convulsive stage. These subshocks or stuns will sometimes produce cardiac irregularities, respiratory distress and collapse. Confusion after a subshock is more marked than after a major fit due to ECT. If three subshocks are given to a patient in one day, the treatment should be stopped. The next day ECT may be given with increased intensity of the current.

TO RECALL

❋ Indications of ECT Treatment are:
- **Major depressive episodes**
- **Involutional Melancholia**
- **Psychotic depression**
- **Unipolar-Bipolar depression**
- **Depression of old age and post-partum depression**
- **Mania**
- **Catatonia**
- **Schizophrenia**

❋ Contraindication
There is no absolute contraindication except in cases of increased intracranial pressure.

❋ Complications are reduced due to modified ECT. There may be impairment of memory, fractures or apnea. All these complications can be totally prevented.

ROLE OF NURSE IN ECT TREATMENT

The psychiatric patients are most frequently hospitalized for ECT treatment. Though some of the outpatients are also given ECT treatment, it is very important that the patients neither see nor hear one another during or after treatment until they are in a reasonably improved condition to understand the effect of therapy.

In a hospital setting where the electroconvulsive therapy is given, the nurse should see to the set-up which includes:

i. Waiting room or resting room
ii. Treatment room or E.C.T. room
iii. Recovery room or after-care room.

(I) WAITING ROOM OR RESTING ROOM

In this room patients are asked to wait or take rest before electroconvulsive therapy. The room should be calm with dim lights, light colour of the walls. Put some flowers to give pleasant feelings to the patient. There should be some magazines to read, so that the patient can divert his mind and reduce anxiety. Lavatory (toilet) should be attached, because the patient needs to empty his bladder and bowels before getting ECT. The nurse should always be available in this room so that the patient and relatives can clarify their doubts. Preanasthetic drugs should be kept ready.

(II) TREATMENT ROOM/ECT ROOM

In the treatment room the nurse needs to do the following preparations:

ARTICLES FOR COMFORT OF THE PATIENT:- The room should be near the waiting room. For privacy a bedside screen, well-padded low-level beds with railings should be placed to prevent injury due to fall.

ARTICLES FOR PREPARATION OF THE PATIENT:- Small pillows to put under the patient's waist to prevent injury. Mouth gag to prevent injury to the tongue during convulsions and to keep the airway Patent. Tongue spatula, endotrachial tube and sterile catheter for suction of the respiratory tract. O_2 cylinder and an ambus bag to give O_2 immediately after the therapy and to give artificial respiration, if required.

ARTICLES FOR THE PROCEDURE:- A trolly with an ECT machine in working order, check all the electric plug points. Jelly or normal saline for putting on electrodes as normal saline is a good conductor of electricity and it facilitates in passing current. Emergency drugs and a resuscitation tray, mouth wipes, B.P. apparatus, sterile syringes and spirit swabs. Adequate light. Doctors and nurses should he present in the ECT room.

(III) RECOVERY ROOM OR AFTER-CARE ROOM

Once the patient responds to a painful stimulus he is transferred to the recovery room. A floor bed with 1 to 1 1/2" padding on the sides for the patient should be kept ready. Observation of vital signs and symptoms such as B.P., temperature, pulse and respiration. Mouth wipes are kept to wipe excessive secretions from the mouth. An extra set of clothes in case the patient has spoiled them with urine or feaces during convulsions. Toilet facilities should be available in the recovery room.

Electroconvulsive therapy equipment should always be available in the psychiatric ward or unit to meet emergency situations. For example, patients with suicidal or homicidal danger and psychotic exhaustion would need ECT therapy immediately.

Once the patient becomes oriented he can be transferred to his ward.

Electroconvulsive therapy involves a significant responsibility of the nursing personnel. Nursing care can be explained as:

i) The patient's care before giving ECT.

ii) The patient's care during ECT, and

iii) The patient's care after ECT.

NURSING INTERVENTION BEFORE GIVING ECT	PURPOSE
* Check that a thorough physical examination (heart including ECG, lungs, bone, blood for Hb, urine for sugar and other tests and albumin, and X-rays) is completed.	To select the patient for ECT therapy.
* Written consent or declaration for the treatment from the nearest relative after explaining the method of treatment and risks. DO NOT TELL THE PATIENT THAT ECT WILL BE GIVEN. The word current may cause fear in the patient. He may be told that "injection" will be given unless he is aware of the treatment. Relatives should be explained in detail.	* For legal protection * Explanation to the relatives will avoid them from shock and fear of therapy.
* The patient should be given nothing orally before treatment. If he is to be treated in an emergency it should be two to three hours after breakfast or meals.	* To prevent vomiting and aspiration after the treatment.
* Remove metallic articles from his or her body; for example, watch, bangles, ring.	* To prevent the electric current passing on unwanted areas. Metal is a good conductor of electricity.
* Remove artificial dentures.	* To prevent it from dislodging and blocking the respiratory passage.
* Remove lipstick, nail polish or any other make-up.	* To check for cynosis. These colours will mask the changes in the patient.
* Loosen the tight clothes like necktie in men and blouse or other tight garments in women, preferably give hospital clothes.	* To help in facilitating respiration and meet any emergency.

Contd.

NURSING INTERVENTION BEFORE GIVING ECT	PURPOSE
* Replace the long acting sedatives with hypnotics.	* To enhance the effectiveness of ECT.
* Encourage the patient to empty his bladder and bowels. He/she should void immediately before the treatment.	* To reduce his/her embarrassment after the treatment. If the bladder is full he may spoil the bed due to a relaxant effect of the drug.
* Encourage the patient to maintain his personal hygiene. Remove oil from hair.	* To help the patient to develop a feeling that he is going for treatment, oil is a bad conductor of electricity.
* Give premedication to the patient, Inj. Atropine and calmpose.	* To reduce anxiety of the patient and achieve effectiveness .
* Take the patient on a stretcher to the waiting room.	* Prepare him or her psychologically that he or she is proceeding for treatment.
DURING ECT	
* The patient is transferred on a trolly from the waiting room to the ECT room on a well-padded bed and placed in a comfortable dorsal position or supine position. A small pillow is placed under the lumber curve.	* To prevent injury, a well-padded bed is given, ECT treatment is given in a dorsal position or supine position.
* Give a short-acting anaesthetic agent. Theopental .25gm to .5gms. I/V, and Scoline (Succinylcholine). 30 to 50 mgm. (Check prescription) The dose of drugs may vary from patient to patient.	* To help the patient to be anaesthetized quickly, to reduce his anxiety and cause less vigorous convulsions, thereby prevent complications.
* Well-padded mouth gag or tongue depressor is placed in between the teeth.	* To prevent biting of tongue or injury to lips.

Contd.

NURSING INTERVENTION DURING ECT	PURPOSE
* Support the shoulder and arms lightly, restraint the thighs with the help of a sheet.	* To prevent fractures. Tight pressure on any of these areas may lead to fracture of humrus or femur.
* Hyperextension of the head with support to the chin by a nurse.	* To prevent jaw dislocation or fracture and for Patent airway.
* Give a few breaths of oxygen to the patient.	* To help the patient to overcome a phase of apnea faster after convulsions.
* Provide electrodes dipped in saline water or jelly for placing on the temporal region.	* Concentrated saline is a good conductor of electricity, thereby it facilitates in producing convulsions.
* Make an observation of grand mal seizures. The presence of the initial tonic stage which lasts for 10-15 seconds, followed by convulsions lasting for 25 to 30 seconds. Then there is a phase of muscular relaxation with stertorous respiration.	* To ensure that there are no stuns or subshocks and the treatment is successful.
* Do suction immediately.	* To keep airway patient and prevent the patient from aspiration pneumonia.
* Restore respiration by giving O_2 by mask, if required.	* To prevent the patient from respiratory and cardiac complications.
AFTER ECT	
* Observe and record the respiration, pulse and blood pressure of the patient.	* To prevent any respiratory or cardiac complication.
* Put the railings and place the patient on a side lying position, wipe the secretions.	* To protect the patient from fall as he may become restless. To avoid aspiration of secretions.

Contd.

NURSING INTERVENTION AFTER GIVING ECT	PURPOSE
* Transfer the patient to the recovery room only when she can answer a simple question i.e. "Open your mouth, Shanti Devi".	* To ensure that the patient has come out of the phase of unconsciousness.
* Record pulse, respiration, blood pressure and the level of consciousness every 15 minutes. Once these vital signs are stabilized, record after 30 minutes till the patient recovers completely. (Refer sample form at the end of this unit).	* To make an early nursing diagnosis of the patient going into complications.
* Allow the patient to sleep for 30 minutes to one hour if he/she wants to sleep.	* To help the patient to overcome physical exhaustion.
* Reassurance to the patient.	* Studies have suggested that these patients are highly suggestible post treatment. So reassurance given will help them to overcome their maladaptive behaviour.
* Reorientation to the ward, toilet and nurse's station.	* To help the patient to overcome confusional state.
* Make a note of any injuries or complaint of pains by the patient—body pain or headache.	* To detect any type of complications, specially fractures.
* Encourage the patient to go for a shower bath and change his/her clothes.	* To give the patient a sense of well-being and freshness.
* Allow the patient to take clear tea, followed by breakfast, if he/she does not vomit.	* To meet the nutritional needs of the patient as he/she has not taken anything orally since morning.
* Help the patient to carry on his daily activity as planned. He should be allowed to go to the day-care room.	* To enable the patient: - to resume his daily work. - to understand that ECT is also a part of the treatment.

Contd.

NURSING INTERVENTION AFTER GIVING ECT	PURPOSE
* Make observation of any change.	* To note the significant change in the behaviour of the patient.

Fig. 17 : Table Describing Nursing Intervention of Patient Prior to ECT, During ECT & After ECT.

TO RECALL

- **Electroconvulsive therapy can be given to patients who are hospitalized as well as to those attending the outpatient department.**
- **Physical set-up includes**
  - **waiting room or resting room**
  - **treatment room or ECT room**
  - **recovery room or after-care room**
- **The nurse's role is to**
  - **check the physical set-up**
  - **care for the patient before, during and after getting ECT.**

INSULIN SHOCK TREATMENT

Insulin shock therapy was introduced by Sakel in 1933 to treat schizophrenia. An injection of a large dose of insulin was given to the patient to produce a state of hypoglycemia. The patient went into a coma within three hours of the injection. Twenty-five percent of glucose I/V or glycagon injection was then given and the patient got up within 10 to 20 minutes. This treatment was given under close medical and nursing observation. Insulin shock is replaced by psychotropic drugs, psychosocial therapies and electroconvulsive therapy (ECT).

PSYCHOSURGERY

The operation of lobotomy, a surgical procedure, consists of severing of the connection between the thalmus and frontal lobe. It was developed by Ega Moniz in 1936. It is used to affect the patient's psychological state, modification of the disturbed behaviour, thought content or mood. Prefrontal lobotomy and transorbital lobotomy are being performed for chronic patients and all those patients who do not respond to psychotropic drugs, electroconvulsive therapy and psychosocial therapy.

TO RECALL

Somatic therapy includes electro-convulsive therapy (ECT), Insulin shock treatment and psychosurgery. ECT is the only treatment which is being practised.

APPLICATION TO NURSING

In therapeutic modalities somatic treatment, specially electroconvulsive therapy is the frequent treatment modality being used for psychiatric patients. Reading of this unit will help the nursing personnel to develop knowledge in the ECT treatment. They will also be able to appreciate the indications and contraindications of the ECT treatment. Besides, they will be able to evaluate the number of treatments to be given to patients, identify the complications or adverse effects due to ECT. A study of the unit will enable the nurse to develop skill in preparing the patient to undergo this somatic therapy effectively. This unit will also help the reader to develop skill in giving care to the patient before and during the ECT treatment. The nurse reader will be able to apply the knowledge in giving effective care to the patient after ECT and prevent complications.

BETTER STUDY SECTION

1. VOCABULARY (USE DICTIONARY)

Amnesia	Postsynaptic
Biotemporal	Primarily
Discorientation	Prophylactically
Divert	Relaxant
Embolism	Reorientation
Episode	Resuscitative
Grimace	Retention
Imaginary	Stimulus
Impairment	Target
Justification	
Planter-flexion	

2. EXERCISE

a) Define Somatic Therapy.

b) List the indications of Electroconvulsive Therapy (ECT).

c) Enumerate the complications of the ECT treatment

d) Make notes on the nurse's role in
   - prepation and care of the patient before getting ECT.
   - care of the patient during ECT
   - care of the patient after ECT.

3. STUDY QUESTION

Shanti Devi, 35 years old woman in severe depression, is going to get her first ECT. Carry on the following activities:

- Explanation to the patient and her relatives.
- Preparation of Shanti Devi for ECT.
- Care of Shanti Devi during and after ECT.
- Preparation of a post-ECT chart.

4. READING REFERENCES

Kolb L.C. and Brodie H.K.H. *Modern Clinical Psychiatry* (10th edition) W.B. Saunders Company, Philadelphia (1982).

Key, J. and Hoffling K.C. *Basic Psychiatric Concepts in Nursing* (4th edition) J.B. Lippincott Company, Philadelphia (1980).

Kalkman M.E. *Psychiatric Nursing.* McGraw Hill Book Co., London (1974).

Karnosh L.J. & Mereness, R.V. *Essentials of Psychiatric Nursing* (6th edition) English Language Book Society (1985).

Matheney R.V. & Topalis M. *Psychiatric Nursing.* (5th edition), The C.V. Mosby Company, London (1970).

Kaplan H.L., Sadock B.J. *Comprehensive Textbook of Psychiatry* (5th edition), Vol. 2 Williams and Wilkins, Baltimore (1989).

Taylor C.M. *Essentials of Psychiatric Nursing* (11th edition) The C.V. Mosby Co., London (1982).

Walker, J.I. *Essentials of Clinical Psychiatry.* J.B. Lippincott Company, London (1985).

SAMPLE CHART OF POST E.C.T.

Name	: Ms. Shanti Devi	Age : 35 years	Sex : F
Diagnosis	: Endogenous Depression	C.R.No. 1234	Bed No. 5
Temp. 37°C	Pulse 80/min.	Resp. 18/min.	B.P. 120/80 mm of Hg.
ECT No. 2	Direct/Modified.	Modified	
Time of ECT :	10.00 AM	Patient Received at :	10.30 AM

Time	Pulse	Respiration	B.P.	Level of Consciousness	Remarks
10.30 AM	78/min.	18/min. regular	120/80 mm of Hg.	Confused	Personal hygiene maintained patient reoriented to relatives and ward. No vomiting.
10.45 AM	80/min	18/min	120/80 mm of Hg.	Fully conscious	Breakfast given, patient is oriented to time, place and person.
11.15 AM	80.min	18/min	120/80 mm of Hg.	Fully conscious	No confusion No headache
12 O'Clock	80/min	18/min	120/80 mm of Hg.	Fully conscious	Patient taken to the day-care centre. Played carrom-board with other two patients, won the game.

Fig. 18 : Table Describing Sample Chart on Post ECT.

COMPREHENSIVE TEST ON CHAPTER VI

I. Define the following terms:

Psychotropic drug ....

Psychosocial Therapy ....

Electroconvulsive Therapy ....

2. Match the following from Column B and place on space given in

Column A			**Column B**
a)	....	Restlessness, difficulties in sitting, still or strong urge to move.	1. Parkinsonism
b)	....	indicated in major depression.	2. Schizophrenia
c)	....	Patient shows akinesia, mask like face, rigidity of muscles, tremors of hands.	3. Extrapyramidal symptoms
d)	....	include, Parkinsonism, akathesia, dystonoia tardive dyskinesia.	4. Serum lithium
e)	....	is characterized by tic of upper body, echokinesis, copralalia and echololia.	5. Cerletti
f)	....	is maintained at 1 mg per litre in the prophylaxis of manic depressive psychosis.	6. Akathesia
g)	....	the first one to work on electroconvulsive therapy.	7. Dystonia
h)	....	is a behaviour therapy.	8. Electroconvulsive therapy
i)	....	is used for patients with suicidal ideas	9. Tourette Syndrome
j)	....	a synonymous to therapeutic community	10. Behaviour modification
k)	....	is replaced with drugs, psychosociotherapy and E.C.T.	11. Watchfulness
			12. Sakel
			13. Insulin shock therapy
			14. Lobotomy
			15. Milieu Therapy.

3. Choose the appropriate word and place in the space given on the left hand side.

Phenobarbital, Anticholinergic, Chlorpramazine, Librium, Haloparidel, Lithium-Carbonate, Trifluperazine, Valium, Pacitan, Tetracyclic.

a) .... is a phenothiazine group of antipsychotic drug.

b) .... is a piprazine group of antipsychotic drug.

c) .... is a butyrophenones group of antipsychotic drug.

d) .... is used to reduce Parkinsonism symptoms.

e) .... is a drug known as antidepressants.

f) .... is a specific drug for mania.

g) .... is a benzodiazepine drug of non-barbiturate group used as an antianxiety drug.

h) .... is a sedative in the barbiturate group of drugs.

4. Choose the best answer and encircle it.

a) Psychoanalysis includes all of these **except:**

i. Free Association

ii. Analysis of Transference
iii. Exploring expressed thoughts
iv. Interpretation of dreams, emotions
v. All of these.

b) Psychosocial Therapy includes all of these execpt:
i. Psychoanalysis
ii. Hypnotherapy
iii. Somatic Therapy
iv. Reality Therapy
v. All of these.

c) Electroconvulsive Therapy is indicated in all of these except:
i. Premorbid Personality
ii. Early morning insomnia
iii. Major depression
iv. Phobia
v. All of these

d) Behaviour therapy includes all of these except:
i. Cognitive therapy
ii. Reciprocal inhibition
iii. Systematic modification
iv. Assertiveness training
v. All of these.

e) Electroconvulsive Therapy is contraindicated in all of these except:
i. Anxiety neurosis
ii. Hysterical neurosis
iii. Fresh Angina Pectoris
iv. Increased intercraicial pressure
v. All of these.

KEY TO COMPREHENSIVE TEST ON CHAPTER VI

1. a) Psychotropic or psychoactive drugs are chemicals that affect the brain and nervous system, alter feelings and emotions. They also affect the consciousness in various ways.

   b) Psychosocial therapy is a process in which a person who wishes to relieve symptoms or resolve problems in living and seek personal growth gets into implicit or explicit contract to interact in a prescribed way with a psychotherapist.

   c) Electroconvulsive therapy is a somatic or physical therapy in which with the help of two electrodes, current is passed through the temporal region in between the two hemispheres of the brain, to produce a grandmal type of seizures.

2. Match the following:
   a) 6
   b) 8
   c) 1
   d) 3
   e) 9
   f) 4
   g) 5
   h) 10
   i) 11
   j) 15
   k) 13

3. a) Chlorpramazine
   b) Trifluperazine
   c) Haloparidal
   d) Anticholinergic
   e) Tetracyclic
   f) Lithium Carbonate
   g) Librium
   h) Phenobarbital

4. a) v
   b) iii
   c) iv
   d) v
   e) v

CHAPTER VII
MENTAL AND BEHAVIOUR DISORDERS

UNIT XVIII

ORGANIC, SCHIZOPHRENIC AND MOOD (AFFECTIVE) DISORDERS

UNIT OUTLINE

Categories of Mental Disorders according to ICD-10

— Organic Mental Disorders

Acute Brain Syndrome-Delirium

- — Definition of Delirium
- — Signs and symptoms
- — Psychopathology
- — Causes of Delirium

Chronic Brain Syndrome-Dementia

- — Definition of Dementia
- — Signs and symptoms
- — Causes of senile Dementia
- — Types of senile Dementia

Korsakoff(Amnesis) Syndrome

Presenile Dementia

- — Alzhemier's disease
- — Pick's disease
- — Parkinson's disease
- — Huntington's chorea

Application to Nursing

— Schizophrenic Disorders

- — Definition
- — Historical development
- — Epidemiology
- — Causes/Etiology
- — Signs and Symptoms
- — Types of Schizoprehnia ICD—10
- — Tabular presentation of types of schizophrenia, age patterns, signs and symptoms
- — Treatment
- — Prognosis
- — Application to Nursing

INTENDED LEARNING BEHAVIOUR

After reading this unit you will be able to:

a) List the major categories of mental disorders according to ICD—10

b) Describe organic mental disorders

c) Identify the patients with delirium and Dementia.

d) Explain the presenile Dementia

e) Define schizonphrenia

f) Describe the causes, signs and symptoms of schizophrenia

g) differentiate various types of schizophrenia.

h) Apply the knowledge while giving nursing care to the patients

i) Define affective/or mood disorders

j) Classify mood disorders according to ICD—10

k) Explain the types of manic episodes

l) Describes the types of depressive episodes

m) Explain involutional melancholia

UNIT OUTLINE

Mood (Affective) Disorders
- **Definition of affective disorders**
- **Classification according to ICD—10**
- **Epidemiology**
- **Etiology**
- **Signs and Symptoms**
- * **Manic Episodes**
  - **Hypomania**
  - **Acute mania**
  - **Delirious mania**
- * **Depressive Episodes**
  - **Mild depression**
  - **Acute depression**
  - **Depressive stupor**
- * **Circular Type**

Treatment of Manic-Depressive Episodes
- **Prognosis**
- **Involutional Melancholia**

Application to Nursing.
Better Study Section.

DESCRIPTION OF MENTAL ILLNESSESS

CONTENTS

INTRODUCTION In Chapter III on Textbook of Psychiatric Nursing emphasis was laid on (i) classification of mental disorders, (ii) Causes of mental disorders; biological, psychosocial and socio-cultural factors contributing towards mental illness, and (iii) Psychopathology of human behaviour.

In this unit, Psychiatric illnesses/Mental disorders will be discussed under the following headings:

Organic Mental Disorders
Schizophrenic Disorders
Mood (Affective) Disorders i.e. Manic Depressive Psychosis

The (International Classification of Diseases) ICD-10 Classification of Mental and Behaviour Disorders is placed in Appendix Page No.465 of this book. From Chapter V (F) of ICD-10 Mental Disorders are categorized. The categories are coded from F00 - F 99.

LIST OF CATEGORIES

F 00 — F .09	Organic, including symptomatic mental disorders
F 10 — F 19	Mental and Behaviour Disorders due to Psychoactive Substance Use
F 20 — F 29	Schizophrenia, Schizotypal and Delusional Disorders
F 30 — F 39	Mood (affective) Disorders
F 40 — F 48	Neurotic Stress-related and Somatoform Disorders
F 50 — F 59	Behavioural Syndromes associated with physiological disturbances and physical factors
F 60 — F 69	Disorders of Adult Personality and Behaviour
F 70 — F 79	Mental Disorders
F 80 — F 89	Disorders of Psychological Development
F 90 — F 99	Behavioural and Emotional Disorders with onset usually occurring in childhood and adolescence
F 99	Unspecified Mental Disorders.

ORGANIC SYNDROMES/ORGANIC MENTAL DISORDERS

DEFINITION

Organic disorders, acute or chronic, involve impairment of brain tissue functions due to such factors as head injury, toxic conditions, encephalitis, systemic infection, brain tumor or cerebral arteriosclerosis. The resulting symptoms include mild to severe impairment of memory, orientation, judgement, general intellectual functions and emotional adjustment.

In DSM III classification this term refers to a "pattern of organic psychological and behaviour symptoms associated with permanent or transient brain disfunction but without reference to etiology."

TYPES OF ORGANIC MENTAL DISORDERS

The organic mental Disorder are divided into two category. They are as under :-

A. Acute Brain Syndrome — Delirium, & (F 05)

B. Chronic Brain Syndrome — Dementia. (F 00— F 03)

A. DELIRIUM

DEFINITION

It is a state of clouded consciousness in which attention cannot be sustained, the environment is wrongly perceived and disturbances of thinking are present. (ICD—10 has categorised Delirium under (F 05).

SIGNS AND SYMPTOMS

Impaired consciousness may vary from slight cloudiness to stupor, disorientation, mental confusion, thinking is distorted, dreamlike content in thinking. Memory, comprehension, factual knowledge, reasoning ability and judgement are impaired. Insight is usually lacking. Mood is liable to swing from apathy to sudden panic. Illusion, hallucination and delusion are present. Inappropriate impulsive, irrational or violent behaviour are present. These changes are transient and reversible.

PSYCHOPATHOLOGY

The main part of the brain responsible for delirious state are: brain stem, autonomic nervous system, limbic system, sensory cortex and pathways. ID and Ego get affected.

CAUSES OF DELIRIUM

i. Head Trauma,

ii. Fever specially common in children

iii. Metabolic

iv. Toxic

v. Other causes such as :

* Drug intoxication or overdosage of drug or drug withdrawal. (For example, Alcohol, Hallucinogen, Bromides).
* The post—operative state.
* Infections especially febrile such as pneumonia, tuberculosis.
* Metabolic disorders such as Vitamin B deficiency, ureamia, liver disease.
* Circulatory disturbance. For example, congestive heart failure, hypertensive encephalopathy.
* Epilepsy.
* Cerebral Tumors.
* Lupus erythematous.
* Respiratory insufficiency.
* Sensory Deprivation.

B. DEMENTIA

DEFINITION

Dementia is a disease of the brain, usually of a chronic or progressive nature in which there is disturbance of multiple higher cortical functions including memory, thinking, orientation, comprehension,calculation, learning capacity, language and judgement. Consciousness is not clouded. Dementia produces decline in intellectual functioning. (ICD—10).

SIGNS AND SYMPTOMS

Recent memory suffers more than the remote memory. Disorientation is progressive, involving time first and ultimately affecting all spheres of life, loss of emotional control, behaviour becomes inappropriate, the patient tends to neglect personal hygiene, indecent in behaviour because of loss of inhibition, sooner or later there is incontinece of bladder and bowels. preseveration in speech. In dementia, the patient may also develop functional reaction such as anxiety, depression or paranoid delusion.

Dementia is often described in terms of deterioration in intelligence and memory but there are other symptoms also such as loss of learning, reasoning, problem solving, personality characteristics and judgement.

CAUSES OF DEMENTIA

Dementia is usually brought on by chronic, progressive, structural or degenerative conditions. Cerebral arterlosclerosis and other cardio-vascular diseases are the commonest causes of dementia. Heredity, hypercholesterolemia, hypertension and diabetes mellitus have been implicated. Degenerative disorders like Alzheimer's disease and Pick's disease. Toxic conditions, such as use of drugs leading to metabolic disturbances or vitamin deficiency, i.e. BeriBeri, Pellagra,Koraskoff or Wernicke's disease. Carbon-monoxide poisoning may also cause dementia. Neurological disorders like head injury, Huntington's chorea may also cause dementia.

SENILE DEMENTIA

Occurring usually after the age of 65 years due to degenerative brain changes as accompanied by a clinical picture of mental deterioration, which may vary markedly in degree.

TYPES OF SENILE DEMENTIA

(I) SIMPLE DETERIORATION : The patient gradually loses contact with environment, typical symptom of poor memory, tendency to reminiscence (recollection of previous experiences especially those of a pleasant nature) intolerance of change, disorientation, restlessness, insomnia, and failure of judgement. This is the commonest senile psychotic reaction constituting about 50 per cent of the entire group of senile dementia.

(II) PARANOID REACTION : The principal characteristic is a gradual formation of delusion. An individual develops the notion that his relatives have turned against him and are trying to rob or kill him.

(III) THE PRESBYOPHRENIC TYPE : Characterised by fabrication in talk, jovial mood, marked impairment of memory. Patients show a peculiar restlessness and excitability.

(IV) DEPRESSED AND AGITATED TYPES : An individual is severely depressed and agitated. Suffers from hypochondrical and nihilistic delusions. Expresses morbid ideas about cancer, syphilis and other diseases. The patient has marked poverty of ideas.

(V) DELIRIOUS AND CONFUSED TYPE : The patient shows severe mental clouding which makes him restless, confused, resistive and incoherent. Completely disoriented to time,, place and person.

All these types of senile dementia deteriorate, and the patient becomes asocial and bedridden. He is reduced to a vegetative life, followed by the complication of a bed-ridden patient and death.

KORSAKOFF (AMNESIS) SYNDROME

Korsakoff is also spelled as Korskov. This type of dementia develops from a delirium tremen which does not completely recover. A major factor in these cases is thiamine deficiency. Other causes may be head injury, brain tumor, cerebral arteriosclerosis. It is distinguished from delirium because the patient's consciousness is not impaired at all. Intellectual ability is also not impaired which is a primary symptom of dementia. The patient may present confabulation, disorientation and retrograde amnesia. The individual lacks in initiative and judgement.

BRAIN SYNDROMES INVOLVED IN PRESENILE DEMENTIA

It resemble that of senile dementia except that disorders occur in a younger age group.

(i) **Alzhemier's Disease:** Usually the age is early 40 to 50 years. Rapid progression with severe brain and mental deterioration, accompanied by overactivity, emotional distress and agitation. Frequent development of aphasia. Death occurs between two and ten years of sickness, usually an average of four years. The patient should be hospitalised. Treatment is symptomatic.

(ii) **Pick's Disease:** It is degenerative disorders of the nervous system. Usually occurs in 45 to 50 years of age. Its onset is slow, involving difficulty in thinking, memory defect and easy fatiguability. Character changes with lower ethical inhibitions. The disease runs between two and seven years when death occurs. The patient should be hospitalised. Treatment is symptomatic.

(iii) **Parkinson's Disease** : Occurs before the age of 30 years. Majority of the cases are reported between 50 and 70 years of age. The disorder is characterized by rigidity and spontaneous tremors of various muscles. Tremors begin on one arm, spread gradually to the same leg and the same side of the body, and then to other limbs. The patient's face is mask-like, speech is not clear. Often the paitent leans forward and walks as if he is running. He becomes dependent, develops apathy and becomes a social. Intelligence is a little affected. L. dopa is the drug which brings a lot of improvement in the patient's symptoms.

(iv) **Huntington's Chorea** : It usually occurs between the ages of 30 and 50 years. It is characterized by a chronic, progressive chorea, there is involuntary, irregular twitching, jerking movements with mental deterioration, leading to dementia and death after 10-21 years of sickness.

EPILEPSY

The word epilepsy is derived from the Greek word 'epilepsia', "Seizure". It is a group of disorders associated with disturbances in the electrical discharges of brain cells, and characterized by transient, recurrent episodes of clouding or loss of consciousness, often accompanied by convulsive seizures or automatic behaviour.

The condition may be (a) symptomatic, that is due to a known condition such as brain inflammation, high fever, brain tumor, vascular disturbances, structural abnormality, brain injury or degenerative changes or (b) idiopathic, that is of an unknown origin or due to a nonspecific brain defect. Genetic predisposition can be found but not in all cases.

SYMPTOMS OF EPILEPSY

Symptoms can be divided into two parts :-

A) Paroxysmal

B) Interparoxysmal.

A) PAROXYSMAL

The site of the origin of clinical symptoms is cerebral disturbance. Some epleptic patients become aware of the occurrence of seizure hours or days before. This is known as 'aura'. It may involve any of the sensory organs. In temporal lobe seizures the 'aura' may be hallucination of taste or smell. In occipital lobe discharge it may be visual hallucination. The patient sees specks of lights in front of the eyes.

There can be motor auras like twitching of muscles or running, psychic 'auras' like sudden disturbance of the use of words.

GRAND MAL EPILEPSY — Consists of four stages:

(i) **Aura** — The patient may fall to the ground with a sudden cry and may injure himself.

(ii) **Tonic stage**—the muscles go into spasm for ten to 30 seconds

(iii) **The clonic stage** — There may be a clonic jerking of muscles. The patient may bite his tongue or lips. Froth appears on his lips. Urine and stool may be passed involuntarily. This stage lasts for three to four minutes.

(iv) **Stage of Coma** — The patient remains in a sleep-like stage for one to two hours or postictal automatism.

STATUS EPILEPTICUS — Sometimes a patient may pass from one seizure to another without recovering consciousness. This involves danger to life. It may be sometimes due to a sudden withdrawal of phenobarbital.

PETTI MAL EPILEPSY — It consists of a momentary loss of consciousness. There may be few or no convulsions. There is no aura. The patient is not aware of attack. He turns pale, suddenly becomes silent or halts in what he is doing, may drop what he is holding. May have twitching of facial muscles. Attack is over within 5-30 seconds. The patient resumes his previous activity as before.

PSYCHOMOTOR SEIZURES — These seizures are episodic disturbances of consciousness (no loss of consciousness) usually without detectable convulsive phenomena, but commonly associated with automatic motor acts. The clouding of consciousness may last for seconds, minutes, hours or exceptionally for days.

EPILEPTIC PSYCHOSIS — It is characterized by a recurrent confusional episode and paranoid delusions.

(B) INTER-PAROXYSMAL

EPILEPTIC PERSONALITY — A personality pattern observed in a minority of individuals with epilepsy and probably due to reaction to the frustrations and anxiety this disease may cause rather than the constitutional factors. These individuals are described as irritable, stubborn, egocentric, uncooperative and aggressive. Also called epileptic characters.

EPILEPTIC DETERIORATION AND DEMENTIA — A progressive mental deterioration occurring in 5 per cent of, or fewer, epileptic patients, especially those who have had seizure all their lives. It may be due to nerve cell degeneration caused by circulatory disturbances during the attacks.

Organic Brain Syndromes also include :

a) Disorders associated with infections; for example, Cerebral Syphillis, Epidemic Encephalitis.

b) Disorders with brain tumors.

c) Disorders with toxins and metabolic disorders; for example, Toxic delirium (discussed in unit) Nutritional deficiencies, Endocrine disturbances, post-partum disturbances.

TREATMENT

The anti-epileptic drugs are bromides which have replaced phenobarbitol (Luminol). Dephenylhydnation (Dilantin, Phenytoin) 60 mgn to 200 mgn/day. Primidone (Mysoline) Acetozolamide (Diamox) 30mg/kg are often necessary for control of seizure.

Trimenthadione (Tridione), Paraldehyde, Chloral hydrate, Amytal specially in status epilepticus.

APPLICATION TO NURSING

Reading this part of organic psychosis and brain disorders will enable the nursing students to develop knowledge of these conditions. It will help her to differentiate between OBS (Organic Brain Syndrome) and other psychotic disorders. It will also help her to prevent many complications in patients while using various types of therapies.

TO RECALL

Organic Psychosis is divided into :
- **Acute Brain Syndrome — Delirium**
- **Chronic Brain Syndrome — Dementia**

Types of Dementia :
- **Senile Dementia**
- **Paranoid Reaction**
- **Preshyophrenic Type**
- **Depressed and Agitated**
- **Delirium and Confused Type**

Kosakoff (Amnesic) Syndrome

Dementia
- **Alzhemier's disease**

TO RECALL

* Pick's Disease
* Parkinson's Disease
* Huntington's Chorea.
* Epilepsy

SCHIZOPHRENIC DISORDERS (F 20 - F29)

INTRODUCTION

It is a group of mental disturbances essentially characterized by a) one or more psychotic features during the active phase, including a bizarre or absurd delusion such as being controlled, b) Somatic, grandiose, religious or nihilistic delusions, c) Delusion of persecution or jealousy with hallucination, d) Incoherence with marked loosening of association, blunted, flat or inappropriate affect, e) Hallucination, f) and grossly disorganized behaviour such as in catatonia. A common term for schizophrenic disorder is schizophrenia.

Psychoses associated with organic brain disorder is organic in nature, the disorders classified functional psychosis are considered primarily psychological in origin. Genetic and other biological causes play a significant role. These functional disorders or psychotic disorders can be classified under three major categories :

a) *Schizophrenia, b) Paranoid disorders consisting of Manic Depressive Psychosis and Involutional Melancholia. Schizophrenia* and paranoid disorders are considered to be **THOUGHT DISORDERS,** while the affective psychosis are dominated by **MOOD DISTURBANCES.**

DEFINITION OF SCHIZOPHRENIA

Schizophrenic disorders, described in ICD-10 Glossary, are characterized in general by fundamental and characteristic distortion of thinking and perception and by an inappropriate affect. Delusion present may be bizarre. Hallucinations, especially auditory, are common. Mood is characteristically shallow and incongruous. Ambivalence may appear.

The American Psychiatric Association defines schizophrenia as, "a group of disorders manifested by characteristic disturbance of thinking, mood and behaviour." Disturbance in thinking is marked by alteration of concept formation which may lead to misinterpretation of reality and sometimes to delusions and hallucinations. Mood changes include ambivalent, constricted and inappropriate emotional responsiveness and loss of empathy with others. Behaviour may be withdrawn, regressive and bizarre."

HISTORICAL DEVELOPMENT OF SCHIZO-PHRENIA

In 1849, John Conolly mentioned that young persons frequently fall in a state of somewhat resembling melancholia without any discoverable sorrow or grief. In 1860, a Belgian Psychiatrist Morel termed it as dementia praecoece while treating a 14-year-old boy, who showed a state of melancholy depression and a hatred for his father even with the idea of killing.

In 1896, Krapeline gave a clinical description of dementia praecox and classified it into three types: Hebephrenic, Catatonic and Paranoid. In 1911, Eugene Bleuler used it as schizophrenia. He described that the harmony of the personality was SPLIT. Bleuler distinguished between primary and secondary symptoms of schizophrenia. Bleuler described the fourth type of schizophrenia and named it as Simple Schizophrenia.

EPIDEMIOLOGY

The incidence of schizophrenia is described under the following headings:

a) OCCURRENCE — It is observed that schizophrenia occurs in all types of societies and all places. Prevalence varies from 0.3 per cent to 1 percent of people who experience a schizophrenic reaction at sometime in their lives.

b) AGE — Rare in childhood. Age varies between 15 and 45 years. Peak age is 30 years.

c) SEX RATIO — Incidence in males and females is almost the same.

d) SOCIAL CLASS — Reviewed literature shows that the incidence of schizophrenia is higher in the lower socio-economic status group in comparison to the upper socio-economic group.

CAUSES/ ETIOLOGY

There is no definite etiology of schizophrenia. In general, the theories of schizophrenia can be described as follows:

A) GENETIC FACTORS

Studies have revealed that monozygotic twins have four times higher chances of developing schizophrenia than the schizophrenia, the chance of the other twin being afflicted is 85.8 per cent. Children of schizophrenic parents are more prone to develop schizophrenia than children of other persons. Approximately 40 per cent of children born to both the schizophrenic parents will be affected. If only one parent either mother or father is schizophrenic, 10 per cent of the children will be psychotic.

B) PSYCHOSOCIAL FACTORS OR PSYCHODYNAMICS

In schizoprehnic psychosis there is:-

(i) **Impaired ego functioning** :- Reality testing and judgement is affected. The intenisty of schizophrenia will depend upon the intense impairment of ego function.

(ii) **Mother infant Relationship** :- There may be a defect in mother-infant relationship. Deprivation of early mothering reduces a child's capacity to socialize. The mother may be present but lack of effective mother-child relationship does withdraw the child from socialization.

(iii) **Pathological Communication:** It has a significant role to play in a child whether to withdraw from the communication or continue. For example, in **Double Bound Communication** the child is not able to discriminate the sort of message being conveyed. The mother says to the child, "Go out and play, but see that you don't fight with anyone." In fact, the other message is, "It is better if you stay inside only," but it is not said. So the child is not able to decide. If he does not go out, the mother will get angry. If he goes out and has a tiff with someone, even then the mother would get angry. So the child withdraws gradually.

(iv) **Pathogenic Family Interactions** :— Transaction between parents or significant people who relate with the child. Parents may be maintaining superficial relationship. Children coming from broken homes are more prone to schizophrenia than those of normal homes as their coping abilities get reduced because of continuous stress.

c) SOCIOCULTURAL FACTORS

Persons who live in low socio-economic families and areas are prone to schizophrenia. For example, a child at a very young age goes for work and is deprived of affection from parents, schooling, playmates. This causes a lot of anger and frustration in the child.

d) ORGANIC THEORY

Theorists believe that schizophrenia is caused due to infection, poison, trauma or metabolic disorders.

e) VITAMIN DEFICIENCY THEORY

A patient with Vitamin B_1, B_6, B_{12} and Vitamin C deficiency may become schizoprehnic.

TO RECALL

— **Definition of Schizophrenia**
It is a descriptive term for a group of psychotic disorders characterized by gross distortion of reality, withdrawal from social interaction, disorganization and fragmentation of perception, thought and emotions.

— **Historical development of schizophrenia**

— **Epidemiology of schizophrenia**

— **Causes or Etiology**
- * **Genetic Factors**
- * **Psychosocial Factors**
- * **Sociocultural Factors**
- * **Organic Theory**
- * **Vitamin Deficiency Theory**

SIGNS AND SYMPTOMS OF SCHIZOPHRENIA

Patients with schizophrenia may present various symptoms. However, Bleuler has made distinction between (i) PRIMARY/Fundamental Symptoms which are present to some extent in every case of schizophrenia and (ii) SECONDARY or Accessory symptoms which may or may not be present.

(i) PRIMARY OR FUNDAMENTAL SYMPTOMS (BLEULER'S FOUR A'S)

a) ASSOCIATIVE DISTURBANCE OR LOOSENESS : It is a thought disorder in which the person does not think logically. Ideas expressed have little or no connection, ideas shift from one point to another very quickly. As a result, thinking appears bizarre, illogic and chaotic. For example, Rani comes, the sky is blue, the doctor fell down, Mahesh must be eating.

b) AUTISM : It is a thought disorder in which the patient is preoccupied with ideas derived from fantasy and day dreaming. The person is unaffected by what is happening in the environment. He or she is emotionally detached from the world or others.

c) AFFECTIVE INCONGRUITY OR DISTURBANCE OR INAPPROPRIATE MOOD : In an effective disturbance the affect/mood of the patient is inappropriate, flat or blunt. For example, the patient may laugh when the situation demands sadness. He expresses no emotions at all for a happy or sad situation.

d) AMBIVALENCE — The schizophrenic patients experience two contradictory or opposing feelings, attitudes or wishes towards the same person, object or situation. For example, a love-and-hate feeling for the same person.

ii) SECONDARY OR ACCESSORY SYMPTOMS

A) Disorders of Perception:

(i) Hallucition — Auditory are most common, visual (seeing angels) tactile (e.g. feeling of crawling ants), gustatory (e.g. bad taste), or olfactory (e.g. bad smell) may also be presented by the patients.

(ii) Illusion — For example, rope is perceived by the patient as a snake falling on him.

B) DISORDERS OF THOUGHT: DELUSIONS — For example, C B I is following me. Delusion of persecution and delusion of grandeur, ideas of reference, depersonalization, incoherence, neolagism and mutism.

C) DISORDERS OF ACTIVITY

- Negativism and automatism
- Stereotype, speech echololia, and verbigeration
- Stereotype activity, echopraxia, mannerism
- Impulsiveness — action performed unexpectedly without consideration of the whole personality. This is due to the result of an ambivalence feeling.

D) DETERIORATED APPEARANCE AND MANNER

Efforts on self-care and grooming may become minimum. Schizophrenic patients have to the reminded of bath, wash and shave and other routine activities.

E) DISTURBANCE IN ATTENTION — The patient is not able to hold attention for a long time. He or she lives in his/her own autistic world.

F) INSIGHT IN SCHIZOPHRENIC: In it, the illness is affected severely. ***(Refer Chapter III, Unit IX for review of Psychopathology of Human Behaviour).***

The type of schizophrenic disorders according to ICD-10

F 20 — 0 Paranoid schizophrenia
F 20 — 1 Hebephrenic schizophrenia
F 20 — 2 Catatonic schizophrenia
F 20 — 3 Undifferentiated schizophrenia
F 20 — 4 Post-Schizophrenic Depression
F 20 — 5 Residual schizophrenia
F 20 — 6 Simple schizophrenia
F 20 — 8 Other schizophrenia
F 20 — 9 Schizophrenia unspecified.

Types of schizophrenia age, pattern of onset and signs and symptoms are described in the tabular form.

TYPES OF SCHIZOPHRENIA, AGE AND PATTERN OF DEVELOPMENT AND SIGNS AND SYMPTOMS

TYPE OF SCHIZOPHRENIA	AGE AND PATTERN OF DEVELOPMENT	SIGNS AND SYMPTOMS
Simple Type	The onset is extremely gradual, begins fairly early in life often during adolescence.	Marked disturbances of interest in human relation, emotions and activity, hallucination and delusions are rare. Associative looseness is present. Goals are not realistic. In early age the patient shows a lot of interest but in the later stage has no interest in school or occupation. Criticism by others may not cause any concern. They keep changing their jobs, described as migratory workers. They become idlers.
Hebephrenic Type	Onset is insidious, age varies between 15—25 years.	More severe disintegration of personality than other types of schizophrenia. Emotionally a person is indifferent. A silly smile, giggling, self-disorbed smile and inappropriate, shallow laughter after little or no provocation are common symptoms. Hallucination (visual) present. Delusions are of fantasy; bizarre nature. There is a tendency to regress, to a state of vegetation. The patient urinates and defecates in the bed, does not attend to personal hygiene. Eats with fingers, masturbates openly. Behaviour of hebaphrenic schizophrenia is indicated as "Silly" behaviour.
Catatonic Type	Onset is very acute or sudden. It occurs in earliest age : 15 to 25 years.	Catatonic patients present two main types of clinical picture : (i) Catatonic stupor, and (ii) Catatonic excitement. *(i) Catatonic stupor* — It follows depression, apathy, the patient becomes uncommunicative, characterised by failing interest, preoccupation in his own thought, emotional poverty and dreaminess. Mute, stuperous

TYPE OF SCHIZOPHRENIA	AGE AND PATTERN OF DEVELOPMENT	SIGNS AND SYMPTOMS
		and mask-like face. Eyes closed or frequently stares fixedly at one point or blankly looks downward. Stands immobile, can sit whole day on the edge of a bed. Catalepsy or waxy flexibility is present. The patient can lie down in the same position for days or weeks if not disturbed. Negativism and somatic disturbances present. The patient refuses to eat occasionally, if he is unobserved he will eat greedily. Dribbling of saliva from the angular region. Holds urine and stool or involuntarily passes urine and stool in the bed. Does not show avoiding sign to painful stimuli. Coming out of stupor the patient will give an account of all the activities, slowly or suddenly, without inhibitions. *(ii) Catatonic Excitement* — The patient may behave in a wild and quite unpredictable manner. He shows an aggressive motor activity, which is not accompanied by an emotional expression — cold approach. The patients are impulsive and may suddenly attack anybody standing nearby. Break or destroy articles. Tear their clothes and remain nude. Flow of speech is from mutisim to flight of ideas, negativism, hallucination (visual and hearing), sleeplessness and dehydration are present. On rare occasions the patient may collapse due to exhaustion. Homosexual-prone and assaultive. The patient is not consistenly joyful as in the case of mania.
Paranoid Type	The onset is gradual most of the time, acute paranoid schizophrenia is also presented. Age after 30 years.	The most common type of schizophrenic psychosis. These patients are extremely suspicious. Delusion of persecution, grandeur and ideas of reference are marked in them. Hypochondrical delusions are also present. "I am having lakhs of rupees, everyone is after my life and talks about me only." Delusions are not joyful-type like in manics. Hallucinations are very common and have association with delusion. The patient hallucinates threatening voices, warning voices and voices directing him what to do. Poor IPR, cold, distrustful and withdrawn from others. Have a chip-on-the-shoulder attitude. "(Oh I don't care," shrugs the shoulder and goes away) Argumentative, sarcastic, resentful to suggestions, gives caustic remarks to others. Disorders of association appears. Depressive delusions are also common.
Acute Schizophrenic Episode	The onset is sudden.	Most types of schizophrenia mentioned above are in an acute or subacute form. The patient presents a dreamlike state with clouding of consciousness. There may be ideas of reference and emotional turmoil, depression and fear. The individual goes under a massive breakdown, gets a fragmented or nightmare type of experience.
Latent Schizophrenia		It is characterised by various symptoms of schizophrenia but lacks in any full blown schizophrenia.

TYPE OF SCHIZOPHRENIA	AGE AND PATTERN OF DEVELOPMENT	SIGNS AND SYMPTOMS
Residual Schizophrenia		It is a chronic form of schizophrenia in which the symptoms persist after the acute phase. But the patient can do his routine work as he has attained a "Social Recovery."
Schizoaffective Type		It is characterized by a mixture of schizophrenia symptoms and manic depressive elements. Mood is hypomanic and ideation is like schizophrenia. If given ECT, only schizophrenia symptoms will be seen post ECT.
Chronic Undifferentiated Type		Schizophrenic symptoms of thought, affect and behaviour are presented by the patient. But the clinical picture is such in that signs and symptoms of many subgroups of schizophrenia are mixed. None is having more dominant symptoms to classify under any group.
Childhood Type	Prior to adolescence.	Preoccupation with fantasy withdrawn and atypical behaviour before puberty.

Fig. 19 : Table Describing the Types of Schizophrenia Age & Pattern of Development and Signs & Symptons.

TREATMENT OF SCHIZOPHRENIC PATIENTS

The selection and method of treatment will depend on the type of schizophrenia the patient is presenting and predominant symptoms. The approach to treatment is as follows :

(a) **Prevention of Schizophrenia** — keeping in mind the etiological factors or causes, the efforts should be made to prevent or reduce the number of schizophrenic conditions.

(b) **Intensive Psychotherapy**—Individual, group, behavioural, supportive and family therapy may be used.

(c) **Therapeutic Community or Milieu** — Therapy will minimize the maladaptive learning in the patient, environmental and physical stress will be reduced to meet his needs.

(d) **Chemotherapy** — Antipsychotic or Neuroleptic drugs may be prescribed. The type of drug, dose and duration depends on the symptoms presented by individual patients. Drugs may be continued after discharge also. Antiparkinsonian drugs are given to reduce E.P.S. (Extra Pyramidal Symptoms).

(e) **Electro-Convulsive Therapy** - The treatment is used for patients with severe schizophrenia. Drugs and psychotherapy are to be continued. *(For all types of therapies refer Chapter VI).*

PROGNOSIS OF SCHIZOPHRENIC PSYCHOSIS

Statistics indicate that approximately one-third of the patients receiving treatment will improve, one-third will not respond and one-third will maintain an unchanged condition. *Poor prognosis indicators* are : history of the previous attack, long duration of illness, gradual onset, and unstable, ill-adjusted personality, an early age of onset, family history and asthenic built of patients.

APPLICATION TO NURSING

Schizophrenia is one of the commonest psychotic disorders seen in the outpatient as well as hospitalized situations. Reading about schizoprehnia will enable the nursing student to build her knowledge on definition of schizophrenia, its types with their difference. She will be able to identify the patients with schizophrenic symptoms, plan for nursing intervention and participation in various types of therapies.

TO RECALL

- **Signs and symptoms of schizophrenia according to Bleuler.**
  - **Primary or fundamental signs and symptoms.**
  - **Secondary or accessory signs and symptoms.**
- **Types of schizophrenia are:**
  - **Simple type.**
  - **Hebephrenic type.**
  - **Catatonic type.**
  - **Acute schizophrenic episode.**
  - **Latent schizophrenia.**
  - **Residual schizophrenia.**
  - **Schizoaffective schizophrenia.**
  - **Chronic undifferentiated type.**
  - **Childhood schizophrenia.**
- **Treatment of schizophrenia.**
- **Prognosis.**
- **Application to Nursing.**

MOOD (AFFECTIVE) DISORDERS

(ICD-10 F 30-39)

INTRODUCTION

Affective disorders are characterized by a severe disturbance of mood manifested as elation or excitement and depression. These are accompanied by one or more of the following : delusion, perplexity (a form of confusion in which the patient is bewildered and uncertain about his thoughts), disturbed attitude towards self, disorder of perception and behaviour. These symptoms appear according to the mood of the patient. In DSM III these disorders include major affective disorders (manic episode, major depressive episode, bipolar disorders). Other specific affective disorders (cyclothymic disorders, dysthymic disorders and atypical affective disorders.)

DEFINITION OF AFFECTIVE DISORDERS

Affective disorders are illnesses in which mood change is the primary and dominant feature.Mood change is relatively persistent and is associated with characteristic changes in thinking, attitude and behaviour. Affective disorders are classified as :

I. Manic Depressive Psychosis, and
II. Involutional Psychotic Reactions.

CLASSIFICATION OF MANIC (DEPRESSIVE) DISORDERS

I. Manic Depressive Psychosis are distinguished in three major types: (i) *Manic Type*, (ii) *Depressed Type*, and (iii) *Circular* Reactions. The patients who present only depression all the the time during their attacks are said to have UNIPOLAR affective illness, while those presenting manic state after depression are said to have BIPOLAR affective illness. ICD-10 classification describes affective disorders as follows :

- F 30 Manic episode
- F 31 Bipolar affective disorders
- F 32 Depressive episodes
- F 33 Recurrent depressive disorders
- F 34 Persistent mood (affective) disorders
- F 38 Other mood (affective) disorders
- F 39 Unspecified mood (affective) disorders.

EPIDEMIOLOGY OCCURRENCE

INCIDENT RANGE :- The incidence range of manic depressive psychosis (MDP) is 3 to 4 patients per 1,000 population.

SEX :- The male/female incidence is 3:2.

SOCIAL CLASS :- It is thought that MDP occurs among people in high social class comparatively.

MARITAL STATUS :- Married people have lesser episodes than the unmarried people; widowhood increases the episode of MDP.

PROFESSIONALS :- It occurs four times more in professionals than non-professionals.

AGE :- There is no specific age for manic depressive psychosis. The first attack may occur between adolescence and 45 years of age. It may occur between 20 and 35 years of age in general. Depression occurs between 35 and 50 years.

ETIOLOGY OR PREDISPOSITION

Genetic Predisposition: There is increasing evidence that genetic plays a strong role in predisposition of MDP . Early studies show that approximately 15 per cent of the brothers, sisters, parents and children of manic depressive psychosis were also suffering from this ailment, whereas expectancy in the general population was 0.5 per cent. It is found that identical twins have higher chances of MDP. Both the twins develop a similar type of MDP reactions.

Neurophysiological Factors : Researchers have found the possibility that imbalance in excitatory and inhibitory processes may predispose MDP. Excitatory functions may cause mania and inhibitory functions may cause depression.

Biochemical Factors : Findings reveal the possibility of metabolic changes in brain pathology with these disorders, particularly the catecholamine imbalance. Increased or decreased catecholamine may cause mania or depression respectively. There may be sleep disturbance also.

Psychological and Interpersonal Factors Predisposing Family and Personality Factors : Mood swings in the parents will lead to maladaptive learning in children. These children may develop a typical premorbid personality pattern. They are described as ambitious, energetic, social, often highly successful. They do not express hostile feelings. These patients are usually endomorphic in their built.

Severe Stress : Patients who have experienced severe stress in their life-time may be predisposed to MDP. But it also depends on how stressful the life events were and what was the reaction of a person to those events.

Feeling of Hopelessness and Use of Defenses : In mania the individual tries to escape his difficulty by "Flight from Reality" like trying to forget an event which is very painful.

Psychodynamics : Psychoanalytical theory explains that a child is placed in a dependent position and ego development is disturbed. The child develops punitive superego or anger is turned inward or into depression. A strong Id, uncontrollable impulsive behaviour is called mania.

Socio-cultural Factors: They also affect a manic-depressive episode. For example, manic reactions are commoner in Africa than depressive episodes. In the United States depression is commoner than mania.

TO RECALL

- **Affective psychosis is a disorder in which mood change is the primary and dominant feature. It has two types:**
  - **Manic Depressive Disorders**
  - **Involutional Malancholic Reactions**
- **Manic Depressive Disorders can be described as**
  - **Manic Episodes**
  - **Depressive Episodes.**
- **Manic Depressive Disorders can be**
  - **Unipolar**
  - **Bipolar**
- **Epidemiology**
- **Etiology or causative factors**
  - **Biological factor**
  - **Psychological and interpersonal factors**
  - **Sociocultural factors**
- **Psychodynamics of affective disorders.**

SIGNS AND SYMPTOMS OF MDP

The signs and symptoms will be described under **Manic Episode and Depressive Episode, Circular type** of Manic Depressive Psychosis. The diagnosis of manic depressive psychosis is based primarily on: (i) Distinct and marked disturbances in affect, in which thinking is consonant (in accordance) with mood, (ii) No intellectual or personality deterioration, (iii) Well-defined attacks, (iv) History of manic-depressive illness in family, and (v) Precipitating psychological factors.

MANIC EPISODES

The classical TRIAD (THREE) symptoms of mania consist of :
(i) Elated, unstable mood.
(ii) Increased pressure of speech.
(iii) Increased motor activity.

Manic types are described as (i) Hypomania, (ii) Acute Mania, & (iii) Delirious Mania.

SIGNS AND SYMPTOMS IN HYPOMANIA

(i) **HYPOMANIA** : It is a mild form of mania.

— The patient shows moderate elation, flightness and overactivity.

— The individual 'simply feels great'.

— The patient shows increased assertiveness, self-confidence and an air of self-assurance.

— Energy is moderately increased.

— Thinking is speeded up. Delusion of grandiosity present.

— Uninhibited in his approach. No matter how inhibited the person was earlier, now becomes free, demanding and surprisingly unconventional in speech and manner.

— Sleep time is reduced, REM (rapid eye movement) time is increased but the patient feels and looks fresh and energetic.

— Appetite may be voracious.

— The patient appears a bright, intelligent and sociable individual.

— Intolerant to criticism.

— Socially aggressive, argumentative, spends money extravagantly, full of ambitious schemes which are never worked out.

— The patient gets bored with routine, lacks sustained interest.

— Hypomanic patients are mischievous. Indulge in jokes with professionals like doctors and nurses. Good humour, it is infectious that means everybody enjoys it.

— Sudden oscillation of mood.

— These patients are erotic, may indulge in sexual excessiveness. Previously a modest young women may become sexually promiscuous.

Signs and symptoms in hypomania are of a mild form.

SIGNS AND SYMPTOMS IN ACUTEMANIA

(II) **ACUTE MANIA** : The signs and symptoms in acute mania are moderately increased and lead towards severity that is Delirious Mania. The signs and symptoms of acute mania are discussed under changes in (a) Affective Tonality, (b) Stream of Thoughts, (c) Psychomotor Activities, and (d) Attention and Judgement.

(A) AFFECTIVE TONALITY

It is the change which occurs in affect or mood of the patient. He shows exhaltation, joyous excitement. The tempo of the whole personality is quickened. The patient's pattern of behaviour reflects his mood. He sings and dances about.

(B) STREAM OF THOUGHT

It is also increased. Rapid association of ideas. Flight of ideas with rhyming, playing with words, clang association are markedly present. His style of phrasing words may be pompous and his speech may assume the character of theatrical declaration (Talking in a theatre on stage.) The patient speaks with crispness, vigour and changes his pitch while speaking. The range of ideas is limited and overvalued. The patient in acute mania is very noisy and hilarious. He is haughty, demanding, revengeful and arrogant. Delusion of grandiosity and paranoid is present. The patient spends extravagantly. Will give a cheque of thousands of rupees to another person.

(C) PSYCHOMOTOR ACTIVITY

There is an overactivity and violent motor excitement in acute mania. The patient decorates himself with trinklets, and improvised beads and medals. He may tear his clothes in small ribbons and decorate himself. He has a suggestion on how to run the institute or the country. He may even destroy bedsheets, out of malice and wants to keep himself busy. Manic patients sleep very little but do not look fatigued. Hallucination may occur but not very common in acute manic patients. They receive cuts and abrasions but do not give importance to it and will not take any treatment.

Appetite is increased but may not have time to eat. So they may lose weight.

(D) ATTENTION AND JUDGEMENT

Attention span is markedly decreased in these patients. Environmental noises disturb them. They misidentify a person and show that they know him. Judgement is markedly impaired.

(III) DELIRIOUS MANIA : It is very rare. The patient is out of contact. His speech is incoherent (word salad). He is constantly and purposelessly active. He may be hallucinating, delusional and extremely dangerous. Without treatment the patient may die of exhaustion.

DEPRESSIVE EPISODES

In depression the classical Triad symptoms are :

(i) Depressed mood
(ii) Slowed or Retarded Thinking, and
(iii) Psychomotor Retardation.

Depressed type of MDP is described as (i) Mild Depression, (ii) Acute Depression, and (iii) Depressive Stupor.

(I) MILD DEPRESSION

The patient is rigid ethically and has moral standards. He is meticulous, and perfectionist, self-depreciatory, sensitive to criticism. In mild depression the patient feels fatigued and staleness. Physical complaints with no organic cause. Blue spells, the patient lacks confidence in himself. Loses his zest and interest for living. Feels inadequate, shows growing aversion to activity. Likes to be left alone and finds difficulty in performing his ordinary duties. Appetite and sleep are decreased. The patient looks stale.

(II) ACUTE OR SEVERE DEPRESSION

In these cases the patient's body is stooped, head flexed, face immobile, forehead furrows, looks fixedly downward. Tongue is coated, marked loss of appetite. Loss of weight, disturbed sleep. Hypochondrical ideas. Feelings—the patient says that he has no feeling, no interest in any activity. Retarded thoughts: the patient's replies are brief and monosyllabic. Expresses in a very low tone, answers with great effort and appears to use a lot of energy to answer questions.Has suicidal ideas. Psychomotor activity is markedly decreased. Is preoccupied in his own thoughts. Gradually these patients progress towards stupor, if not treated.

(III) DEPRESSIVE STUPOR

It is the most intensive form of depression. The patient presents with acute dementia, mute, sensorium is clouded, and he is intensively preoccupied. He has dream-like hallucination and marked ideas of death.

CIRCULAR TYPE

The circular type is characterised by an alteration of manic and depressed phases. Occasionally, the progression may be towards delirious mania or depressive stupor.

Manic Depressive Psychosis is unipolar and bipolar as described earlier. Patients suffering from bipolar are younger, more men than women, and have history of relatives with bipolar diseases. Bipolar patients respond well to Lithium-Carbonate therapeutically and poorly to Imipramine, whereas unipolar patients respond better to Imipramine and poor to Lithium.

TREATMENT OF MANIC & DEPRESSIVE DISORDERS

The patient with Manic-Depressive Psychosis needs to be hospitalized. A severely depressed patient with an idea of suicide requires constant medical care. Similarly, the patient displaying symptoms of mania requires hospitalization. The treatment includes antidepressants Tricyclic, Tetracyclic and MAO inhibitor group. Lithium-carbonate is a drug of choice in mania. The blood serum level is to be maintained. *(Refer Unit XV of Chapter VI)*

Psychotherapy can be effectively used for depressed patients. Individual, group and family psychotherapy is effective. Milieu therapy is effective for depressive and manic patients.

Before giving any type of psychotherapy, manic patients are to be given psychotropic drugs.

Electro-convulsive therapy is effective for depressive patients, especially if the patient is not responding to antidepressants. ECT is given to depressed patients where rapid, remission of symptoms is required. A combination of chemotherapy and psychotherapy is effective rather than a single-approach treatment.

PROGNOSIS : For a single attack prognosis is good. Recurrence is very common. Studies reveal almost 90 per cent recover from attack. About 5 per cent of cases become chronic. Recovery is quicker in the younger age group. About 10 to 15 per cent patients may die by committing suicide.

INVOLUTIONAL MELANCHOLIA

Involutional melancholia is a mental disorder occurring in the late middle life or during the menopausal period characterized by severe depression and less often by paranoid thinking. Other symptoms are agitation, apprehension, feeling of despair and worthlessness, persistent insomnia, chronic fatigue and loss of appetite. They also show persecutory delusion, hypochondrical and nihilistic delusions.

These symptoms are believed to be a psychological reaction to physical changes and external stresses.

The treatment of choice is Electro-Convulsive Therapy. Antidepressants are also helpful.

APPLICATION TO NURSING

This content on mood (affective) psychosis will enable the students to understand the predominant difference between functional psychosis and affective psychosis. Reading about MDP will help her to plan her nursing intervention based on the symptoms presented by the patient.

TO RECALL

* **Triad signs and symptoms of manic disorders are (i) elated or unstable mood, (ii) Increased pressure of speech and (iii) Increased motor activity. These symptoms vary in (a) Hypomania, (b) Acute mania, and (c) Delirious mania.**
* **Triad signs and symptoms of MDP depressive type are (i) Depressed mood, (ii) Slowed or retarded thinking, and (iii) Psychomotor retardation. Symptoms vary in depression according to its severity that is (a) Mild Depression, (b) Acute Depression, and (c) Depressive Stupor.**
* **Circular Type MDP is characterized by an alternative of manic and depressed phases.**
* **Treatment includes antidepressants, antipsychotic drug, Lithium- Carbonate, Psychotherapy, ECT, and Milieu therapy.**
* **Prognosis**
* **Involutional Melancholia**
* **Application to nursing**

APPLICATION TO NURSING

Reading this unit on organic mental disorders, schizophrenic disorders and mood (affective) disorders is very important for student nurses. It will help them to learn various types of mental illnesses classified under these mental disorders. The students will be able to apply the knowledge in planning the nursing intervention of patients with various mental disorders. It will also give them a detailed insight into the disease, including therapeutic modalities used.

BETTER STUDY SECTION OF UNIT XVIII

1. VOCABULARY (USE DICTIONARY)

Study the word you do not know from the following text:

Agitation	Hypercholesterolemia
Ambivalent	Indecent
Amnesic	Indicators
Assertiveness	Inhibitor
Bewildered	Melancholic
Chaotic	Morbid

Degenerative
Deprivation
Elation
Errotic
Excitatory
Extravagantly
Fantasy
Predispose
Transient
Unconventional

2. ASSIGNMENT

Review Chapter III on Classification of Mental Disorders, Causes and Psychopathological Behaviour.

3. STUDY QUESTIONS

(1) Define the following terms :
Organic Mental Disorder
Schizophrenic Disorder
Mood/Affective Psychosis

(2) List the categories of schizophrenia according to ICD-10 (Refer to the unit content)

(3) List the categories of Mood Disorders

(4) Make a tabular chart on four common types of schizophrenia: simple, hebaphrenic, paranoid, catatonic,explaining onset, age and signs and symptoms

4. READING REFFRENCE

— ***The ICD-10 classification of Mental and Behaviour Disorders, Clinical Description and Diagnostic Guidelines.*** Oxford University Press, Delhi, Bombay, Calcutta, Madras, WHO 1992.

— Kapoor, Bimla, ***A Textbook of Psychiatric Nursing,*** Kumar Publishing House, Delhi (1992).

— Kolb L. and Brodie H.K. ***Modern Clinical Psychiatry*** (10th ed), W.B. Saunders Company, (1982).

UNIT XIX

NEUROTIC, PERSONALITY AND SEXUAL DISORDERS

UNIT OUTLINE

— NEUROTIC DISORDERS

- Definition of Neurosis
- Causes and Etiology
- Classification of Psychoneurotic disorders
- Anxiety Neurosis
- Hysteria
  - — Hysterical Neurosis/ Conversion Reaction
  - — Dissociative Reaction
    - * Psychogenic Amnesia
    - * Multiple Personality and Depersonalization
    - * Psychogenic Fugue
    - * Sleep walking/ Somnambulism
- Phobic state
- Obsessive Compulsive Neurosis
- Neurotic Depression
- Neurasthenia
- Hypochondriasis
- Treatment of Neurotic Disorders

Difference between Psychosis and Neurosis

PERSONALITY DISORDERS

- Types of Personality Disorders
- Psychopathic Personality

SEXUAL DEVIATION AND DISORDERS

- Normal sexual disorders.
- Abnormal sexuality.
- Sexual Deviation.
- Sexual Problems with Social and legal Aspects.
- Treatment

Application to Nursing.

Better Study Section.

INTENDED LEARNING BEHAVIOUR

After reading this unit you will be able to :

a) Define Neurosis
b) Classify psychoneurotic disorders
c) Describe anxiety neurosis
d) Explain Hysterical Neurosis/ Conversion Reaction and Dissociative Reaction
e) Describe obsessive Compulsive Neurosis
f) Differentiate between Psychosis and Neurosis
g) Describe personality disorders
h) Explain various sexual disorders
i) Apply the knowledge while nursing the patients in psychiatric units/ community.

NEUROTIC DISORDERS

INTRODUCTION

In modern medicine and nursing, psychological factors are increasingly regarded as significant in all types of illnesses. There are significant aspects of human mind and drives i.e. the neurological system, and adjustment mechanisms. Disturbances to any such factors may lead to pathological conditions of mind. The non-professional may term Neurosis as 'Nervousness' and Psychosis as 'Insanity'.

Neurosis or Psychoneurotic personality disorders arise from an effort when the person tries to deal with a specific, private, internal psychological problem and a stressful situation. This problem or stressful situation the person is unable to solve or overcome without tension or anxiety. The effect of anxiety is regarded as a common source of neurosis.

DEFINITION OF NEUROSIS

Neurosis is defined as a mild-to-moderately severe illness of the personality, in which the ego function of reality testing is not gravely (intensively) affected and maladjustment to life is limited.

According to Longman Dictionary of Psychology and Psychiatry, "Neurosis is a functional mental disorder characterized by a high level of anxiety and other distressing emotional symptoms such as morbid fears, obsessive thoughts, compulsive acts, somatic reactions, dissociative states and depressive reactions. The symptoms do not involve gross personality disorganization, total lack of insight or loss of contact with reality. It is generally viewed as an exaggerated, unconscious method of coping with the internal conflict and anxiety they produce. Also called PSYCHONEUROSIS in DSM III.

CAUSES OR ETIOLOGY OF NEUROSIS

(i) BIOLOGICAL FACTORS

Inherited predisposition has little role to play. But biological and psychological factors together may precipitate neurosis. For example, a hypersensitive person with family background in which attention is given to very small things will have anxiety in everyday life. So an anxious environment at home by parents or other family members may contribute to neurosis.

(ii) PSYCHOLOGICAL FACTORS

In neurosis maladaptive learning, use of anxiety defences, blocked personal growth, pathogenic inter-personal relationship, stress and decompensation play an important role.

MALADAPTIVE LEARNING : This is when an individual is not able to learn the correct or proper adaptive technique to solve the problem of life. For example, a person who has not prepared well for examination avoids it by telling her parents that she is feeling very sick or having abdominal pain. Such an individual is not able to achieve a level of maturity. It can be explained as follows:

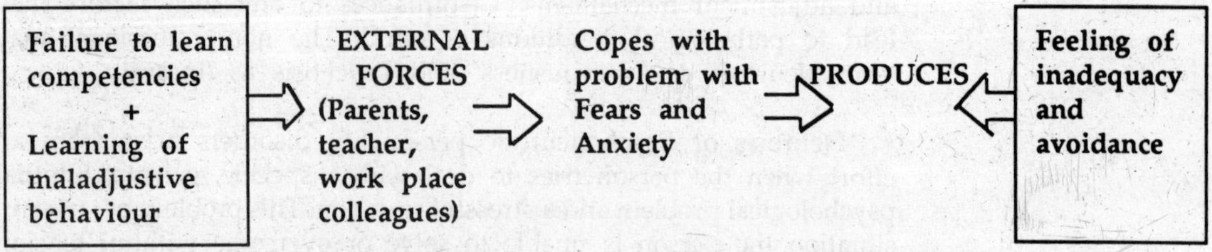

Fig. 20 : Explaining the Maladaptive Learning and Effect on Behaviour.

ANXIETY DEFENSE : This is introduced as a causative factor by Freud. He described that threatening inner desires and impulses produce anxiety in a person. To overcome them the person uses ego defence mechanisms such as Denial, Repression and Undoing. He may use them repeatedly. It can be described as follows:

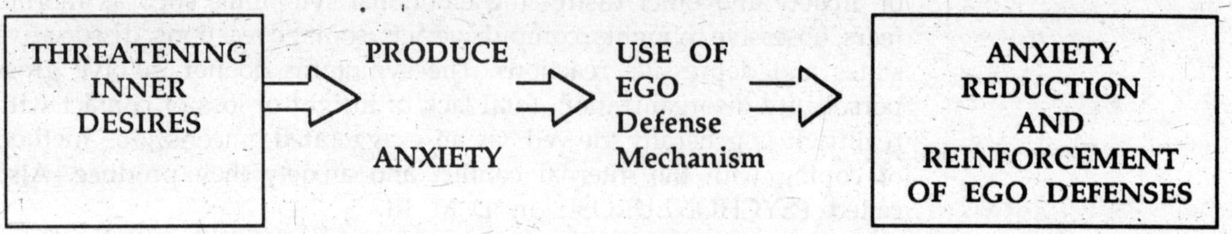

Fig. 21 : Explaining the use of Reinforced EGO Mechanism Leading to Neurotic Behaviour.

BLOCKED PERSONAL GROWTH: Personal growth may be blocked due to various factors. It may be that a person does not get needed opportunities. For example environmental factors such as values of society may not let the girl, go out and work. Then there is faulty socialization where the thinking is only towards factors of satisfying the basic needs. Chronic alienation for lack of a stimulating environment may block the personal growth. This gives a feeling of inadequacy to a person when he/ she is exposed to an environment which is demanding.

PATHOGENIC INTERPERSONAL PATTERNS Pathogenic interpersonal pattern in the family develops a feeling of inadequacy and despair in an individual. Distorted interpersonal relationship where honesty and mutual support are not demonstrated by family members also cause a feeling of inadequacy in a person.

STRESS AND DECOMPENSATION : Various types of stressors cause a lot of pressure on an individual, specially where the chance of compensating is less. A widow who has to fight to live in society, bring up her children, earn money and go to work, with no psychological support, feels under stress all the time.

(iii) SOCIOCULTURAL FACTORS

Socioculturally conversion hysteria is common in low socio-economic-status people with less education, while anxiety and obsessive compulsive neurosis are common in upper socio-economic status people.

TO RECALL

Neurosis is defined as mild-to-moderately severe illness of personality, in which the Ego function of reality testing is not affected much and maladjustment to Life is Limited.

ETIOLOGY

- **Biological factors**
- **Psychological factors**
- **Sociocultural factors**

CLASSIFICATION OF PSYCHONEUROSIS

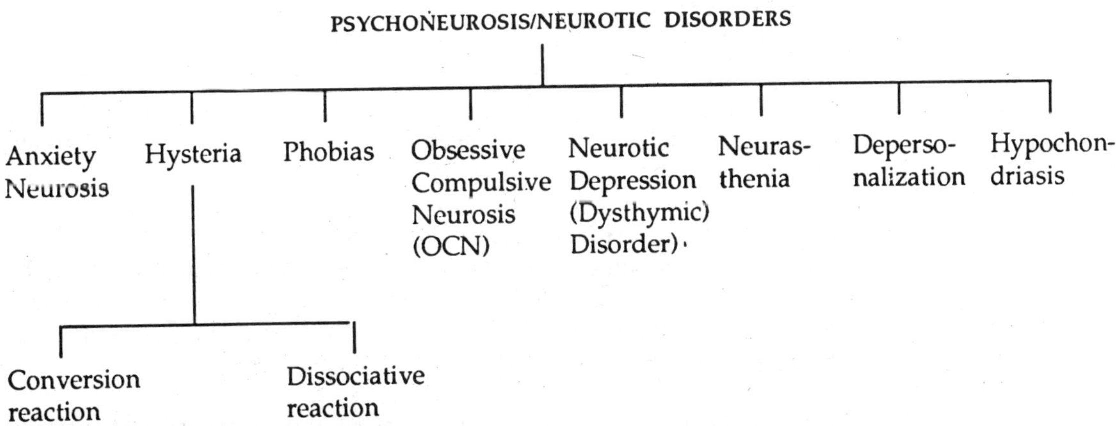

Fig. 22 : Flow Chart Describing the Clinical Conditions of Psychoneurosis.

ANXIETY NEUROSIS

It is a psychoneurotic disorder characterized by persistent apprehensiveness, a feeling of an impending disaster and free floating fear, it is a generalized sense of fear that is not directed to a particular object or situation. It is accompanied by symptoms as: difficulty in making decision, insomnia, loss of appetite and heart palpitations. Source of anxiety is an unresolved conflict, forbidden impulses or disturbing memories which threaten the individual. **Anxiety Neurosis** will be discussed in detail in *Chapter VIII under Nursing Management.*

HYSTERIA

Hysteria is a neurotic disorder characterized by suggestability, emotional outbursts, histrionic behaviour (i.e. attention-seeking behaviour) repressed anxiety, and transformation of an unconscious conflict into physical symptoms such as paralysis, blindness, and loss of sensation. It includes various somatoform disorders. In the text these two conditions will be discussed : (i) Conversion reaction and (ii) Dissociative reaction.

CONVERSION DISORDER :

Hysterical neurosis: Conversion hysteria is a psychoneurotic disorder in which repressed inner conflicts are unconsciously converted or transformed into physical symptoms that have no organic basis, e.g. paralysis, blindness, loss of sensation, or seizures. Conversion reaction is also called somatoform disorders. Conversion symptoms are used for **Primary Gain,** that is the patient gets relief from anxiety by not going through the threatening situation, for example not going for an interview, and **Secondary** gain by getting sympathy and attention from others. "Oh poor Mahesh, he could not go for an interview, though he had prepared himself so well." Conversion reaction will be discussed in detail in *Chapter VIII under Nursing Management.*

DISSOCIATIVE REACTION

Hysterical neurosis; dissociative reaction or state Dissociative reaction is a group of disorders characterized by a sudden, temporary state of consciousness, i.e. (i) Psychogenic Amnesia; (ii) Multiple Personality (iii) Depersonalization, (iv) Psychogenic Fugue and Sleep Walking Disorder or Somnambulism.

(i) PSYCHOGENIC AMNESIA : There is sudden failure to recall one's own identity and in some cases, one's past life but without forgetting the basic habits and skills. There is no organic cause. Recovery of memory often occurs spontaneously within a few hours. In resistent cases hypnotherapy may be used.

PSYCHODYNAMICS : Amnesic patients basically are egocentric, emotionally immature, highly suggestible personalities. They have faced actually unpleasant situations and want to run away unconsciously.

(ii) MULTIPLE PERSONALITY : There may be a temporary alteration in the identify of a person. Dual or multiple personalities is the disorder in which two or more personalities exist in one individual. One personality at a time is dominant and works at a conscious level at one time. The other personality of an individual may be at an unconscious level. The original personality is unaware of this subpersonality. For example, Radha, mother of two children, may be a very sophisticated, cultured, homely type of woman. Does not go for dance and hotel parties. The other side of Radha which is Ann may predominate at sometimes without her knowledge. She dresses up in tight jeans with her hair tied up in a short ponytail, goes to a hotel, dances with everyone and smokes. On reaching home, she changes and goes back to the attire of Radha. When asked, she completely refuses to accept and is not able to recall that she could ever behave like the one being mentioned. So Ann is a subpersonality of Radha.

PSYCHODYNAMICS : In a multiple personality, its conflicting parts of develop into autonomous or actual parts.

(iii) DEPERSONALIZATION : It is a state of mind in which self of an individual appears to him as unreal. The individual feels estranged from himself and the world around him. A feeling that one's extremities are changed in size, a feeling that the external world is unreal. The individual has a sense of being mechanical. Depersonalization may occur as a clinical feature in several mental disorders such as depression, hypochondriasis, dissociative states, temporal to be epilepsy and early schizophrenia.

PSYCHODYAMICS : It is often interpreted as an unconscious attempt to escape from threatening situations.

(iv) The other type of dissociative disorders are classified under alteration in motor behaviour: (A) Psychogenic Fugue and (B) Sleep-walking disorders.

(A) PSYCHOGENIC FUGUE: Derived from French word Fyoog—'Flight'. It is an amnesic dissociated state in which the individual flees or runs away from home, forgets his entire past but not the basic skills. So he starts his new life with a new name. After recovery he will able to recall all the events prior to the state of fugue but not the events during this state.

PSYCHODYNAMICS : Fugue state could be an unconscious desire to escape from threatening or distasteful situations. It can be treated through hypnotherapy or abreaction.

Brief fugue may occur in epilespsy or state of catatonic excitement sometimes.

(B) SLEEP-WALKING DISORDERS OR SOMNAMBULISM : This disorder occurs repeatedly when the individual sits up, picks up his bed, goes and eats, sitting on a dining table, opens the door and goes. Sleeps on the floor in the courtyard/verandah. When woken up with great difficulty, sleep walker will stare blankly and unres-ponsively. The episode will not be remembered by him the next morning.

PSYCHO DYNAMICS : It is thought that a patient uses symbolic escape from some conflicting situation. The acts which the person cannot carry on at the conscious level come on during sleep.

PHOBIA STATE

PHOBIA : Phobia is an exaggerated pathological fear of a specific type of stimulus or a situation. People may have fear of height, fear of pain, fear of animals, fear of dirt or bacteria. The fear that a person feels is in the presence of a particular object of experience. Some of the terms used for describing fears are Agrophobia, Algophobia, Clustrophobia *(Refer Chapter III Unit IX).*

PSYCHODYNAMICS : This may be due to a conflict in people symbolizing a particular type of phobia. It is also felt that anxiety is displaced on a less threatening object. A person gets attention from the significant people as they protect him or her from these situations.

OBSESSIVE COMPULSIVE DISORDERS

Obsessive Compulsive Neurosis (OCN) is a neurotic disorder in which obsessions or compulsions are a significant source of distress, and interfere with the individual's ability to function. Obsessions are persistent, recurrent ideas and impulses (thoughts of committing violence, ideas of doubt). Though these thoughts appear senseless to an individual, these force themselves on his/her consciousness and cannot be ignored or suppressed. Compulsions are repetitive, stereotype acts (e.g. hand washing, counting, checking, touching) which must be performed by an individual to relieve tension even though they are recognized as senseless by the person.

Obsessive compulsive neuroris will be discussed in detail in *Chapter VIII under Nursing Management.*

NEUROTIC DEPRESSION

Neurotic depression is also called reactive or exogenous depression. It will be discussed in detail, differentiating it from Endogenous or

Psychotic depression, in *Chapter VIII under Nursing Management.*

NEURASTHENIA

Derived from the Greek word "neurasthenia, nerve weakness," it is a neurotic condition marked by fatigue, insomnia, aches and pains, irritability, depression and difficulty in concentrating. A person shows lack of capacity for enjoyment (anhedonia). It may follow exhaustion.

DEPERSONALIZATION

It is a state of mind in which the self appears unreal. The individual feels estranged from himself and also from enternal world. Patients' thoughts and experiences are dreamlike in character. Depersonalization is observed in disorders such as depression, hypochondriasis, dissociative states, temporal lobe epilepsy and early schizophrenia.

HYPOCHONDRIASIS

Hypochondrical Neurosis is also called somatoform disorder characterized by unrealistic interpretation of physical signs or symptoms as abnormal. An individual preoccupies himself with a fear or belief that he has a serious disease which persists and interferes with his social and occupational functioning,though the medical result shows no physical disorder.

TO RECALL

Psychoneurosis or neurotic disorders are classified as:

- **Anxiety neurosis**
- **Hysteria**
  - **Conversion reaction**
  - **Dissociative reactions**
  - **Temporary alteration in the state of consciousness e.g. psychogenic amnesia**
  - **Temporary alteration in the identify of a person e.g. Multiple**
  - **Personality and depersonalization**
  - **Temporary alteration in motor activity e.g. psychogenic fugue & somnambistism or sleep walking disorder somnambulism.**
  - **Phobias**
  - **Obsessive compulsive neurosis**
  - **Neurotic depression or dysthymic disorder**
  - **Neurasthenia**
  - **Depersonalization**
  - **Hypochondrias**

TREATMENT OF NEUROTIC DISORDERS

In psychoneurosis or neurotic disorders psychotherapy is the basic line of treatment. Individual psychotherapy: psychoanalysis, abreaction and uncovering can be used. Behavioural psychotherapy is effectively used in these patients for modifying their faulty behaviour. Behaviour modification, desensatization, cognitive behaviour therapy, assertiveness therapy implosive or flooding and positive reinforcement can be used in most of the psychoneurotic disorders. *(Refer Chapter VI Unit XVI).* Family therapy and group therapy will also help the patient as well as family members to create a therapeutic environment.

Drugs are used sparingly for these patients. If the patient is highly anxious and depressed sedative (usually barbiturates) and minor tranquillizers can be used. But these drugs should be for a very short duration as they can cause physical dependence in the patients. Somatic therapy/ECT is usually not helpful.

PROGNOSIS

Very few patients go to chronic disorder. Ninety per cent of them benefit from proper help. Prognosis is good in patients with history of the type of premorbid personality, family support, short duration of illness, favourable socio-cultural patterns. Very rarely the patients develop psychosis or antisocial behaviour.

TO RECALL

- **The treatment in psychoneurosis is basically psychotherapy. Drugs are used with caution. Electro-convulsive therapy does not have much effect.**
- **Prognosis is difficult to assess.**
- **Favourable factors help in good prognosis.**

Units XVIII & XIX included the content on psychosis and neurosis. It is significant to summarize the difference between psychosis and neurosis.

DIFFERENCE BETWEEN PSYCHOSIS AND NEUROSIS

	PSYCHOSIS	NEUROSIS
a)	**Definition** Psychosis is defined as a very serious illness of the personality which involves impairment of ego functions. Reality testing is markedly impaired. There are signs of grave maladjustment to life.	It is a mild-to-moderate illness of the personality. Ego function and reality testing are not affected much. Maladjustment to life is limited.
b)	**Causes** Psychosis is caused by organic factors and psychological factors or any-one of these.	Neurosis is mainly due to psychological factors. There are various stressors which cause psychoneurotic changes in an individual.
c)	**Psychodynamics** Psychosis is the result of a weak ego. Development of the ego has been inhibited by a symbiotic parent-child relationship. Previous repressed and suppressed conflicts come up. Behaviour is often a representation of ID aspect of personality.	In neurosis there is partial impairment of ego functioning. Neurotics attempt to use suppression and repression to overcome the anxiety due to conflicts.
d)	**Clinical Features**	
	(i) **Ego Functions** — Impaired ego functions, reality testing are decreased or lost. Confusion and insight in the illness are lacking.	Ego function is not affected much, reality testing and insight into the illness are present.
	(ii) **Affect** — Psychotics show affect chan-ges in terms of elation, depression, apathy, ambivalence and inappropriate affect.	The affect is appropriate to the situation, person or object. At times neurotics are tense and unhappy due to fear or loss.
	(iii) **Perception** — Marked illusion and hallucination are presented by psychotic patients.	— Hallucination and illusion not present.
	(iv) **Thought Changes** — Delusions,	Patients do not present any of these

PSYCHOSIS	NEUROSIS
flight of ideas, preservation or circumstantiality and other thought changes are seen in patients with psychosis.	changes in thinking.
(v) **Behavioural Changes** — Overactivity, impulsiveness, retardation, withdrawal, are markedly present. These patients do not socialize. Vocational, social and sexual adjustment are markedly impaired. Routine activities get markedly affected.	There may be overactivity and impulsiveness due to anxiety. Vocational, social and sexual adjustment, are impaired but not markedly. The patient can carry on routine activities.
(vi) **Judgement** is impaired and at times very poor.	Judgement is not impaired in these patients. They can discriminate between right and wrong.
(vii) Memory, attention and intelligence are affected markedly.	There is no effect on memory, attention and intelligence.
(e) **Defense Mechanisms:** Psychotics often use defenses such as denial, regression, introjection and identification.	Neurotics use repression, displacement, isolation, reaction formation, undoing, substitution and conversion as defense mechanisms.
(f) **Treatment**—Psychotic patients usually require hospitalization. Psychotropic drugs, psychotherapy and electroconvulsive therapy in combination are used. Milieu therapy and group therapy are also effective.	Very rarely neurotic patients require hospitalization for physical exhaustion, for example in obsessive compulsive neurosis and hysterical neurosis. Preferably, neurotics are treated in the out-patient department. Barbiturate sedatives, or minor tranquillizer are given for a very short duration. Psychotherapy — mainly behaviour therapy — is very effective.
(g) **Prognosis** — Prognosis in psychotic patients is not very good. If it is the first attack or acute psychosis, recovery may be good, recurrence is very common.	Prognosis is good. Recurrence is very less.

Fig. 23 : Table Describing the Difference Between Psychosis and Neurosis.

PERSONALITY DISORDERS

INTRODUCTION

The personality pattern of behaviour is generally recognized by early adolescence. These changes persist throughout life, causing difficulty to the individual and members of the family. Certain types of personalities are known to be predisposed to certain types of mental disorders.

TYPES OF PERSONALITY DISORDERS

The types of personality disorders are Cyclothymic-personality, Hypomanic personality, Melancholic personality, Schizoid personality, Obsessive compulsive personality, Hysterical personality, Passive-aggressive personality, Explosive personality, Inadequate and denial personality *(Refer to Chapter III, Unit IX)* for detailed discussion on the types of personality disorders. Psychopathic personality is discussed in this unit as it was omitted in *Unit IX.*

PSYCHOPATHIC PERSONALITY

Psychopathic personality is one of the other types of personality disorders. It is also described as antisocial reaction. The behaviour pattern, which is more common in males than females, starts before the age of 15 years with such behaviour as lying, stealing, fighting truancy (absence from school), vandalism, theft, drunkenness or substance abuse. It continues after the age of 18.

It is a character disorder marked by impulsive, egocentric (self centred), unethical behaviour, rejection of authority and discipline, extreme irresponsibility, absence of genuine loyalty to individuals or groups. It includes a mixed group of individuals, unprincipled businessmen, shyster (distrustful) lawyers, quack doctors, imposters, drug pushers and a sizable number of prostitutes and some delinquents and criminals.

TREATMENT

Psychotherapy, specially behaviour therapy, is helpful for these patients. Negative reinforcement is helpful.

TO RECALL

* Personality disorders are recognized in early adolescence.
* Psychopathic personality is also called antisocial reaction.

SEXUAL DEVIATION AND DISORDERS

INTRODUCTION

Sexual behaviour, normal or abnormal, is termed according to the society, the culture in which the person lives. Sexual behaviour is considered in the context of the whole personality of the individual. Emotion and personality disorder do produce a pathological symptom in the sexual behaviour of an individual.

A sexual problem that appears trivial to the professional may be of great concern for an individual. Many a time the individual is not able to tell about the exact complaint due to cultural factors. He or she may complain in terms of aches, pains and generalized weakness. But the individual gradually talks about his problems with the therapist. There are certain sexual behaviours which are not abnormal like masturbation is normal upto some age and frequency. This unit will include:

i) Normal sexual behaviour
ii) Abnormal sexuality
iii) Sexual deviations
iv) Other sexual problems with social and legal aspects.

NORMAL SEXUAL BEHAVIOUR

MASTURBATION

It is defined as sexual satisfaction by manipulation of sex organs especially the penis and clitoris. It is also called Autoerotism or Onanism.

ORALISM

Oralism or oral sexual intercourse is defined as pleasure obtaining from mouth genital contact. It may be homosexual or hetrosexual. Very rarely used for sexual satisfaction.

ANAL INTERCOURSE

Sexual pleasure obtained by intercourse per anus. It is common amongst male homosexuals. Uncommonly used in heterosexual relationship. It is also called ***Sodomy*** or ***Buggary.***

ABNORMAL SEXUALITY

IMPOTANCE

Impotance occurs only in males, and may be defined as weak, unsustained or complete lack of erection resulting in unsuccessful sexual performance. The condition is usually psychogenic. May take the form of premature ejaculation, limited interest in sex and coitus without ejaculation.

FRIGIDITY

It is a female sexual disorder in which there is partial or complete lack of sexual enjoyment or satisfaction in the female.

DYSPAREUNIA AND VAGINISMUS

Dyspareunia is painful or difficulty in sexual intercourse and vaginismus is involuntary painful spasm of the vagina prior to sexual intercourse.

HYPERSEXUALITY

It is a an excessive desire for sexual activity. It may occur in both men and women.

PROMISCUITY

It is transient, casual sexual relations with a variety of partners.

SEXUAL DEVIATIONS

A sexual deviation, perversion or paraphilia is defined as any sexual behaviour that is regarded as significantly different from the standard establishment of local culture or subculture.

HOMOSEXUALITY

It is defined as a desire for sexual contact with a person of one's own sex. Homosexual behaviour between women is termed as lesbianism.

EXHIBITIONISM

It is a common deviation which is defined as compulsive and deliberate exposure of the genitals in public, mostly by males. Women drive more pleasure than males in displaying their parts of the body.

VOYEURISM (SCOPOPHILIA)

It is obtaining sexual satisfaction or gratifi-cation through observing sexual organs and sexual activities of others, usually women.

TRANSVESTISM OR TRANSVESTITISM

It is defined as the pathological impulse to wear the clothes and accessories of the opposite sex. Cross dressing.

TRANS-SEXUALITY

It is a psychosexual disorder consisting of a persistent sense of discomfort and desire to change one's sex. A male transsexual is a person who wants to get rid of his genitals, feels and acts like females, but is biologically male. Hermaphrodites have a biological abnormality of intersex (both sex) but the sex role is appropriate to his predominant sexual characteristics.

SADISM AND MASOCHISM

Sadism is a sexual deviation in which gratification is obtained by inflicting pain or humiliation on a sexual partner. Masochism is a disorder in which the individual derives pleasure from pain inflicted by others or in some cases by himself.

PEDOPHILIA

It is a psychosexual disorder in which sexual acts or fantasies with prepubertal children are the exclusive method of achieving sexual satisfaction. Children are of the opposite sex; sexual activity often consists of looking and touching rather than intercourse.

BEASTIALITY

Sexual excitement or gratification through intercourse or other sexual contact with animals.

FETISHISM

It is a psychosexual disorder in which non-living objects are repeatedly or exclusively used in achieving sexual satisfaction. Fetishes are most often feminine undergarments, shoes, occasionally hair or nails.

FROTTAGE

It means sexual pleasure obtained by rubbing or pressing against the object, usually the buttocks of a fully clothes woman. It commonly takes place in crowded places where these things go unnoticed.

OTHER SEXUAL PROBLEMS WITH SOCIAL AND LEGAL ASPECTS

INCEST

Incest refers to sexual activity between members of the same family like father and daughter, mother and son, sister and brother. It may involve close relatives like uncles. Incest is prohibited in all cultures.

RAPE

Rape is defined as a forced sexual intercourse by a man with a woman, who is not his wife, against her will or without lawful consent.

SEDUCTION

The woman is induced to consent in sexual intercourse by bribe, or deceit but not force or threat of force.

PROSTITUTION

It is a sex service based on the payment of money or exchange of other property or valuables.

PORNOGRAPHY

It may be defined as writing or pictorial art whose sole aim is to arouse the sexual passions of the reader or viewer.

TREATMENT

Intensive psychoanalytical psychotherapy may help. Behaviour psychotehrapy with negative reinforcement may help to some extent. Many patients are helped by counselling and supportive psychotherapy to achieve better conscious control and self-discipline.

TO RECALL

* **Sexual deviation and disorders are termed abnormal according to the society, the culture in which the person lives.**
* **Types of sexual behaviour deviations:**
  - **Normal sexual behaviour**
  - **Abnormal sexuality**
  - **Sexual deviation**
  - **Other sexual problems with social and legal aspects.**

APPLICATION TO NURSING

This unit has described neurotic disorders, personality disorders, sexual deviation and disorders. It will enable student nurses to identify patients with various neurotic disorders. The students will also be able to differentiate whether the patient is suffering from psychotic or neurotic disorders which will help them to plan nursing interventions effectively. The content of this unit will help the student-nurse to identify the clients with personality and sexual disorders in community and hospital settings. Early identification by student-nurses of these deviant-behaviour clients can be prevented from going in severe mental disorders.

BETTER STUDY SECTION OF UNIT XIX

1. VOCABULARY

Alteration	Inflicted
Decompensation	Maladjustment
Distressing	Pathogene
Genuine	Spontaneously
Humiliation	Suppressed
Impending	Trivial

2. ASSIGNMENT

Read Chapter III on Etiology and Symptomatology of Mental Illness and Chapter VI on Therapeutic Modalities.

3. STUDY QUESTIONS

(1) Define the following terms:
Neurosis
Anxiety Neurosis
Hysteria
Hypochondriasis
Phobic State

(2) Make a tree chart of classification of Neurotic Disorders

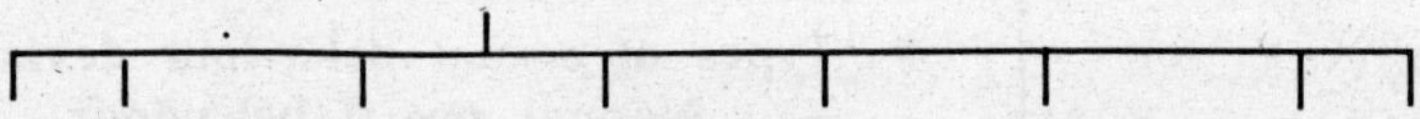

(3) Write the difference between Psychosis and Neurosis.

(4) List some of the sexual disorders which have social and legal implications.

4. READING REFERENCES

Cavener J. & Brodie H.K. *Signs and Symptoms in Psychiatry*. J.B. Lippincott, Philadelphia.

Kapoor, Bimla. *A Textbook of Psychiatric Nursing*. Kumar Publishing House, Delhi (1992).

Kaplan Harold & Sodock B.J. *Comprehensive Textbook of Psychiatry* (5th edition.) Williams & Wilkins, London (1989).

UNIT XX

PSYCHOPHYSIOLOGICAL DISORDER, CHILDHOOD DISORDERS, SUBSTANCE/ DRUG ABUSE AND PSYCHIATRIC EMERGENCIES

UNIT OUTLINE

Psychophysiological Disorders
- Definition
- Etiological factors
- Psychodynamics
- Types of Psychophysiological Disorders
- Treatment

Disorders of Infancy, Childhood and Adoloscence
- ✻ Developmental Disorders
  - — Mental Retardation
- ✻ Disruptive Behaviour Disorders
  - — Attention-Deficit Hyperactive Disorder
  - — Conduct Disorder - Delinquency
- ✻ Anxiety Disorders
  - — Separation anxiety disorders
  - — Avoidant Disorders
  - — Overanxious disorders
- ✻ Eating Disorders
  - — Anorexia nervosa
  - — Bulimia nervosa
  - — Obesity
  - — Pica
  - Rumination Disorder of Infancy

General Identify Disorders of Childhood
- ✻ Transsexualism
- ✻ Gender identity disorder
  - — TIC Disorders
  - — Elementary disorders
- ✻ Functional enuresis
- ✻ Functional encopresis

INTENDED LEARNING BEHAVIOUR

After reading this unit, you will able to.

a) define psychophysiological disorder.

b) describe the types of psychophysiological disorders.

c) classify the childhood disorders.

d) explain the childhood disorder in terms of:
- ✻ development disorders
- ✻ disruptive behaviour disorders
- ✻ anxiety disorders
- ✻ eating disorders
- ✻ general identity disorders of child hood.

e) explain TIC, elementary, speech and autistic disorders.

f) define the terms used in drug abuse.

g) explain the causative factors of drug abuse

h) list the drugs and their subcategories.

i) apply the knowledge while working in a community and a hospital.

j) identify the psychiatric emergencies.

k) plan for the nursing interventions.

UNIT OUTLINE | INTENDED LEARNING BEHAVIOUR

— Speech Disorders
 * Stuttering
— Autistic Disorders
— Childhood Schizophrenia

Substance Abuse/Drug Abuse

Definition of Terms
— Drug
— Drug Abuse
— Drug Dependence
— Physical Dependence
— Psychic Dependence
— Tolerance
— Cross Tolerance
— Withdrawal

Prevalence of Substance Abuse

Causative Factors

Commonly abused substances/Drugs
— Types
— Effects
— Withdrawal Symptoms
— Treatment

Diagnostic Criteria for Psychoactive Substance Abuse/Drug Abuse

Psychiatric Emergencies
— Definition
— Types of Psychiatric emergencies
 * Overactive patient
 * Underactive patient
 * Suicide
 * Other psychiatric emegencies
 — AIDS related psychiatric emergency
 — Adolescent Emergency
 — Puerperial sepsis

Application to Nursing.

Better Study Section.

PSYCHOPHYSIOLOGICAL DISORDERS

INTRODUCTION

Psychophysiological or psychosomatic disorders are characterized by physical symptoms resulting from psychological factors usually involving one system of the body. As the word indicates Psychophysiological-*Psycho+Physiological.* Changes occurring in Psyche and Physiology of the client, changes occurring on Physiology due to Psyche or vice-versa. DSM III termed it as psychological factors affecting physical conditions.

DEFINITION

Psychophysiologic disorders represent a group of ailments in which emotional stress is a contributing factor to physical problems involving an organ system under involuntary control. The most often affected systems are : respiratory, cardiovascular, gastrointestinal, genitourinary, musculoskeletal and integumentary and endocrine.

ETIOLOGICAL FACTORS

It is difficult to point out a single cause of psychosomatic illness. But emotional factors affect the physical illness such as

(I) ATTITUDE TOWARDS PHYSICAL ILLNESS : Some patients use denial of the actual physical condition, but some will be too much involved in the symptoms of sickness. The interaction of psychological, social and biological symptoms has direct relationship with the appearance or disappearance of physical symptoms.

(II) SOCIAL ENVIRONMENT AROUND THE PATIENT: If the social environment is such where quicker recovery is expected, the patient may show more of physical symptoms and recovery may be delayed.

(III) PERSONALITY TRAITS: Individual who is always tense, under pressure, is more prone to psychosomatic disorders than the person who is not being anxious type.

(IV) FAMILY DYNAMICS: It has a major role to play. For example, a child observes the attention-seeking mechanisms, the ways of secondary gains he gets may predispose him towards psychosomatic illnesses.

PSYCHODYNAMICS

Psychophysiological disorders are thought to be due to an unresolved dependency conflict. These conflicts are expressed somatically, with physiological changes. People possessing some type of personality traits are predisposed to a certain disease process e.g. those who are dependent develop asthma, depression, cancer, aggressiveness, coronary artery disease. For example, on the arrival of relative mother develops severe headach. She gets the attention of her husband and guests. On the other hand, relatives cook food for the whole family (secondary gain).

MAJOR TYPES OF PSYCHOPHYSIOLOGICAL DISORDERS

(I) PSYCHOPHYSIOLOGICAL DISORDERS OF GASTRO-INTESTINAL SYSTEM:

Peptic ulcer, irritable bowel syndrome (IBS), Ulcerative colitis, obesity, anorexia nervosa. Anorexia nervosa is a condition that primarily affects women in adolescence or young adulthood and involves a profound weight loss, preoccupation with ideas related to food and weight, behavioural disturbances, distorted perception of body image and problems related to self-concept and personal identity.

(II) PSYCHOPHYSIOLOGICAL DISORDERS OF CARDIOVASCULAR SYSTEM :

Coronary artery disease, angina pectoris, myocardial infarction. After cardiac surgery patients who utilized the illness to avoid anxiety-provoking situations have delayed recovery and hypertension.

(III) PSYCHOPHYSIOLOGICAL DISORDERS OF THE ENDOCRINE SYSTEM :

Diabetes mellitus, hyperthyrodism etc.

(IV) PSYCHOPHYSIOLOGICAL DISORDERS OR THE GENITOURINARY SYSTEM :

Nonspecific urethritis, chronic prostatitis, menstrual disorders, dysemenorrhea, amenorrhea, marked menopausal symptoms etc.

(V) PSYCHOPHYSIOLOGICAL DISORDER OF THE MUSCULOSKELETAL SYSTEM:

Rhumatoid arthritis, backache etc.

(VI) PSYCHOPHYSIOLOGICAL DISORDERS OF THE RESPIRATORY SYSTEM :

Hyperventilation, Cronchial asthma.

(VII) PSYCHOPHYSIOLOGICAL DISORDERS OF INTEGUMENTARY SYSTEM :

Neurodermatitis, eczmea, psoriasis, alopecia, trichotillomania (Hair pulling etc.)

(VIII) PSYCHOPHYSIOLOGICAL DISORDERS : (Miscellaneous)

Accident proneness, visual disturbances, tinnituts, tension headach; migraine (migraine is a headach that usually is severe, recurrent, often limited to one side of the head and likely to be accompanied by nausea, vomiting and diarrhoea or constipation).

TREATMENT

Physical examination should be conducted for the patient to exclude any organic cause. Psychotherapy is effective. Medical treatment should be given to the patient.

TO RECALL

- ✱ **Psychophysiological disorders represent a group of ailments in which emotional stress is a contributing factor to physical problems.**
- ✱ **Etiological factors**
- ✱ **Psychodynamics**
- ✱ **Psychosomatic or psychophysiological disorders of various systems.**

DISORDERS OF INFANCY, CHILDHOOD AND ADOLESCENCE

INTRODUCTION

Nursing personnel encounter various childhood and adolescent problems while working in a hospital as well as a community setting. The development of these problems could be due to (i) genetic factors like mongolism or mental retardation, lack of prenatal, natal and postnatal care. (ii) Nutritional factors or physical disease or brain damage can lead to psychiatric disorders, (iii) Psychological factors; relationship with parents, personality traits, interpersonal relationship, unstable mood, difficulty in adapting to an environmental change. All these factors affect the temperament of a person. (iv) Environmental factors are the main cause of behaviour disorders in children. The family, school, playground, neighbourhood help in shaping the child's development. Family environment also has a lot of influence. For example, scapegoating where anger, frustration, hostility of all the persons is placed on one person. Sometimes too much of responsibility given to a child also causes behavioural problems. A child whose mother is sick or depressed will also affect his/her behaviour.

To summarize the developmental phase from infancy to childhood is a significant period to prevent a number of behaviour and other problems listed in this unit.

CLASSIFICATION OF CLINICAL DISORDERS

DSM III-R classified the disorders in infancy, childhood and adolscence as follows:

(i) ***Development disorders :*** Such as mental retardation, pervasive developmental disorders and specific developmental disorders.

(ii) ***Disruptive behaviour disorders:*** Such as hyperactive and conduct disorders.

(iii) ***Anxiety disorders of childhood or adolescence :*** Such as separation anxiety, avoident behaviour and overanxious disorders.

(iv) ***Eating disorders:*** Anorexia nervosa, Bulimia nervosa, Pica, and rumination disorders of infancy.

(v) ***General identity disorders of childhood :*** Such as transsexualism, gender identity disorders of adolescence or adulthood.

(vi) ***Tic disorders.***

(vii) ***Elimination disorders.***

(viii) ***Speech disorders.***

(ix) ***Other disorders.***

DEVELOPMENTAL DISORDERS

MENTAL RETARDATION

It is a disorder characterized by a significantly subaverage general intellectual function, an I.Q. of 70 or below, with impairment in adaptive behaviour, including thinking, learning, social and occupational adjustment. It is menifested during the development stage. *(Mental retardation discussed in detail in Chap. VIII)*

DISRUPTIVE BEHAVIOUR DISORDER

ATTENTION - DEFICIT HYPERACTIVE DISORDER

It is also called hyperkinetic syndrome. It is a childhood disorder with onset before age seven, involving (a) Inattention that is failure to finish things, not listening, distractability, difficulty in concentrating on school work or play activity, (b) Impulsivity that is acting before thinking, shifting from activity to activity, difficulty in organizing work and taking turns in games, needing extra supervision. (c) Hyperactivity as in excessive running about or climbing things, inability to stand still and being always on the "Go".

CONDUCT DISORDERS

Conduct is the behaviour of the total individual as expressed in psychological as well as physical activity, also behaviour that conforms to the standards established by the person's social group. Conduct disorders marked by repetitive, persistent, aggressive conduct in which basic rights of others are violated. For example, physical violence against persons or property like vandalism, rape, breaking and fire setting, mugging, assault, purse snatching.This is also known as delinquent behaviour.

ANXIETY DISORDERS

"Anxiety disorders" is a group of disorders in which anxiety is either the predominant disturbance or is experienced in facing a dreaded object or situation or in resisting obsessions or compulsions.

SEPARATION ANXIETY DISORDER

It is a disorder characterized by excessive anxiety lasting at least two weeks, during which separation from an attachment figure occurs or is going to occur. The disorder involves such reactions as worry about possible harm to these figures, fear of being lost or kidnapped, refusal to go to school, sleep alone, or stay alone, repeated nightmares, physical complaints on school days, tempertantrums, crying or pleading and social withdrawal, sadness, apathy or difficulty in concentrating.

AVOIDANT DISORDERS

It is a disorder lasting at least six months between the ages of two-and-a half and 18 years and involving persistents, excessive avoidance from strangers. Timidity and withdrawals are severe enough to interfere with peer relationships, although warm and satisfying relationship, with family members and other familiar figures are generally maintained.

OVERANXIOUS DISORDERS

It is a generalised and persistent anxiety or worry among children or adults, shown in several of the following symptoms: Unrealistic worry about future events, preoccupation with appropriateness of the past behaviour, overconcern, excessive need for reassurance about worries, somatic complaints, marked self-consciousness or feeling of tension.

EATING DISORDERS

Eating disorders are generally more prevalent amongst the adolescent girls and women. Some of the common disorders amongst preadolescents are discussed as follows:—

ANOREXIA NERVOSA

It is a persistent lack of appetite by refusal of food, often accompanied by amenorrhea, vomiting, severe weight loss, and wasting (cachexia). The condition occurs most frequently in adolescent girls, and is often explained as an urge to remain "as thin as a boy", thereby escape the burdens of growing up and assuming a female sexual and marital role. Characteristically, they feel fat even when dangerously thin, deny their illness and in some cases develop an active hatred and disgust for food.

BULIMIA NERVOSA

Bulimia is derived from a Greek word Boulimia ("hunger of an ox."). Bulimia is an eating disorder involving repeated taking a large quantity of food and drink in a short time (binge eating) This episode is due to a stressful situation, depressed mood and self-depreciation. The food will be consumed by the individual in large quantities and she will induce vomiting for fear of gaining weight. Bulimia may also occur due to some of the endocrine disorders, but it is more often attributed to psychological factors such as relief from stress, an attempt to get a childhood feeling of security or substitution of food for affection or sex.

OBESITY

It is a psychogenic condition characterized by an excessive desire to eat (Bulimia) and excessive weight (at least 20 per cent above age and sex standard norms). Overeating could be due to tension, use of food as a substitute satisfaction for food and sexual desires. Overemphasis by parents about food.

PICA

It is an eating disorder found primarily in young children and pregnant women, and marked by a persistent craving for unnatural, non-nutritive substances such as plaster, paint, hair, starch or dirt. Occasionally, hysterical patients eat such substances as ash, salt, or vinegar. Schizophrenic patients sometimes complain of a peculiar taste in their mouth and the strange taste may be experienced as an aura or a warning signal before an epileptic attack.

RUMINATION DISORDER OF INFANCY

It is a rare disorder in which infants between three and 12 months of age repeatedly regurgitate all food, with ejection or reswallowing but without nausea. These infants may develop extreme weight loss and malnutrition.

GENERAL IDENTITY DISORDERS OF CHILDHOOD

Transsexualism discussed in sexual deviations of this unit. **Gender—identity disorder of childhood:**

It is a psychosexual disorder consisting of a persistent feeling of discomfort and inappropriateness concerning one's anatomical sex. This condition arises before puberty. The child has a desire to be, or insists that he or she is of the opposite sex. The child does persistently the activities of the opposite sex.

TIC DISORDERS

It is a repeated involuntary contraction of a small group of muscles as it continuosly clearing the throat, shrugging the shoulders or grimacing. These automatisms may be either psychogenic as a tension-reducing behaviour. It can be neurogenic as after-effects of enciphalitis. TOURETT'S disorder is also described as a life-long disorder of an unknown origin, which usually starts with eye spasm before the age of 13, involving vocal tics such as grunts, barks, sniffs and in most cases an urge to utter obscenities.

FUNCTIONAL ENURESIS

It is a repeated involuntary voiding of urine (bed wetting) during day or night after the age of five years when the child has learnt to have developed control of the bladder. This condition may be due to improper toilet training, delayed bladder development or a stressful situation such as hospitalization or entering the school.

ELEMENTARY DISORDERS

FUNCTIONAL ENCORPESIS

It is a repeated voluntary or involuntary passage of faces in day or night time in one's clothings after the age of four years and is not due to physical disorder. This condition may be due to strict toilet training, a stressful situation as in entering school or birth of a sibling. It is clearly purposeful. It may be regressing to infancy or early childhood to get the attention of the mother.

SPEECH DISORDERS

STUTTERING

It is a frequent repetition or prolongation of sounds, syllables or words with hesitation and pauses that disrupt speech. The disorder occurs in about 1 per cent of children. Mild cases usually recover spontaneously; chronic stutterers experience difficulty where communication is required. It is also called stammering.

OTHER DISORDERS

AUTISTIC DISORDER

Infantile autism is a severe disorder appearing before 30 months of age, and characterized by (a) a pervasive lack of responsiveness to other people. The child shows disinterest, failure to cuddle, lack of eye contact, mask-like face, indifference to affection, (b) Communication also gets affected. Communication development is only of immature grammar, echolalia, reversal of "you" and "I"; inability to name objects. Bizarre behaviour such as resistance to even minimum changes, extreme attachment to selected objects such as a piece of string, a rubber band, clapping or staring at moving objects. Approximately 50 per cent of autistic children have an I.Q. below 50. These children have overactivity, distractibility, poor concentration, sudden unprovoked anger or fear.

CHILDHOOD SCHIZOPHRENIA

In childhood schizophrenia some of the common symptoms are; inability to respond emotionally, frustration-tolerance level is low, autistic thinking, the child is not able to relate to others. Disordered motor activity. The child may adopt a bizarre posture, extreme restlessness, sudden kicking and screaming. Refusal to talk or to eat. Loss of interest in play or continuously plays with one toy only. Head banging and an irregular sleep pattern.

PSYCHODYNAMICS

It could be due to mother-child relationship. It could also be due to extremely frightening or threatening experience in the early life of the child.

TEMPERTANTRUM

It is a violent outburst of anger occurring between the ages of two and four. The child exhibits behaviour as screaming, kicking, biting, hitting and head banging. The cause may not be that intense to provoke these symptoms. Tempertantrum is thought to be due to tension and frustrations. Some of the other types of disorders are : reading disorders, developmental arithmetic disorders, developmental articulation disorders.

TREATMENT

Individual psychotherapy, group therapy, play therapy, family therapy, behaviour therapy, use of day hospitals.

TO RECALL

Disorders of infancy, childhood and adolescence are:

- **— Development disorders mental retardation.**
- **— Disruptive behaviour disorders hyperkinetic syndrome, conduct disorders.**
- **— Anxiety disorders separation anxiety, avoidant disorders, overanxious disorders.**
- **— Eating disorders — Anorexia nervosa; Bulimia nervosa, obesity, pica, rumination disorders of infancy.**
- **— General identity disorders.**
- **— Tic disorders**
- **— Functional enuresis,encopresis**
- **— Speech disorders**
- **— Stuttering**
- *** Other disorders**
- *** Autistic disorder**
- *** Childhood schizophrenia**
- *** Tempertentrum.**

APPLICATION OF NURSING

The text of this unit provides the basic concepts of disease patterns in a psychiatric setting. Reading of this unit will enable the student nurse to form nursing diagnosis of whether the patient is having organic disorders, functional psychosis i.e. schizophrenia, affective psychosis i.e. manic depressive psychosis, neurotic disorders, psychyolphysiological disorders. The nursing student will be able to identify the personality disorders in a patient, any sexual deviation affecting the personality of the patient. Reading of this material will help the community health nurse in identifying childhood disorders and to care for the family as well as children with a psychological approach. The content will also enable the student nurse to use the appropriate psychotherapeutic approach for her patients.

This unit provides the baseline information for the nurse to plan nursing interventions for patients suffering from various mental illnesses. The nursing/managements will be discussed in *Chapter VIII.*

SUBSTANCE/DRUG ABUSES

INTRODUCTION

Man had used psychoactive drugs for a very long period, not only to enhance pleasure and relieve discomfort but also to facilitate the achievement of social, religious and ritualistic aims. Earlier, the range of available psychoactive substance was not large. Also in the past, the use of psychoactive or "mind-altering" drugs was limited largely to persons who had an "elder person's" role in the community. These drugs were taken more by men than women.

Only a certain proportion of those who took these drugs for recreational purposes became dependent on them. But now drug addiction is a social problem. It is the problem of society, family and individual. It is widely recognized that non-medical use of dependence-producing drugs involves dynamic interactions among three major factors:

a) the properties of the drug taken and the manner of use.

b) the characteristics of the user, and

c) the nature of the immediate and larger socio-cultural environment in which the drug use occurs. Drug addicts or 'junkies', as they are called by peers, take in drugs for a number of reasons ranging from — to relax, to forget problems, to be sociable at parties. Some use because it is fun, or drugs help them to feel better when they are under stress, some use because of pressure of friends. Some even use the drugs for experimental purposes.

In the following content certain terms such as etiology, classification, treatment and application to nursing will be described. Nursing management will be dealt with in detail in *Chapter VIII.*

DEFINITION OF TERMS

In examining the human problems associated with the use of drugs outside approved medical practice, the following concepts and definitions are explained:

DRUG

It is derived from a French word' drogue'. A medicinal substance used in the treatment of disease. (Taber's Dictionary).

DRUG ABUSE/SUBSTANCE ABUSE (ACCORDING TO LONGMAN DICTIONARY).

A term applied to the pathological use of drugs or alcohol with impairment in social and occupational functioning (e.g. failure to meet family obligations, erratic or criminal behaviour, missing work or school) and a minimal duration of disturbance of at least one month.

DRUG DEPENDENCE/SUBSTANCE DEPENDENCE

A state psychic, sometimes also physical, resulting from taking a drug, characterized by behavioural and other responses that always include a compulsion to take a drug on a continuous or periodic basis in order to experience its psychic effects and sometimes to avoid the discomfort of its absence. Tolerance may or may not be present. A person may be dependent on more than one drug.

PHYSICAL DEPENDENCE

Physical dependence occurs when the drug user's body becomes so accustomed to a particular drug that he can function normally only if the drug is present in his body chemistry. Without the drug the user may experience symptoms of mild discomfort to convulsions. These symptoms will only be relieved by readministration of the same drug or of another drug or a similar pharmocological quality. Physical dependence is a powerful factor in reinforcing upon continuing the drug use.

PSYCHIC DEPENDENCE

Psychic or psychological dependence occurs when the drug is central to a person's thought, emotions and activities. It is difficult for the person to stop thinking of the drug which causes intense craving for it and its effect. It is reduced only on readministration of the drug like in physical dependence.

TOLERANCE

It is "an adaptive state characterized by a diminished response to the same quantity of a drug or by the fact that a larger dose is required to produce the same degree of pharmacodynamic effect." (WHO Bulletin, 1965).

CROSS TOLERANCE

The ability of one drug to produce the effect of another when the body has developed a tissue tolerance for effect of the first substance. A person who has developed dependence upon alcohol can substitute with another drug to prevent withdrawal symptoms and vice versa.

WITHDRAWAL

It is an organic mental disorder following cessation (stopping) or reduction in the intake of a substance such as alcohol, an opioid, amphetamines, tobacco or sedatives that have previously been used regularly to induce intoxication. Withdrawal symptoms vary in intensity depending upon the substance or drug, but they usually include some degree of anxiety, restlessness, insomnia, impaired attention and irritability. Withdrawal symptoms will be discussed under each category of addictive drugs.

PREVALENCE OF DRUG ABUSE

Findings and recommendations made in a report of the National Committee on Drug Addiction (1977) focused on the following dependence-producing drugs and other substances commonly misused in India.

1) Cannabis and its products (e.g. Bhang, Ganja and Charas).
2) Hallucinogen e.g. LSD (Lysergic Acid Diethylamide).
3) Tranquillizers, hypnotics and sedatives (e.g. diazepam methaqualone and chloral hydrate).
4) Barbiturates (e.g. phenobarbital and secobarbital).
5) Amphetamines (e.g. dextro-amphetamine and methyl amphetamine).
6) Tobacco.
7) Other narcotic drugs (e.g. opium, pethidine, morphine, heroin and cocaine, and
8) Alcohol.

Nationwide information on the incidence and magnitude of the problem of alcoholism and drug dependence is not available. However, a large number of studies have been conducted in the country. For example, in 1964 a study team on prohibition estimated that drinking was common among 12 per cent of the working class families in India. The use of intoxication among factory/industrial workers is quite high. For instance, a study conducted on industrial workers in Delhi brings out that amongst users alcohol is most common, followed by cannabis and opiates. That college and university campuses in the country have a sizable prevalence rate which was brought out by several researchers (Khan and Singh, 1979, Murthy and Kapoor 1981).

ETIOLOGY OR CAUSES

There seems to (1982) be no unitary theory to explain drug dependence. Wilson and Kneisl have classified the theories of drug dependence as psychological, sociological and physiological. Causative factors for narcotics and other substance abuse can be studied under the following headings:

i. Interpersonal and Psychosocial
ii. Socio-economic
iii. Cultural and Ethnic
iv. Youth culture
v. Pharmocological
vi. Ecological

(I) INTERPERSONAL & PSYCHOSOCIAL FACTORS

Drug dependents have difficulty in their relationship with members of their families. Psycho-analytically, they are described to be regressed and fixated at the oral stage of psychosexual development. Wursmer (1972) has stated that families where the parents are self-centred and are preoccupied with success and prestige may lead their children in drug addiction. These children may feel personal insecurity, show rebellious attitude towards authority, escape from a difficult situation, critical behaviour due to self-doubt and absence of a strong and efficient ego.

(II) SOCIO-ECONOMIC FACTORS

In the early sixties, writers emphasized that the drug addiction problem is due to low socio-economic status. The difficult life style, poverty and hopelessness lead to frustration and then to drug addiction. Broken families, unloving parents where there is no meaningful relationship are also contributory factors. However, the trend of drug addiction is increasing in middle socio-economic status people also.

(III) CULTURAL AND ETHNIC FACTORS

Literature reveals that in the United States minorities such as black, Spanish and native Indian are high-risk potential because they are disproportionately poor. So frustration leads them to drug. The slum youth take model of drug addicts, whose level they try to reach.

(IV) YOUTH CULTURE

Adolscents try to follow the peer group. They also try to be a part of the group, use the drugs and get addicted.

(V) PHARMOCOLOGICAL FACTORS

Some substances/drugs are likely to cause an addictive effect more than others. For instances, opium produces tolerance and physical dependence more in comparison to other drugs.

(VI) ECOLOGICAL FACTORS

Freedman (1972) suggests that people and their drug environment are interwoven. To achieve a sense of belongingness some youth may join the group of drug abusers. Social groups are another environmental pressure for drug addiction.

TO RECALL

TERMS USED IN DRUG DEPENDENCE

- Drug
- Drug abuse
- Drug dependence
- Physical dependence
- Psychic/psychological dependence
- Tolerance
- Cross-tolerance
- Withdrawal

Prevalence of drug abuse.

Etiology or Causative Factors

- Interpersonal factors
- Socio-economic factors
- Cultural and ethnic factors
- Youth culture
- Pharmocological factors
- Ecological factors

CLASSIFICATION OF DRUGS

COMMONLY ABUSED SUBSTANCES/DRUGS

The drugs which are commonly abused can be classified as follows:

I. *Narcotics*

II. *Sedatives & Depressants*

III. *Stimulants*

IV. *Psychedelics and Halluncinogens*

V. *Minor Tranquillizers.*

NARCOTICS

Narcotics are referred to as 'hard stuff' by drug abusers. Narcotic analgesics are drugs that are highly addictive. These drugs alleviate physical pain, induce relaxation, produce euphoria or a sense of well—being, alleviate anxiety and tension. These drugs can be classified as:

(a) Opium and its derivates such as opium, morphine, heroin, codeine (brown sugar, junk, H, horse, smack chase, shyam)

(b) Synthetic Narcotics such as methadone.

EFFECTS OF NARCOTICS

When opium is taken in the form of injection, the user feels a sense of pleasure, gratification towards hunger, pain and sexual urge. The dose required for this effect may also cause restlessness, nausea and vomiting. When taken orally, the effects are felt more gradually. Physical effects include nausea, vomiting, insensitivity to pain, contractions of pupils, increased urination, constipation, sweating, itchy skin and slowed breathing. When the drug is taken in large doses, pupil contract to pinpoint, skin becomes cold, moist, bluish and breathing may completely stop, resulting in death. Heroin use is particularly risky, because purity of content and dose is not ascertained. Heroin, when used in combination of alcohol, can cause death. Chronic users may develop lung problems. Injection abcesses due to use of unsterilised needles; tetnus and brain damage infective endocarditis, osteamylitis may also occur.

WITHDRAWAL SYMPTOMS

Whenever opium is withdrawn abruptly, abstinence or withdrawal symptoms appear. Withdrawal symptoms and patients' reaction are explained in the following table :

Withdrawal Symptoms within 12 to 24 hours if the dose is not repeated.	Yawning, lacrimation, and rhinorrhea, sneezing and prespiration. Followed by these symptoms anorexia, dilated pupils, tremors and gooseflesh appears.
Withdrawal Symptoms after 36 hours, if the dose is not repeated.	Uncontrollable twitching of muscles, cramps in the legs, abdomen and back, the patient is intensely restless, unable to sleep, increase in pulse and B.P., vomiting and diarrhoea are frequent.
48 hours from the last dose.	Symptoms become more intense.

72 hours from the last dose.	Symptoms remain at the height of intensity.
5 to 10 days.	Symptoms gradually subside.
Reaction of the patient during withdrawal symptoms.	As the withdrawal symptoms develop, the patient becomes restless, pessimistic, rude, fault-finding, exhibits increased psycho-motor activity. Has a feeling of weakness. He may curse, cry, be impulsively destructive. He may show gestures of attempting to commit suicide. To some degree the patient can control his symptoms. If during the withdrawal the patient doesn't exhibit any symptoms or is peaceful, he may be possessing the drug.
Treatment	It is mainly concerned with developing a rapport with the client. Gradual withdrawal of the drug and maintenance treatment with methadone. However, recurrence is very common.

Fig. 24 : Table Explaining Duration Absence of Drugs and Reaction on Patient.

SEDATIVES/ DEPRESSANTS

Depressants and sedatives are drugs which slow down or depress the functions of the central nervous system. The drugs which come under this group are :

a) Ethyl Alcohol or Ethonol such as toddy, bear, arrack, whisky, brandy and rum.

b) Sedatives and hypontics such as barbiturates; pentobarbital (nembutal) amobarbital (amytal) seconbarbital (seconal) phenobarbital (luminal). Hypontics include doriden, hypentex, nitresum, dornin, nindral and dalmane.

(c) Ethyl Alcohol is a central nervous system depressant. Reduces tension and facilitates social interaction. It is known as spirit among the users.

A. ETHYL ALCOHOL OR ETHONOL

EFFECTS OF ALCOHOL : Small doses of alcohol can produce euphoria, drowsiness, dizziness, flushing, release of inhibition and tension. Larger doses produce an aggressive and violent behaviour, staggering of gait, double vision. Excessive consumption of alcohol within eight to 12 hours may produce headache, nausea, shakiness and vomiting. Very large doses may cause respiratory centre depression and death. Regular consumption of alcohol causes cirrhosis of liver, peptic ulcer, pancreatitis. It also disrupts the social, family and working life of the person.

WITHDRAWAL SYMPTOMS : The withdrawal symptoms include sleeplessness, sweating and poor appetite, tremors, convulsions, hallucinations and even death.

TREATMENT : Alcoholism is regarded as a social problem. So a rapport needs to be established with the alcohol user and members of his family. Social support from the family is required because alcoholics have a dependent personality. Behaviour psychotherapy and group psychotherapy are effective, specially the Alcoholics Anonymous group. In this group the attitude of each member towards the addict is tolerant and constructive. There is a desire to help each other. An opportunity for self-expression is provided and experiences are shared with the same intensity. Each one has experienced the social isolation, the rejection from friends and family members so they are able to help each other better.

The antabuse therapy or disulfiram (tetraethylthiuram disulfiram) under constant medical supervision is given. Calcium carbamide (Temposil) also produces results similar to disulfiram. Calcium carbamide is more acceptable to the patient as it produces lesser hypotension and ECG changes in comparison to disulfirm.

B. SEDATIVES AND HYPNOTICS

These drugs slow down or depress the functions of the central nervous system. They reduce tension, induce relaxtion and sleep. The user also has a feeling of euphoria. These drugs are known as "Red Devil" amongst the users.

EFFECTS OF SEDATIVES AND HYPNOTICS

— **Acute barbiturate intoxication.** Frequently occurs in those patients who usse it with a suicidal intent and sometimes accidental occurrence. Some of the people who use these drugs for insomnia are partially confused and in the resultant confusion they automatically take an excessive amount accidently.

— **Mild Intoxication** The patient is confused. If drowsy, he can be easily aroused. Judgement is defective and the nystagmus (constant involuntary movement of the eyeballs) is transient, with no decrease in respiration and B.P.

— **Moderate Intoxication** Drowsiness is marked. The patient can be aroused with vigorous stimulation. Constant nystagmus, respiration is slow.

— **Severe Intoxication** Coma, absence of all reflexes. Periodic respiration and symptoms of shock.

WITHDRAWAL SYMPTOMS : Restlessness, anxiety, insomnia, delirium, convulsions and even death.

TREATMENT — Treatment is conservative for all the patients. Gastric lavage in acute intoxication is given. The patient should be kept awake. Caffeine, sodium benzoate 0.5 gm I/M or 10 to 40 mgm of amphetamine sulfate by mouth or I/M. O_2, fluid and electrolyte levels need to be maintained.

STIMULANTS

Stimulants are drugs which stimulate the central nervous system. These drugs are: (i) Amphetamines, (ii) Cocaine.

(I) AMPHETAMINES

The amphetamines group of drugs increase a feeling of alertness and confidence, a decreased feeling of fatigue. Users can stay awake for long periods. These drugs decrease appetite and produce a feeling of euphoria. The amphetamine drugs are Benze-drine (amphetamine), Dexedrine (dextroamphetamine), Methedrine (methamphetamine).

Effect of Amphetamines : These drugs cause a sense of well-being and exhilaration. Abuses are common among thrill-seeking adolscents and long among those needing a "lift" from depression. Snorting (inhalation) or injection of the substance produce a sudden, intense "flash" termed as 'speed run". Many inject amphetamine in combination with barbiturates, heroin or cocaine. Chronic users are unable to move or speak, pulse is rapid, increase in B.P. and temperature. Severe intoxication causes shallow respiration, circulatory collapse, increased insomnia and anorexia. Chronic users may develop malnutrition and amphetamine psychosis.

Withdrawal Symptoms: On withdrawal of the drug the psychotic symptoms disappear. However, paranoid state, hallucinations (auditory and the visual) disorganization of thoughts occur. Personality disorganization, depression, impaired ability to concentrate may be present.

Treatment : Withdrawal of the amphetamines is usually not psychological painful to the patient.

(II) COCAINE

Effect of Cocaine, like opium, is taken by sniffing, swallowing or injecting. It causes an euophoric state for four to six hours, brings sefl-confidence and increased flow of ideas, pressure of speech and activity. During the period of stimulation a person may have an increased capacity to work.

Withdrawal Symptoms : Loss of social approval and self-respect. The client is preoccupied only in getting the drug. There are no physical symptoms.

PSYCHEDELICS AND HALLUCINOGENS

Hallucinogens are drugs which dramatically affect perception, emotions and mental processes. They destroy senses and can cause hallucinations. Sensory images are similar to nightmares. They are commonly described as "mind expansion" drugs. The hallucinogens and psychedelics drugs are :

* Cannabis such as marijuana, gganja, charas, hashish, bhang. Cannabis is obtained from the Hemp Plant, known as Savita Indica in India.
* Marijuana — Any part of the plants.
* Ganja — Leaves of the cultivated plant.
* Charas/Hashish` — Resins/exudate of the flowers of the plant.
* Bhang — Dried leaves with flowers.
* Mescaline.
* DOM/STP (dioxyamphytamine).
* DMT (diethyltropton).
* Psilocybin (psychotogenic mushrooms).
* LSD (Lysergic acid diethylamide).

EFFECTS

These drugs increase perception, colours appear brighter. Change in perception of time and distance occurs. Thinking and concentration become difficult, memory is impaired. Extreme mood swings, anxiety and aggression may occur. Confusion because of drugs may cause accidents. Depression may occur due to prolonged use of drugs.

LSD (LYSERIGC ACID DIETHYLAMIDE)

It is the most potent hallucinogen leading to addiction. So LSD will be discussed further in more detail. LSD is an odourless, colourless and tasteless drug. The intoxication can be caused even with less than a grain of salt. It was discovered by the Swiss chemist, Hoffman, in 1938.

EFFECTS OF LSD

These agents produce intense perceptions with kaleidoscopic visual hallucinations. The person may see flowers in colours that he has never seen before. Thoughts appear novel and illusionary. A person using these drugs may have a phenomenon called "humanity identification'. The individual develops a feeling of love, affection and kindness towards all humankind. A feeling of being out of control of one's emotions and thoughts. Some of the users experience panic states having a terrifying experience or a haunting experience of loneliness, depression, depersonalization and visual hallucination. LSD intoxication may lead to homicide or suicide acts. The LSD "trips" are not always pleasent. Persons undergo 'bad trips' frequently. The users may jump from high places, set themselves to fire and die. May feel monsters are talking to him and may come and kill him.

Flashbacks may occur amongst the drug users. The person may experience the same type of hallucination that he had experienced during the use of LSD.

TREATMENT

These drug (LSD) users may develop psychosis for which hospitalization is required for antipsychotic treatment. For 'bad trip' flashbacks and psychological dependence psychotherapy is very effective.

PHECYCLIDINE (PCP)

Originally introduced as an anasthetic. It is also an halluconogen.

MINOR TRANQUILLIZERS

Minor tranquillizers lead to drug abuse. Libirium (chloradiazepoxide hydrochloride), Miltown (meprobamate) and valium (diazepam) are a few of the examples. These drugs alleviate tension and anxiety. They also induce relaxation and sleep.

DIAGNOSITC CRITERIA FOR PSYHOACTIVE SUBSTANCE ABUSE DSM-III-R.

Kaplan et al have described DSM-III-R diagnostic critera for psychoactive substance in a comprehensive textbook of psychiatry/V.

DIAGNOSTIC CRITERIA FOR PSYCHOACTIVE SUBSTANCE DEPENDENCE

A. At least three of the following:

(1) substance often taken in larger amounts or over a longer period than the person intended.

(2) persistent desire or one or more unsuccessful efforts to cut down or control substance use.

(3) a great deal of time spent in activities necessary to get the substance (e.g. theft), taking the substance (e.g., chain smoking) or recovering from its effects.

(4) frequent intoxication or withdrawal symptoms when expected to fulfil a major role obligation at work, school, home (e.g. does not go to work because hung over, goes to school or work "high", intoxicated while taking care of his or her children), or when substance use is physically hazardous (e.g., drives when intoxicated).

(5) important social, occupational, or recreational activities given up or reduced because of substance use.

(6) continued substance use despite knowledge of having a persistent or recurrent social, psychological, or physical problem that is caused or exacerbated by the use of the substance (e.g. keeps using heroin despite family arguments about it, cocaine-induced depression, or having an ulcer made worse by drinking).

(7) marked tolerance; need for markedly increased amounts of the substance (i.e. at least a 50% increase) in order to achieve intoxication or a desired effect, or a markedly diminished effect with continued use of the same amount.

Note: The following items may not apply to cannabis, hallucinogens, or phencyclidine (PCP);

(8) characteristic withdrawal symptoms (see withdrawal syndromes under psychoactive substance-induced organic mental disorders).

COMMONLY ABUSED SUBSTANCE/DRUGS:

Drugs	Types	Route
1. Narcotics	a. Opium and its derivates such as: * Opium, morphine, heroin * Codeine.	a. Oral, parenteral
	b. Synthetic narcotics— such as Methadone.	b. Smoking
2. Sedatives/Depressants	a. Ethyl alcohol or Ethonal such as toddy, beer, arrack, whisky, brandy and rum.	a. Oral
	b. Sedative and hypnotics such as Barbiturates: — Pento barbital (Nembutal) — Amboarbital (Amytal) — Secobarbital (Seconal) — Phenobarbital (Luminal)	b. Oral & Parenteral
	c. Hypotics such as: — Doriden — Hypentex — Nitresum — Dorrin — Nindral — Dalmane	c. Oral
3. Stimulants	a. Amphetamines group of drugs such as: — Benzedrine (amphetamine) — Dexedrine (dextroamphetamine) — Methedrine (methamphetamine)	Oral
	b. Cocaine	

Drugs	Types	Route
4. Psychedelics and Hallucinogens	a. Cannabis such as — Marijuana — Ganja — Charas — Hashish — Bhang	a. Oral, Smoking
	b. Mescaline	b. Oral
	c. DOM/STP (Dioxyamphytamine)	c. Oral
	d. DMT (Diethyltropton)	d. Oral
	e. Psilocybin (Psychetogenic mushrooms)	e. Oral
	f. LSD (Lysergic Acid Diethylamide)	Oral
	g. PCP (Phenyclidine)	Oral smoking inhalation, Parenteral.
5. Minor Tranquillizers	— Librium (Chlordizepoxide Hydrochloride) — Miltown (Meprobanate) — Valium (Diazepam)	Oral & Parenteral.

Fig. 25 : Table Describing the Type of Drug, its Classification and Route.

TO RECALL

A. Commonly abused Substances/Drugs:

DRUG	TYPES
1. Narcotics	(a) opium and its derivates—such as: ✱ opium, morphine, heroin ✱ codeine. (b) Synthetic narcotics—such as Methadone
2. Sedatives/ Depressants	(a) Ethyl alcohol or Ethonal—such as toddy, beer, arrack, whisky, brandy and rum. (b) Sedatives and hypnotics such as Barbiturates:

TO RECALL

	— Pento barbital (Nembutal) — Amobarbital (Amytal) — Secobarbital (Seconal) — Phenobarbital (Luminal) Hypnotics such as: — Doriden — Hypentex — Nitresum — Dorrin — Nindral — Dalmane.
3. Stimulants	(a) Amphetamines group of drugs such as: — Benzedrine (amphetamine) — Dexedrine (dextroamphetamine) — Methedrine (methamphetamine) (b) Cocaine
4. Psychedelics and Hallucinogens	(a) Cannabis such as — Marijuana — Ganja — Charas — Hashish — Bhang (b) Mescaline (c) DOM/STP (Dioxyamphetamine) (d) DMT (Diethyltrupton) (e) Psilocybin (Psychetogenic mushrooms) (f) LSD (Lysergic Acid Diethylamide) (g) PCP (Phenyclidine) — Librium (chlordizepoxide hydrochlo ride) — Miltown (meprobanate) — Valium (Diazepam).

B. Effects of the drugs.

C. Withdrawal Symptoms.

D. Treatment.

E. Diagnostic Criteria for Psychoactive Substance Dependence based on DSM-III-R Diagnostic Critera.

PSYCHIATRIC EMERGENCIES

INTRODUCTION

A psychiatric emergency is a disturbance of behaviour, affect and thought for which immediate treatment is judged to be necessary by
(a) the patient, because of his discomfort
(b) the family, friends and authority because of the signs shown by the patient, and
(c) the nurses and physicians because of the prognosis, for some of the disturbance, if untreated, can be fatal.

DEFINITION

Psychiatric emergency is defined as a sudden onset (days or weeks) of an unusual (for that individual), disordered or socially inappropriate behaviour caused by an emotional or physiological situation. For example, suicidal feelings or attempts, overdose, acute psychotic reaction, acute alcoholism, or acute anxiety.

TYPES OF PSYCHIATRIC EMERGENCIES

Psychiatric emergencies are usually described as:
— **Overactive patients.**
— **Underactive patients.**
— **Suicidal**
— **Other psychiatric emergencies.**

OVERACTIVE

These patients are overactive to an extent that they can be dangerous to themselves and to others. Less inhibited, thought process is accelerated. Conditions in which overactivity is presented:
—Acute excitement
 * schizophrenia
 * mania
— Acute Anxiety
— Organic disorder
— Drug reaction
— Acute Psychosis
— Alcoholic Disorders
— Drug withdrawal

Some of the conditions are described in the following text :

A. VIOLENT

These patients are disturbed, unmanageable and psychotic.They are irrational, uncooperative, delusional, paranoid, assaultive and hallucinating patients. Treatment for them is to sedate with cholroprmazine 100 mgm I/M. Use a quiet, calm, firm and unhurried approach.

B. ANXIOUS

These patients are agitated and panicky. They are rational and cooperative but restless, prespire profusely, flushed face with a rapid pulse and respiration, dilated pupils, reflexes are quickened. These symptoms may be present in a prepsychotic, psychotic or neurotic state. Treatment is to look for the cause or situation which may be organic or psychological, calm the patient. Sedation is followed by psychotherapy.

C. DRUNK

The drunken patient is brought to the hospital with a flushed face and a staggering gait. He may be comatose. Treatment is symptomatic. The patient should be examined for any injuries, subdural hematoma. Exclude the comatose stage from diabetes, acidosis. Maintain fluid and electrolytic balance, attend to the nursing needs of the patient.

D. DRUG WITHDRAWAL

As already mentioned in this unit, opiate group of drug withdrawal causes restlessness, anxiety, psychological dependence, a craving for the drug, yawning, increased lacrimation, diarrhoea, dilated pupils, muscle twitching, increased B.P., pulse and respiration, insomnia and restlessness. Use substitute therapy with methadone.

Barbiturate-type withdrawal is characterized by agitation, insomnia and convulsions. Admit the patient and give pentobarbital as prescribed by the psychiatrist.

Nursing the patient with overactivity may lead to a feeling of disgust or fear as he is unpredictable. Through aggressive behaviour the patient is expressing the need for security. The nurse should be confident.

Isolate the patient in a safe environment. Attend to all stat instructions. Send for the doctor. When the patient finds nurses and doctors helping him, he becomes cooperative.

Get extra help, for the patient may try to run away.

Avoid restraining the patient but, if necessary, restraining may be done.

While communicating the nurse should be calm in her approach. Avoid arguments. Avoid giving a long explanation.

Nursing problems with these patients may be, inadequate nourishment. Provide finger food which they can hold and eat quickly. Give plenty of fluids and develop a therapeutic nurse-patient relationship.

UNDERACTIVE PATIENT

In such a patient activity is reduced to an extent that he just lies on the bed motionless, does not speak, remains mute, psychomotor retardation is marked.

The conditions in which underactivity may occur are:

a. Depression.
b. Catatonia — stupor.

A. DEPRESSION

The symptoms presented are melancholy, tearfulness, self-accusation, psychomotor retardation, impairment in ordinary activities like house work, or job. Decrease in appetite, sex, sleep. The patient may express a desire to attempt suicide.

B. CATATONIA — STUPOR

The patient is mute and motionless. Catalepsy present. He may look stuporous, but very alert and dangerous otherwise.

These conditions will be discussed in nursing management under *Chapter VIII.*

ATTEMPTED SUICIDE

Suicide is the act of killing oneself. In psychiatry a suicidal attempt is considered to be one of the psychiatric emergencies. In psychiatric nursing, suicide threats and gestures are always taken seriously. Half-hearted attempts for suicide may be desperate cries for help and the individual may succeed by accident. It may be a symptom of depression, schizophrenic withdrawal, turning of hostility inward to the self, an attempt to make others feel guilty, a reaction to personal guilt, means to obtain release from unbearable pain, failure, grief or fear of old age, in occasional cases an act of revenge.

MYTHS ABOUT SUICIDE

(a) It is felt that a suicide threat is just a bid for attention and should not be taken seriously. *It is not right.* If the client has expressed a desire to attempt suicide, he should be taken seriously.

(b) It is harmful for a person to talk about suicide. His attention should be diverted.

No, patient should be allowed to talk about suicide plans. It will provide him/her with mental catharsis. The client may have second thoughts about suicide and find pleasure in living.

(c) Only psychotic persons commit suicide. *It is not true.* People suffering from other types of disorders also commit suicide. Many of the patients said to be suffering from psychosomatic illness, illness associated with activities in males and disfigurement in females may lead to suicidal attempt. Other factors are disruption in relationship and loss of prestige or status (Despal 1968).

(d) Another myth is that a nice home, good job or an intact family prevent suicide. There may be *other stresses* outside these factors which lead a person to commit suicide.

(e) Myth that a failed suicide attempt should be treated as manipulative behaviour. *No. not always.* The client may plan his future attempt with more lethal ways.

EPIDEMIOLOGY

It is difficult to know the incidence of a suicide attempt. In India, one out of 12 attempts to commit suicide was found to end fatally. The national suicide rate, according to the Police Department, is 8-9/1000 annually.

A) SOCIALLY

(i) There are low suicidal rates among people in developing communities in which hope and optimism are high: Warm cultures such as Irish, Italians. Culture in which there is strong disapproval of suicide is found, among others, in Italy, Spain and Ireland, where the Catholic Church is highly influential.

(ii) High Suicidal Rate in societies where there is too much of social unrest, pessimistic outlook, nothing to look forward to. Culture that is uncaring and cold. Societies where an individual performance is expected such as Japan, Russia, and Germany.

B) DEMOGRAPHICALLY

Single persons and married persons without children show a higher incidence of suicide in comparison to married persons with children. *Men* commit suicide three times more than women. *Women attempt* suicide three times more than men. *Suicide* is more common in the *middle age.* Males above 45 years and females beyond 55 years do it. It is also slightly higher in adolescents than the general population. In India *(Sethi et al 1975),* 80 per cent of those who committed suicide were between 16 and 30 years. The male female ratio was 3:2, 85 per cent hailed from unitary families, 63.3 per cent were single.

C) CLINICALLY

The suicide rate is higher among people who have attempted suicide before. Persons who have experienced loss of an important person. People who are recovering from depression, persons with physical illness particularly when the illness involves an alteration of the body image or life style. Persons who abuse alcohol and drugs develop a decrease in their impulsive control.

a) Self-Destructive People are those who actually do commit suicide, those who attempt suicide, those who are chronically self-destructive.

ESTIMATION OF LETHALITY AND DEGREE OF SUICIDE

HIGH LETHALITY PLAN	LOW LETHALITY PLAN
— Continued death stress	— Hypochondriases
— Psychosis	— Male over 40
— Marked depression	— Homosexuality
— Previous attempt	— Mild depression
— Suicide note	— Chronic maladjustment
— Violent method	— Bankrupt
— Chronic disease	— No apparent secondary gains.
— Recent surgery or childbirth	
— Recent serious loss	
— Alcoholism	
— Drug dependence	
— Use of gun	— Wrist cutting
— Jumping from a high building	— Inhaling domestic gas
— Hanging	
— Drowning	— Use of non-descriptive drugs.
— Carbon-monoxide inhalation	
— High doses of Barbiturates	
— Car Crash.	

Nursing care will be discussed in *Chapter VIII.*

OTHER PSYCHIATRIC EMERGENCIES

(I) ACQUIRED IMMUNE DEFICIENCY SYNDROME (AIDS)

AIDS-related psychiatry emergency includes change in behaviour secondary to illness. The onset of symptoms is gradual, like systemic infection, hypoxia, electrolyte imbalance. Dementia reaches from moderate to severe within two and three months of its onset. Along with organic symptoms, depression, anxiety, suicidal attempts, delusion, denial to disease and treatment are alarming. Sexual promiscuity leads to the risk of infecting others. Hypochondriasis, mutism, agitation, restlessness, mania are associated psychiatric emergencies.

Management of the suicide risk is most significant.

(II) ADOLESCENT CRISIS

Adolescent crisis may be due to suicidal ideation or attempts, drug use, decline in school performance, pregnancy, abortion, eating disorders, and psychoses. Depression may be very serious.

(III) PUERPERAL PSYCHOSIS

Child birth as a major life event can precipitate schizophrenia, depression, reactive psychosis and mania. Suicide risk is decreased during pregnancy but it is increased in the post-partum period. Management depends on the nature of symptoms.

TO RECALL

— Psychiatric emergency is a disturbance of behaviour, affect and thought.
— Types of psychiatric emergencies
a) Overactive patient
— Violent
— Anxious
— Drunk
— Drug withdrawal
b) Underactive patient
— Depressed
— Catatonic stupor
c) Suicide
— Definition
— Myths of suicide
— Epidemiology
* Social factors
* Demographic factors
* Clinical factors
* Self-destructive people
d) Estimation of degree and lethality of suicide.
e) Other Psychiatric Emergencies
— AIDS-associated psychiatric emergency.
— Adolescent crisis.
— Post-partum psychosis.

APPLICATION TO NURSING

Reading of the content of *Unit XX* will help the student nurses to learn the common psychophysiological disorder. The etiological factors and psychodynamic involved in the psychophysiological disorders. Disorders of infancy, childhood and adolescence will help the nursing students to help children, adolescents and parents in school health services and community outreach services. Substance/drug abuse learning will help the nursing personnel to develop an insight into the correct terminology, drugs and withdrawal symptoms. As nurses they would be equipped with knowledge and skill to help the clients, family and community to fight this dragon of death that is drug abuse. Reading of psychiatric emergencies will enable the nursing student to identify conditions in which the nurse has to care for the patients more briskly. She will be able to prevent suicidal attempts of the patient due to close observation.

BETTER STUDY SECTION OF UNIT XX

I. Vocabulary (Use dictionary)

Abruptly	Alopecia	Altering
Amenorrhea	Assaultive	Bankrupt
Conflict	Craving	Demographic
Disproportionately	Gooseflesh	Gratification
Irrational	Lethal	Myth
Phenomenon	Rebellious	Ritualistic
Somatically	Stupor	Tinnitus
Violent.		

2. Assignment

Make reading notes on:

(i) Psychophysiological and childhood disorders.

(ii) Other psychiatric emergencies not included in this unit.

3. Study questions

(i) List the two common disorders under the following headings:

a) Disruptive behaviour disorders.

b) Eating Disorders.

(ii) Give two examples of the following:

— Narcotics	—	—
— Sedative/Depressants	—	—
— Stimulants	—	—
— Hallucinogens	—	—
— Underactive Patients	—	—
— Overactive Patients	—	—
— High Suicidal Patients	—	—
— Low Suicidal Patients	—	—

4. Reading References

Coleman, J.C. ***Abnormal Psychology and Modern Life.*** (5th ed.) Scott Forsman and Company, Illinois (1970).

Kapoor, Bimla. ***A Textbook of Psychiatric Nursing.*** Kumar Publishing House, Delhi (1992).

Kaplan Harold & Sadock, B.J. ***Comprehensive Textbook of Psychiatry*** (5th ed.) Williams and Wilkins, London (1989).

Kneisl, C.R. & Wilson, H.S. ***Psychiatric Nursing.*** Addison-Wesley Publishing Company, Mento Parle, California, (1979).

Solman, P., Patch V.D. ***Handbook of Psychiatric.*** La Jolla, California, Boston, Massachusetts (1974).

COMPREHENSIVE BIBLIOGRAPHY OF CHAPTER VII

— Coleman J.C. ***Abnormal Psychology and Modern Life.*** (5th ed.) Scott Foresman and Company, Illinois (1976).

— Shives L.R. ***Basic Concepts of Psychiatric - Mental Health Nursing*** (2nd ed.) J.B. Lippincott Company, Philadelphia (1990)

— Keys J. Hoffling C. ***Basic Psychiatric Concepts in Nursing*** (4th ed.) J.B. Lippincott Company, Philadelphia (1980).

— Kolb L. and Brodie H.K. ***Modern Clinical Psychiatry.*** (10th edi.) W.B. Saunders Company, 1982.

— Walker J.I. ***Essentials of Clinical Psychiatry.*** J.B. Lippincott Company Philadelphia (1985)

— Soloman P. and Patch V. ***Handbook of Psychiatry*** (3rd ed.) La Jolla, California (1974).

— Kapoor, Bimla. ***A Textbook of Psychiatric Nursing.*** Kumar Publishing House, Delhi (1992).

— Chapman A.H. and Almeida E.M. ***The Interpersonal Basis of Psychiatric Nursing.*** G.P. Putnam's Sons, New York (1972).

— Henderson and Gillespie's. ***Textbook of Psychiatry for Students and Practitioners.*** (10th ed.) Oxford University Press, London (1975).

— Kalkman M.L. & Davis A.J. ***New Dimensions in Mental Health Psychiatric Nursing*** (4th ed.) McGraw Hill Book Company, New York (1974).

— Cavener J. & Brodie H.K. ***Signs and Symptoms in Psychiatry.*** J.B. Lippincott Company, Philadelphia.

— Kaplan Harold & Sadocck B.J. ***Comprehensive Textbook of Psychiatry.*** (5th ed.) Williams and Wilkins, London (1989).

— Taylor C.M. ***Essentials of Psychiatric Nursing.*** (11th ed.) The C.V. Mosby Company, London (1982).

— Wilson. H.S & Kneisl C.R. ***Psychiatric Nursing.*** (Second Edition) Addison Wesley Publishing Company California (1982)

COMPREHENSIVE TEST OF CHAPTER VII

1. Select one of the best answers and encircle it.

1. Causes of Delirium are:
   a) Head trauma b) Metabolic Disorders c) Infections
   d) a and c e) a, b and c.

2. Primary symptoms of schizophrenic disorders are:
   a) Associative looseness b) Autism c) Affective incongruity
   d) Ambivalence e) All of these.

3. The triad symptoms of Manic Episode are:
   a) Elated, unstable mood b) Increased pressure of speech
   c) Increased motor activity d) Delirious state e) a, b, and c.

4. Neurotic Disorders occur mainly due to:
   a) Biological factors b) Maladaptive learning c) Stress factors
   d) None of these e) a, b and c.

5. Addiction seems to result from:
   a) Availability b) Opportunity. c) Individual predisposition
   d) Social isolation e) All of these

6. Withdrawal symptoms of opium include all of these except:
   a) Yawning b) Dilated pupils c) Anorexia
   d) Constipation e) Rhinnorrhea

7. All of these are sexual disorders except:
   a) Exhibitionism b) Homosexuality c) Incest
   d) Masturbation e) All of these

II. Match the statements given in Column A with the terms in Column B. Write the alphabet in the space given in Column A.

Column A	Column B
1. A state of clouded consciousness in which attention can't be sustained, perception and thinking are distorted.	A. Korskoff syndrome

2. Characterized by physical symptoms resulting from psychologic factors.	B. Senile Dementia
3. Occurs usually after the age of 65 years due to degenerative changes of brain with marked mental deterioration.	C. Delirium
4. Characterized by suspiciousness, delusion of persecution and grandiosity.	D. Schizophrenic Disorders
5. Occurs due to thiamine deficiency with no impairment of consciousness.	E. Paranoid disorders
6. Characterized by distoration of thinking, perception, inappropriate effect, shallow effect and ambivalence.	F. Hypomania
7. Characterized with behaviour as stealing, lying, fighting, truancy, substance abuse.	G. Neurosis
	H. Neurosthenia
	I. Psychopathic Personality
	J. Psychosomatic disorders

III. Encircle 'T' if you find the statement is True and 'F' if the statement is false.

1. Dementia is a loss of memory.	T	F
2. Simple schizophrenia does not present with hallucinations and delusion.	T	F
3. Hebaphrenics do not have disintegration of Personality.	T	F
4. Threat of suicide is a psychiatric emergency.	T	F
5. Anorexia nervosa is presistent lack of appetite and refusal of food.	T	F
6. Tempertantrum needs no special attention and care.	T	F
7. Psychotic and neurotic disorders are treated with ECT and psychotherapy.	T	F
8. Drugs taken just for fun don't lead to addiction.	T	F
9. Most non-alcoholic drug abusers use more than one agent.	T	F
10. Flashback may occur amongst any type of drug users.	T	F

IV. List Five Types of Dementia :

1. 2.

3. 4.

5.

V. Enlist four types of schizophrenic disorders:

1. 2.

3. 4.

KEY TO CHAPTER VII

1. 1. e
   2. e
   3. e
   4. e
   5. e
   6. d
   7. d

II. 1. C
   2. J
   3. B
   4. E
   5. A
   6. D
   7. I

III. 1. F
   2. T
   3. F
   4. T
   5. T
   6. F
   7. F
   8. F
   9. T
   10. F

IV. i. Senile — Deterioration
   ii. Paranoid Reaction
   iii. Presbyphrenic type
   iv. Depressed and agitated type
   v. Delirious and confused type

V. i. Paranoid (Delusional) Schizophrenia
   ii. Catatonic schizophrenia
   iii. Hebaphrenic schizophrenia
   iv. Simple schizophrenia

CHAPTER VIII
NURSING INTERVENTIONS OF MENTAL AND BEHAVIOUR-DISORDERED PATIENTS

UNIT XXI
NURSING PROCESS

UNIT OUTLINE

Definition of Nursing Process.
Steps of Nursing Process.
Assessment & Identification of Needs
- Data Collection
- Analysis of Data
- Nursing Diagnosis.

Planning
- Determining Priorities
- Setting Goals
- Selecting Nursing Actions
- Writing Nursing Care Plan.

Implementation.
Evaluation.
Advantages of Nursing Process.
Better Study Section.

INTENDED LEARNING BEHAVIOUR

After reading this unit, you will be able to :

a) Define Nursing Process.
b) List the steps of Nursing Process.
c) Explain information to be obtained during the assessment phase.
d) Describe the aspects of planning.
e) Develop skill in identifying independent and dependent nursing actions.
f) Identify the importance of the evaluation phase.
g) Explain the advantages of nursing process.

CONTENTS

INTRODUCTION

The basic approach to the Nursing Care Process is a patient-centred or problem-solving approach. It includes the following steps:

* Assessment and identification of needs
* Plan of action
* Implementation of the plan
* Evaluation

DEFINITION

Nursing process is based on a problem solving approach to nursing. It is an organized, systematic method of giving individualized nursing care to the patient. It consists of assessment and identification, planning, implementation and evaluation.

STEPS OF NURSING PROCESS

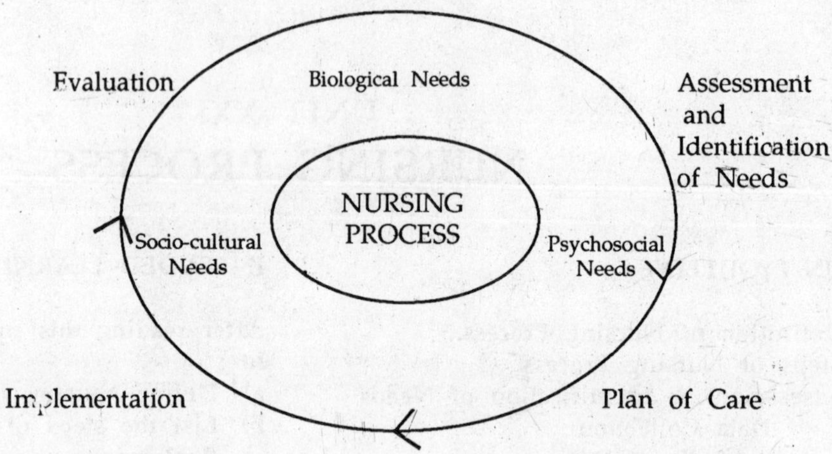

Fig. 26 : Inter-relationship of the Steps of Nursing Process.

ASSESSMENT AND IDENTIFICATION OF NEEDS

Assessment is the first step of the nursing process. It is the systematic and purposeful collection of data on the health status of the patient and the interpretation of the collected data. Assessment includes (A) data collection, (B) data analysis, and (C) nursing diagnosis or identification of nursing problems.

A. DATA COLLECTION

Data are collected by means of an interview, history taking, observation of symptoms and examination of the patient.

Data include:

(i) Identification Data:
Such as name, age, sex, marital status, educational status, occupation, economic status.

(ii) Subjective Data:
Information obtained from the client/friend/relative on the patient's problem, what he/she is experiencing such as taking history of the patient's mental illness.

(iii) Objective Data:
Information obtained from observation, physical examination and clinical investigation. For example, data collected through a mental status examination, observation of the patient's behaviour after giving drugs.

(B) ANALYSIS OF DATA

The data collected are critically examined, utilizing the scientific knowledge. The patient's strength, limitations, adaptive and maladaptive behaviour are identified. Based on the analysis, nursing diagnosis is made.

C. NURSING DIAGNOSIS

A statement of the patient's actual and potential problems in which nursing intervation brings a change in his/her health.

Example	Nursing Diagnosis	Medical Diagnosis
Physical	* Slumped posture * Extreme slowness in * performing activity.	Depression
Emotional	* Apathy * Hostility	-----Do-----
Social	* Low self-esteem * Mistrust of others.	-----Do-----

PLANNING

As soon as the patient's problem are identified or nursing diagnosis made, planning of nursing care begins. The planning consists of (A) Determining priorities (B) Setting goals, (C) Selecting Nursing Actions, and (D) Developing/Writing the Nursing Care Plan. In planning the care, the nurse can involve the patient, family and members of the health team.

A. DETERMINING PRIORITIES

On the basis of an analysis, the nurse decides which problem requires priority attention or immediate attention.

B. SETTING GOALS

Goals stated indicate as to what is to be achieved if the identified problem is taken care of. These can be immediate, or short-term and long-term goals.

C. SELECTING NURSING ACTION

The nursing action/technique chosen will enable the nurse to meet the goals or desired objectives. For example, the short-term goal for a depressed patient is "to pursue him/her to take bath". Nursing action may be: "The nurse firmly directs the patient to get up and finish his bath before 8 o'clock". On persuasion the patient takes bath.

This is an example of selection of the nursing action.

D. WRITING NURSING CARE PLAN

Writing or recording of the problems, goals, and nursing actions is a nursing care plan.

IMPLEMENTATION

Implementation is a step when planning is put into action. It is actual giving of comprehensive nursing care to the patient, that is, therapeutic, physical, psychosocial, recreational, spiritual, and discharge plan. To implement the actions, nurses need to have intellectual, interpersonal and technical skills.

Nursing actions are of two types:

(i) Dependent Nursing Action: Action derived from the prescription of the physician; for example, giving medicine.

(ii) Independent Nursing Action: This is based on nursing diagnosis and plan of care, like pursuing the patient to attend to personal hygiene.

EVALUATION

The continuous or ongoing phase of the nursing process is evaluation. This can be done by checking — Have I done everything for my patient ? Is my patient better after getting the planned care ? Evaluation is a feedback mechanism for judging the quality of care given aganist the actual care to be given. Evaluation of the patient's progress indicates what problems of the patient have been solved, which need to be assessed again, replanned, implemented and re-evaluated.

ADVANTAGES OF THE NURSING PROCESS

Nursing process helps to:

i) Collect relevant data for which the patient/client has been hospitalized.

ii) Plan the expected outcome/objectives which will help provide and evaluate the nursing care.

iii) Give quality nursing care based on judgement.

iv) Provide an opportunity in directing the nursing car to the team members and students.

v) Give nursing care systematically and logically.

vi) Provide continuity of the nursing care to the patient.

vii) Provide an opportunity to use decision-making.

viii) Provide a feedback so that quality of the patient care can be maintained.

TO RECALL

- ✱ Definition of Nursing Process.
  Nursing process is defined as an organized systematic method of giving individualized nursing care to the patient.
- ✱ Steps of Nursing Process
  - — Assessment and Identification of Need
    - : Data Collection
    - : Data Analysis
    - : Nursing diagnosis
  - — Planning of Nursing Carte includes:
  - ✱ Determining priorities
  - ✱ Setting goals
  - ✱ Selecting nursing actions
  - ✱ Writing nursing care plan
- ✱ Implementation
  - — Dependent nursing action
  - — Independent nursing action
- ✱ Evaluation
- ✱ Advantages of Nursing Process

APPLICATION TO NURSING

This unit is core of nursing interventions. Reading of the unit will enable the students to relate that the nursing process is basically a problem-solving approach. It has various steps, assessment and identification of needs, plan of actions. Implementation of action and Evaluation. This unit will provide a basic concept for giving effective nursing care to the patients.

BETTER STUDY SECTION OF UNIT XXI

1. Vocabulary (Refer dictionary)

Adaptive	Obtained
Approach	Priority
Critically	Pursue
Determining	Slumped
Identification	Systematically
Logically	

2. Assignment

Make a list of independent and dependent roles which you are performing in any ward.

3. Study questions

a) List steps of the nursing process

b) List the information obtained during the assessment phase of the nursing process

c) Write four advantages of the nursing process

4. Reading reference

Kapoor, Bimla, *A Textbook of Psychiatric Nursing*, Kumar Publishing House, Delhi (1992)

Kratz, Charlottee R. *The Nursing Process.* Baillier Tindall (1979)

Marriner A. *The Nursing Process — A Scientific Approach to Nursing Care.* The C.V. Mosby Company, Saint Louis (1975)

Orem, Dorthea E. *Nursing Concept of Care.* McGraw Hill Book Company, London (1980).

UNIT XXII
NURSING CARE PLANS FOR PATIENT WITH MENTAL DISORDERS

UNIT OUTLINE

Nursing Patient with Schizophrenic Disorders
- * Definition
- * Etiological Factors
- * Psychodynamics
- * Nursing Diagnosis
- * Nursing Care Plan

Nursing Patient with Delusional (Paranoid) disorders
- * Definition
- * Related Disorders
- * Etiology
- * Psychodynamics
- * Nursing Diagnosis
- * Nursing Care Plan

Nursing Patient with Excitement
- * Definition
- * Etiology
- * Associated Conditions
- * Psychodynamics
- * Nursing Diagnosis
- * Nursing Care Plan

Nursing Patient with Depression
- * Definition
- * Etiology
- * Associated Conditions
- * Difference between Psychogenic and Reactive Depression
- * Psychodynamics
- * Nursing Diagnosis
- * Nursing Care Plan

Nursing Patient with Withdrawn Behaviour
- * Definition
- * Associated Conditions
- * Psychodynamics
- * Nursing Diagnosis

INTENDED LEARNING BEHAVIOUR

After reading this unit, you will be able to:

a) Identify the needs of a schizophrenic patient
b) Develop short-term and long-term goals
c) Plan Nursing Intervention
d) Implement and evaluate nursing care
e) Identify the nursing needs of the patients with delusional disorders
f) Plan Nursing Care based on Psychodynamics
g) Develop skill-giving care to the patient with paranoid disorders
h) Identify the associated conditions of excitement
i) Identify the nursing needs of the patients with excitement
j) Develop skill in attending the patient with excitement
k) Identify associated conditions of depression
l) Differentiate between Psychogenic and Reactive Depression
m) Develop skill in giving care to the patient with depression.
n) Develop skill in giving care to the patient with withdrawn behaviour.

* Nursing Care plan

Nursing Patient with Suicidal Ideation/ Attempt

* Definition
* Myths about Suicide
* Epidemiology
* Etiology
* Psychodynamics
* Nursing Diagnosis
* Nursing Care Plan

Nursing Patient with Anxiety

* Definition
* Types of Anxiety
* Description of mild, moderate, severe and panic forms of anxiety
* Associated conditions of anxiety
* Etiological factors
* Psychodynamics
* Nursing Diagnosis
* Nursing Care Plan

Nursing Patient with obsessive Compulsive Neurosis

* Definition
* Etiology
* Associated Conditions
* Psychodynamics
* Nursing Diagnosis
* Nursing Care Plan

Nursing the Patient with Conversion Disorders (Hysterical Neurosis—Conversion Type)

* Definition
* Classification of somatoform disorders
* Definition of conversion disorders
* Signs and Symptoms
* Psychodynamics
* Nursing Diagnosis
* Nursing Care Plan

Application

Better study section

o) Develop skill in identifying the patient with suicidal ideation.

p) Plan nursing intervention for the patientwith suicidal ideation.

q) Build knowledge on identifying the patient with anxiety.

r) Develop skill in caring for the client/ patient with various degrees of anxiety.

s) Nurse the patient with obsessive compulsiveneurosis based on psychodynamics

t) Describe the somatoform disorders

u) Explain the nursing intervention of the patient with obsessive compulsive neurosis

v) Develop skill in nursing the patient with conversion disorders.

NURSING PATIENT WITH SCHIZOPHRENIC DISORDER

INTRODUCTION

Schizophrenic Disorder is a group of mental disturbances essentially characterized by (a) one or more psychotic features during the active phase, including bizarre or absurd delusions such as being controlled, (b) somatic, grandiose, religious or nihilistic delusions, (c) delusion of persecution or jealousy with hallucination, (d) incoherence with marked loosening of association, blunted, flat or inappropriate effect, (e) hallucination, and (f) grossly disorganized behaviour such as in catatonia.

DEFINITION

According to ICD - 10 (F-20), schizophrenic disorders are characterised in general by fundamental and characteristic distortion of thinking, perception and inappropriate or blunted affect. Delusion are bizarre in nature. Hallucinations, especially auditory, are the commonest. Thinking is vague and speech sometimes incomprehensible. Mood is characteristically shallow and incongruous, ambivalence, negativism, stupor or catatonia may be present. The onset may be acute or insidious with a seriously disturbed behaviour.

ETIOLOGICAL FACTORS

The etiological factors can be:

* Genetic factors
* Psychosocial factors
* Pathological communication
* Pathogenic family interaction
* Socio-cultural factors

(Refer Unit XVIII)

PSYCHODYNAMICS

In schizophrenic psychosis there is impaired ego functioning. Reality testing and judgement are affected. As the reality is affected, a person regresses to the previous development at stage. Due to increased regression the *ego* and *superego* are further weakened and *id* predominates. Deprivation of early mothering reduces the capacity of the child to socialize.

NURSING DIAGNOSIS

The most common nursing diagnosis of schozophrenic patients for planning nursing care will be as follows:

* Altered thought — Delusion
  — Associative looseness
  — Autism
* Altered affect — inappropriate or blunt affect
* Altered perception — Hallucinations, illusions
* Activity disturbances
* Impulsiveness
* Impaired judgement and attention
* Sleep disturbance

* Low self-concept
* Decreased socialization
* Impaired communication
* Impaired insight
* Self-care deficits (in physical needs, cleaning, shaving, bathing, nutritional need; eating.)

Sample nursing care plans on various symptoms are presented in the following content. Short-Term Goal is read as (STG), Long-Term Goal is read as (LTG). These developed nursing care plans will vary according to an individual patient's needs. Keeping the holistic care of the individual, nursing care plans are discussed under the following nursing needs.

I. THERAPEUTIC NEEDS

II. PSYCHOSOCIAL NEEDS

III. PHYSICAL NEEDS

IV. RECREATIONAL NEEDS

V. SPIRITUAL NEEDS

VI. DISCHARGE PLAN.

NURSING CARE PLAN OF SCHIZOPHRENIC PATIENT

NURSING NEEDS	GOALS	PLANNING	IMPLEMENTATION	EVALUATION
1	2	3	4	5
THERAPEUTIC NEED				
(i) Compliance to treatment.	STG To help the patient to recover. LTG To enable the patient to: — learn the importance of treatment — decrease/ eliminate his symptoms — recover from disease.	* Plan the drug therapy with doctor and relatives. * If physical therapy, ECT is to be given, it should be discussed with relatives and patients. Individual and group psychotherapy needs to be planned and given.	* Give the drugs prescribed by the psychiatrist. * Keep 5 R in mind. * Observe for side-effects. * Record any change in the patient after medicine. * Record and report early and late side-effects of antipsychotic drugs. * Explain ECT therapy to the relatives. * Explain to the patient he will be getting an injection.(for ECT) * Interact with the patient at one-to-one level. * Allow him to speak about his illness.	* Patient participates in his treatment. * Asks how many more injections (ECT) are required.

* *STG (Short Term Goal)*
LTG (Long Term Goal)

1	2	3	4	5
PSYCHOSOCIAL NEEDS				
To decrease disturbed thoughts.	STG To help the patient communicate his problem effectively. LTG To help the patient to: — develop effective communication ability. — develop skill in integrating his thoughts and speaking. — reduce his fantasies which may be leading to looseness of thought and autism	Plan to: * establish positive relationship, help the patient develop trust in the nurse. * provide a planned opportunity for interaction.	* Sit next to the patient. * Teach the patient when appropriate (when the patient) is feeling sad, crying). * Talk to the patient about his problem. * Don't criticise the patient (you should not have scolded your child). * Interact with the patient as planned. * Make conversation simple. * Encourage the patient to talk.	Develops trust in the nurse and others in communicating. Reduction in fantasies.
To reduce delusions.	STG To help the patient to accept reality. LTG To help the patient to: accept reality identify relationship of the delusional content with behaviour.	* Plan to identify the relationship of reality and delusion. * Ignore the delusions expressed by the patient.	* Listen to the patient's delusion and find out its relationship with his behaviour. * Ignore the delusions of the patient and tell other staff also to	Decrease need to use delusions.

1	2	3	4	5
	— decrease need to use delusions.		do the same. * Do not probe into the delusional material/content in the initial phase. * Assure and provide a safe environment.	
To decrease or break hallucinations (gradually)	STG To help the patient to concentrate on his tasks and care. LTG To enable the patient to: — lead a productive life. — reduce his anxiety. — develop relationship with others.	* Plan to talk to the patient to find out the reason for anxiey. * Develop therapeutic relationship with the patient. * Do not give any importance to the voices or visual objects.	* Select a separate room for interaction. * Talk in a trustworthy and comfortable environment so that his anxiety is reduced. * Talk about all other things but not the hallucinations. * Don't give any importance to the voices while interacting with the patient, refer them as "so-called voices" or " those voices" just don't bother.	Gains insight into his illness, Hallucinations decrease.
To improve communication.	STG To decrease anxiety associated factors while interacting.	* Build rapport with the patient. * Use an active friendly ap-	* Don't ignore the patient. * Initiate the conversation.	Develops confidence in communicating relevantly with others.

1	2	3	4	5
	To promote self-confidence. LTG To enable the patient to: — verbalize the problem. — provide mental catharsis. — develop self-confidence. — gain pleasure through conversation.	proach. * Try to listen to the patient * Provide a comfortable and trustworthy environment. * Use various communication techniques.	* Allow the patient to talk and be an active listener. * Provide a separate place for talking. * See that there is no disturbance while talking to the patient. * Use pinpointing, clarifying, reflecting, summarizing techniques of communication. * Don't probe, argue or criticise the patient. * Allow silence for some time.	
To improve socialization	STG To help the patient to have a sense of belongingness. — To help him to improve his self-confidence LTG To enable the patient to: — enhance his self-concept — feel comfortable in a group. — increase social interaction with	* As these patients are withdrawn, an environment should be created for socialization. * Plan socialization with other patients who are not overactive, so that sefl-confidence of the patient is enchanced. * Select a group where the patient is also able to	* Speak in short, clear sentences * Allow the patient to sit with others. * Take initiative to talk to the patient. * Tell him to come out of the bed and talk to his neighbour patient. * Allow him to talk to one patient, then two and then four and gradually in the group.	The patient starts making positive comments on himself. Develops a feeling that he is also of some worth.

1	2	3	4	5
	others (group relation).	interact and talk and does not feel that he is being deminated.	* In the group, the patient should be given a chance to talk. * Pat the patient or encourage his good performance in the group. * Tell other patients to come and play with him. * Allow him to spend more time with others.	Enjoys interaction with others.
To enchance self-concept.	STG To help the patient feel worthy and competent. LTG To enable the patient to: — develop a sense of worthiness — feel less dependent on others — take up social roles.	* Plan activities in which the patient is able to show his worth. * Help the patient to do most of his activities himself. * Help the patient to remain clean. * Plan activities so that the patient can socialize, and take up the role of a leader.	* Provide simple activities like calling all the patients for day activities and making them sit. * Tell the patient to see all the patients leave the day-room clean and tidy. * Allow him to check if all the patients had their food.	The patient feels more confident of himself.
To improve attention and judgement	STG To improve the span of attention. LTG To enable the patient to: — enhance attention	* Activities of such kind where attention is required for a long time. * Provide an oppor-	* The patient may be asked to play Ludo with the nurse. * Write about what	Concentrates and attends to the activities, participates in giving opinion on family issues.

1	2	3	4	5
	and concentration. — improve judgement — develop decision-making ability.	tunity where judgement can be made. * Certain problems (simple) can be placed before him and he may be asked to take a decision. (These problems should not be difficult; if the patient fails, his self-concept will go low).	he did yesterday. * Provide new activities to hold attention of the patient. * If two patients are fighting to go to the bathroom at a time, he may help them in deciding.	
To improve family support.	STG To help in adjusting a mentally ill patient in the family. To help the family to participate in the care of the patient. LTG To enable the family to: — feel responsible in the care of the patient. — learn skills in handling the problems of patients. — help the patient to be socially productive. — develop realistic	* Plan for the relative to be available with the patient during hospitalization. * Plan care activities in which the relatives can participate actively. * Education of the relatives about the kind of illness the patient is suffering from and his social productive abilities.	* Make sure that one relative is always with the patient. * Teach the relative to persuade the patient to maintain his personal hygiene, take diet, participate in day-care activities and to accept the treatment. * Explain about the types of jobs the patient can perform. * Encourage the relatives to keep supporting.	* The patient feels wanted by the family members. * Looks forward to his discharge. * Makes future plans with his family members.

1	2	3	4	5
	goals in recovery of the patient.		* Don't over-protect, criticise and show rejection. * Tell them about the type of sickness the patient is suffering from (verbal, written material and meeting with other patients and their families can be arranged).	
PHYSICAL NEEDS				
Provide protection	STG To prevent harm to others and self. LTG To enable the patient to: — protect from self injury — prevent from causing harm to others as these patients are impulsive.	* Provide a safe environment. * Set limits on the patient's behaviour. * Discourage his acts of violence.	* Avoid keeping a glass, knife, blade or any sharp instrument with the patient. * Tell the patient that he will not be allowed to see T.V. if again he tries to slap his brother. * Don't allow him to go and play in the day care which he likes the best.	* The patient identifies that his behaviour is unacceptable and makes effort to have more self—control.
To assist in personal hygiene care.	STG To improve his personal appearance. To help the patient to have a	* Ensure that the patient takes his bath and attends to personal hygiene, brushing,	* Be with the patient or tell his relative to be with him, if required. * Tell the patient to	* Starts maintaining cleanliness.

1	2	3	4	5
	sense of well being by being clean. LTG To enable the patient to: — have a sense of well-being. — maintain self-respect. — promote his self-concept — maintain his self-identity. — feel accepted by others.	shaving, going to toilet, bathing, changing his clothes.	get up from the bed. * Encourage him to go and brush his teeth. * Persuade him to go for bowel evacuation as the patient may retain feaces. * In the case of a male patient, tell him to shave his beard.	
			* Send the patient to the bathroom and wait outside or tell the relative to wait till the patient finishes up bath. * Tell him to wear his own clean clothes daily.	Takes pride in his appearance.
To improve sleep pattern.	STG To help him to get up fresh and active LTG To enable the patient to: — develop a regular sleep pattern — enhance self-concept by being active.	* Try to provide a calm and comfortable environment. * The patient should be allowed to have less of sleep in the day time. * Plan of activities should be made	* Patients should be encouraged to go to sleep by 10.30 P.M. * Switch off the main lights. * Put on the bed-side floor lights. * If any patient is having a disturb-	The patient has longer hours of sleep, feels less tired.

1	2	3	4	5
	— improve socialization as the patient feels fresh after good sleep.	for the day time.	ing behaviour, isolate him. * Give a glass of hot milk to the patient. * Give enough activities during the day time. * Discourage the patient for frequent naps in the afternoon.	
Nutritional Care	STG To increase the patient's energy level. To help him develop interest in eating. LTG To enable the patient to: — improve his physical health — accept the need for an intake of fluids and food. — develop interest in eating — cope with any other physical stress such as infections.	* Diet may be given according to the choice of the patient. The patients are not interested in eating so encourage them to eat. * Sometimes they are unable to eat, so somebody should help them to eat. * May be afraid of eating because of delusions of suspiciousness.	* Plan an adequate and balanced diet with the patient on the previous day. * If the patient eats from hospital ask him what all he would like to take from the food trolly. * Serve food in a neat and attractive manner in the patient's own utensils. * Provide a clean environment before serving food. * Persuade the patient to eat himself.	The patient's appetite improves. Starts eating food with minimum persuasion.

1	2	3	4	5
			* Tell the relatives to taste the food, if the patient is afraid of taking it due to his delusion.	
RECREATIONAL NEEDS	STG To divert the attention of the patient from his sickness. To help him feel that he is recovering. LTG To enable the patient to: — lead towards a normal pattern of life. — develop a sense of recovery and achievement. — promote his self-concept. — improve socialization.	* Provide the activities of his interest. * If the patient is too aloof, give those activities by which he can socialize. * Provide the activities which give him a sense of achievement. Failure may reinforce worthlessness.	* Ask the patient what all he likes to do or his hobbies. * Choose a few according to the availability of place and equipment for recreation. * Tell him to play carromboard with two to four people. * Encourage him to play badminton so that his energy is utilized. * Don't allow any competition in the beginning. * If the patient is good in some activity allow competition and help him to achieve success. * Pat him when he wins a competition.	Enjoys life routine. Finds meaning in his activities.

1	2	3	4	5
SPIRITUAL NEEDS				
	STG To provide freedom to the patient to practise a pattern of living. LTG To enable the patient to: — develop a sense of satisfaction and freedom. — have a sense of recovery. — demonstrate less disgust towards life.	* Provide a place for the patient to practise his beliefs. * Provide opportunities for religious activities.	* Allow/encourage the patient to say his prayers daily. * Provide a separate corner in the ward/unit for the patient to come and pray. * Celebrate with the patients X-mas, Diwali, Iohri, Guru Purab, Holi and other religious functions. * Don't force the patient if he does not want to participate in other religious activities.	* The patient feels confident of his life.
DISCHARGE PLAN.				
	STG To help the patient to lead a meaningful life: — in the family — in the community. LTG To enable the patient to: — be socially productive. — take up family roles. — not to become a burden on the family and society.	* Activities should be planned according to the symptoms of the patient from the day he/she is admitted. * Help the patient to take up social and family roles whenever required.	* Encourage the patient to meet his relatives. * Encourage family members to take his opinion on important issues of the family. * Send the patient on parole (trial visits). * Follow—up at his job, if required.	* The patient develops a sense of recovery.

TO RECALL

Nursing Patient with Schizophrenia
— Definition
— Etiological factors
— Psychodynamics
— Nursing diagnosis
— Nursing care plan
I Therapeutic needs
II Psychosocial needs
  * Decrease disturbed thoughts
  * Reduce delusions
  * Decrease Hallucinations
  * Improve Communications
  * Improve Socialization
  * Enhance Self concept
  * Improve attention and judgement
  * Improve Family support
III Physical needs
  * Prevent from injury
  * Personal hygiene needs
  * Improve sleep
  * Nutritional needs
IV Recreational needs
V Spiritual needs
VI Discharge plan

NURSING PATIENT WITH DELUSIONAL (PARANOID) DISORDERS

INTRODUCTION

Paranoid is a commoly used term for suspicious behaviour. DSM-III has described it as paranoid disorders but now DSM-III-R has replaced it with delusional (paranoid) disorders because delusions are the primary symptoms of disorder.The themes of delusion include erotomanic (one is loved by another), grandiose (one who believes in possessing greatness or a famous relationship), jealousy (false belief that a friend is unfaithful), persecutory (the theme of delusion is that he is the victim of someone's plot), somatic (one's body parts are malfunctioning or infested with worms). So the term delusional and paranoid will be used interchangeably as described in DSM-III-R.

DEFINITION

Paranoid disorders are characterised by moderately impaired reality testing, affect and sociability. Delusions may be persecutory, grandiose, erotic, jealous or somatic. Emotions and behaviour are appropriate to the delusional system. For example, if a patient has a persecutory delusion, he may be looking for clues, eyes will be suspicious, movement will be guarded, will avoid eating from others' hands.

RELATED DISORDERS

The disorders in which paranoid/delusional disorder occur are briefly described in the following text :

* Schizophrenia—paranoid type.
* Delusional disorders (discussed)
* Paranoid personality disorders.
* Paranoia
* Psychoactive substance/drug abuse
* Organic mental disorders
* Hearing loss in elderly
* Immigrants, refugees, prisoners-of-war, leaving home for the first time.

SCHIZOPHRENIC DISORDERS — PARANOID TYPE.

According to ICD-10 (F20.0), paranoid schizophrenia is the commonest type of schizophrenia. The clinical picture is dominated by delusions usually accompanied by hallucinations (auditory). The common paranoid symptoms are:

a) Delusions of persecution, reference, bodily change, jealousy.
b) Hallucinatory voices threatening the patient with command or auditory hallucinations without verbal form, such as whistling, humming or laughing.
c) Halluncination of smell or taste, or sexual or other bodily sensation,

visual hallucinations are rare.

Affect is less blunted but mood disturbances such as irritability, sudden anger, fearfulness and suspicion are presented. (Delusional Disorders discussed in the introduction.)

PARANOID PERSONALITY DISORDERS

Persons with a paranoid personality suspect that other people will harm them. For example, a person may be suspicious of his wife, coworkers or some of his neighbours. These people are very efficient because they do work with perfection. The person with a paranoid personality is tense, insecure, rigid, secretive and seclusive. He finds people untrustworthy.

PARANOIA

It is a rare chronic psychosis in which systematized delusions develop. gradually without hallucination. Delusions are mostly from grandeur, suspiciousness to ideas of reference.

PSYCHOACTIVE SUBSTANCE/DRUG ABUSE

High doses of amphetamines and use of cannabis may cause persecutory delusions. Use of hallucinogens may also lead to delusions during the withdrawal state. Chronic alcoholic states lead to a paranoid delusional state.

ORGANIC MENTAL DISORDERS

In senile dementia of the paranoid reaction type, the principal characteristic is a gradual formation of delusion, the individual develops a notion that his relatives are going to rob him or kill him. Drug intoxication may lead tö delirium and a delusional state. Epilepsy, myxeodema may also lead to a delusional state.

HEARING LOSS IN ELDERLY

Delusional states may also be caused by hearing loss in elderly due to a sensory handicap.

IMMIGRANTS,REFUGEES,PRISONERS-OF-WAR,LEAVING HOME

Immigrating refugees and prisoners of war may also develop delusional states due to stress, alienation and insecurity. Leaving home for the first time may also lead to (paranoid) delusional states.

ETIOLOGY OR CAUSATIVE FACTORS

Refer to Chapter VII — Unit XVII.

PSYCHODYNAMICS

Delusional (Paranoid) disorder patients use projection as a major defense mechanism to overcome rejection, inferiority and inadequacy. Projection is directed towards feelings resulting from delusion about CBI, people are following, a gang is against him. Regression is marked, reality testing inadequate. Ego function is better preserved so that the delusional material/content can be readily understood. These people develop with lack of trust which leads to suspiciousness due to a hostile environment during early parenting. High expectations cause stress on the child. These children set unrealistic goals due to which they have failures. They are poor in interpersonal relationship because of delusions.

NURSING DIAGNOSIS

The most common nursing diagnoses of delusional (paranoid) disorders for planning nursing care are:

* Increased anxiety.
* Impaired communication and interpersonal interaction.
* Altered thought.
* Impaired perceptions.
* Impaired socialization/social isolation for lack of trust, security, delusion of persecution.
* Increased hostility.
* Disturbed sleep patterns.
* Self-care deficit (eating, bathing, poor personal hygiene.)
* Restricted movements.
* Sense of inadequacy and powerlessness
* Family stress.

NURSING CARE PLAN OF DELUSIONAL DISORDER PATIENT

NURSING NEEDS	GOALS	PLANNING	IMPLEMENTATION	EVALUATION
1	2	3	4	5
I THERAPEUTIC NEEDS				
Ensure that the patient takes medicine	STG To reduce delusions and false perceptions of the patient. LTG To enable the patient to: — reduce his symptoms. — develop the habit of taking medicine in time. — accept the treatment — appreciate the need of taking treatment.	* The patient is suspicious of taking medicine from everyone due to his persecutory delusions. May avoid taking medicine. * The nurse must plan that the patient. takes medicine. * Provide opportunities for the patient to clarify his doubts on his treatment	* Allow the same nurse to give him medicine. * If any medicine is changed, explain the purpose. * Allow the patient to come to the treatment room while taking out medicine. * If the patient asks why the colour of B. Comp. is changed, explain that as B.Comp. is not available, Multi Vitamin is being given. * Observe for the side-effect of drugs. * Explain to the patient that treatment will reduce hearing of voices and confusion.	* Comes to treatment room and asks for medicine.

1	2	3	4	5
II. PSYCHOSOCIAL NEEDS				
To reduce anxiety.	STG To help him develop trusting relationship with others. LTG To enable the patient to: — feel less threatened in new relationships and situations. — develop trust on others. — develop an effective interpersonal relationship.	* Diminish the social isolation that arouses suspicion in the patient that something is wrong. * Try to use the same language and answer even though the patient asks repeatedly. * Help the patient to interact initially with those patients and relatives in whom he has developed trust. * Reduce anxiety-producing situations.	* Don't put the patient in isolation * Allow the patient to move around freely. * Walk with the patient while talking, if the patient is too anxious/ suspicious to sit at one place. * Answer questions briefly and to the point. * Be consistent in clarifying doubts of the patient. * P. Today also I am getting a red medicine which is for cough. * N. Yes, it is for your cough. Repeat the same medicine the next day,if required). * Use simple and clear sentences. * Don't force the patient to develop a new contact in the beginning. It	* Shows reduced anxiety. * Moves about freely. * Tries interacting with few people (Decrease in social isolation)

* *P (Patient)*
N (Nurse)

1	2	3	4	5
			may arouse more anxiety. * Encourage him to participate in his therapies.	
To decrease delusions	.STG To reduce anxiety LTG To enable the patient to: — develop an insight into the problem. — be more realistic. — come out of his delusional system. — develop a meaningful relationship with others. — reduce suspiciousness and ideas of reference.	* Provide an environment in which he can talk about his delusions. * Expressing his grandiosity delusion which may not be acceptable to the group,allow him to interact with others. * Plan for developing trust with the patient which is basics of IPR. * Try to provide an environment which is less suspicious.	* Establish a therapeutic relationship with the patient. * Use a matter-of-fact attitude as the patient is hypersensitive, suspicious and uses projection.. * Show mild concern at his delusions. * Help the patient to interact with others and share feelings. * Don't attack delusions. It may cause social isolation, but don't support also. * Talk in loud clear words. * Inform the change in activities. * Avoid talking to others by looking	* Takes initiative in talking to others * Blaming others is decreased. * Demonstrates trust in one/two significant people. (Nurse, father, mother).

1	2	3	4	5
			at the patient.	
To encourage movement.	STG To develop confidence and trust. LTG To enable the patient to: — feel less threatened in the environment — move about freely. — decrease his suspiciousness and persecutory delusion.	* Plan for the allowing more of territorial space. * Restriction of movement will cause suspiciousness that something is wrong and a feeling of being trapped. * May go and confirm if somebody is hiding to kill him.	* Allow the patient to move around freely. * Walk with the patient if he wants security. * Allow him to peep into the bathrooms or behind the doors of rooms or bathroom.	* Walks with confidence. * Admits that he is not scared in the ward.
To promote accurate perception	STG To reduce social isolation. ETG To enable the patient to: — see things more realistically than imaginary. — reduce his auditory and visual halluncination. — develop confidence that the environment is safe.	* Provide an opportunity for the patient to express his hallucination. * Provide an opportunity to develop a trusting relationship. * Provide a secure environment to the patient.	* Allow the patient to talk about his hallucination. * Focus on reality, avoid reinforcing his delusion and hallucination. * Avoid saying that you are wrong. * Explain I don't think, see and hear, but I understand you, see and hear to what you say. * Gradually, the patient may be asked to find out	* Hears and sees an imaginary thing less frequently. * Feels comfortable in the environment

1	2	3	4	5
			from others also of what he hears and sees whether they also hear and see the same.	
To improve communication	STG To reduce anxiety. — To develop self-confidence. LTG To enable the patient to: — improve his self-concept. — divert from his delusions and hallucination. — Improve communication skills	* Provide an environment which is less anxiety-producing and helps in communication as these patients are poor in IPR * Provide opportunities by which the patient's self-concept is enhanced. * Planning the therapeutic communication in a way in which he does not talk much about hallucination and delusions.	* Allow the patient to initiate conversation. * Have a matter-of-fact attitude during conversation (Refer to *Chapter VI, Unit XVI)* * Provide opportunities to lead the group or ask the patient to help send all the relatives out of the ward before the rounds. * Use various communication techniques such as reflecting, pinpointing, clarifying, analysing beliefs.	* Interacts with others without doubt. * Restlessness and anxiety are reduced. * Respects others.
To improve socialization.	STG To help the patient trust others to improve socialization. LTG To enable the	* Milieu should be therapeutic in which the other patients and relatives give impor-	* Avoid provoking or agitating questions. * (Did you say hospital is not	* Moves out of the bed.

1	2	3	4	5
	patient to: — reduce his social isolation. — interact with group members. — develop an insight into his problems by interacting with others. — develop self-confidence.	tance to the patient and not to his symptoms. * Environment plan should be such in which the patient identifies that certain behaviour of his needs to be improved/changed/deleted.	giving proper food.) * Avoid arguing with the patient, his/her suspiciousness will be reinforced. * Inform the patient about the change of routine like ward rounds, time of giving medicine.	* Sits with others.
			* Provide opportunities which reinforce a trusting relationship and environment. * Don't laugh at delusions expressed by the patient. All the team members should use a matter-of-fact attitude.	
			* Ignore the delusion of suspiciousness. * Talk loudly in clear words. * Answer why's of the patient (Why this medicine ? Why am I called ?).	* Goes to the day-care room.

1	2	3	4	5
To provide security	STG To help the patient feel safe. LTG To enable the patient to: — develop a sense of security. — reduce a feeling of inadequacy. — enhance a feeling of trust.	* The patient keeps looking for a clue in the environment because of his/her delusional state * Provide an environment in which he feels comfortable and safe. * The patient develops a feeling that if somebody comes to harm him he will not be able to protect himself. * Looks for safe people and environment.	* Allow the patient to change his cubicle. * Close the windows if the patient so desires. * Be with the patient, hold his hand, if required. * Touch the patient sparingly. * Allow the relative of the patient's choice to stay. * Take him around and show the security in the ward. * Make the environment less congested with equipment/furniture.	* Feels comfortable. * Makes a statement "I wonder why I was so afraid."
III. PHYSICAL NEEDS				
To attend nutritional needs	STG To help the patient maintain weight. To improve his physical health. LTG To enable the patient to: — take adequate food. — improve his	* Try to provide food from the food trolly from where other patients are taking. * Due to a marked persecutory delusion the patient refuses the food. * Plan serving the food along with	* Allow the patient to come to the food trolly and take food. * Provide whole foods—Apple, bananas, orange, egg (boiled), biscuits. * If food is brought from home, tell the	* Takes his food regularly. * Comes to check his weight.

1	2	3	4	5
	weight. — build up physical health.	other patients.	relatives to taste it first. * Ensure that the patient takes adequate food. * Plan out diet for the next day with the patient. * Eating together in a group will reduce suspiciousness. * Maintain a weight record.	
To ensure personal hygiene.	STG To help the patient feel fresh and have a sense of well-being. For aesthetic sense. LTG To enable the patient to: — develop regular bowel habits. — maintain personal hygiene. — develop self-cofidence.	* Supervise that the bathroom and toilets are clean. * Plan bath for the patient when there is no hurry, a knock at the door may reinforce delusion.	* Let the patient examine the bathroom and toilet. * Encourage the patient to spend some time in the toilet and bathroom. * Inform the patient that a relative or the nurse is standing outside. * Keep talking in between so that the patient is not in a hurry to come out due to his persecutory delusions. * Tell the patient not to lock the door.	* Takes bath regularly * No complaints of constipation.

1	2	3	4	5
To improve sleep	STG To help the patient have good sleep. LTG To enable the patient to: — feel secure. — develop a regular sleep pattern — remain active during day time.	* Plan that the patient has regular sleep—with a secure environment. * Sleep is reduced because of delusions.	* Encourage the patient to do activities during day time. * Allow a relative to stay with the patient. * At night if the patient wants to sleep near the nurse's station, allow him. * Be with the patient. * Leave the lights on if other patients do not feel disturbed.	* Sleeps for longer-hours. * Admits that "he had sound sleep today".
To protect from injuries.	STG To prevent the patient from physical harm to self and others. LTG To enable the patient to: — restrain from injuring self and others.	* Due to his suspicious delusion the patient may harm others. * Provide a protective environment to others. * Due to voices of control the patient may harm himself.	* Observe the patient's behaviour * Restrict and explain his hostile act if he has. * Explain to relatives about possible attacks when the patient may perform. * Check the patient's mental status. * Assess his level of hostility towards	* Hits at the pillow when angry. * Verbalizes his hostile feeling

1	2	3	4	5
		Plan constant observation.	a particular person. * Inform the person not to be scared but how to protect himself. * Explain to family members and others about the temporary symptom of the patient.	
IV RECREATIONAL NEEDS				
To provide recreational activities	STG To divert the patient's mind from his delusions. LTG To enable the patient to: — develop a sense of well-being. — find a meaning in his life. — lead towards a normal life pattern. — improve his self-concept.	* Planning of activities to divert the patient's mind from delusion and provide him with a sense of achievement.	* Give him solitary recreational activities of his choice such as reading, painting. * Allow him to play and sit with people whom he likes. * Gradually encourage the patient to play with others. * Tell the patient to go out and bring all the patients. * Send the patient alone/or with one patient to the store to take out recreational articles for all the patients.	* Shows confidence in managing things independently. * Appreciates success of others.

1	2	3	4	5
			* Allow others to win so that his grandiosity gradually decreases.	
V. SPIRITUAL NEEDS				
To provide spiritual needs	STG To help the patient to follow his routine. LTG To enable the patient to: — develop his routine activities. — get satisfaction in life. — reduce a feeling of inadequacy.	* Plan activities for the ward where all the patients attend to spiritual needs in the morning and evening. * Plan the discussion on religious and other spiritual issues. * Invite religious people like priest (Pandits), Father (of Church), Maulvi (Muslim priest) and Granthi (Sikh priest) to talk to patients.	* Encourage all the patients to go in the prayer room after/before breakfast. * Be present during religious discussions. * Make it voluntary for the patient to attend religious talks.	* The patient calls enveryone to join in the prayer room. * Sometimes leads the prayer meeting.
VI. DISCHARGE PLANS				
	STG To help the individual to adjust in family LTG To enable the patient to: — develop self-confidence.	* Plan gradual independence for the patient. * Activities with the family can be planned. * Involve family members in	* Allow the patient to go out for a cup of tea. * Send the patient for parole at home. * Discuss with the patient and family members after	* The patient wants frequent parole.

1	2	3	4	5
	— feel as normal as before the episode of sickness. — be acceptec by others because of his changed behaviour. — reduce stress for his family member.	managing the patient at home. * Plan discussion with family members, the patient and the social worker.	the visit. * Tell the patient to work out his activities at home and work place. * Explain to relatives to involve the patient in routine activities and take his suggestions for family issues. * Encourage the patient and relatives to discuss their worries and anxieties after discharge. * Educate family members and the patient the importance of continuity of follow-up and medicines.	* Enquires about what medicine he has to take at home and how. * Ensures days of follow-up and the doctor whom he has to visit.

TO RECALL

Nursing Patient with Delusional Disorders
Definition of Delusional Disorders
Related disorders:

- Schizophrenia — Paranoid type
- Delusional disorders
- Paranoid personality
- Paranoia
- Psychoactive substance, drug abuse
- Organic mental disorder
- Other conditions—
  - ❋ Hearing loss in elderly
  - ❋ Immigrants, refugees and prisoners of war.
  - ❋ Leaving home first time.

Psychodynamics
Nursing Diagnosis
Nursing Care Plan

I. Therapeutic need
II. Psychosocial need
- reduce anxiety
- decrease delusions
- encourage movement
- promote accurate perception
- improve communication and IPR
- Improve socialization
- Provide security

III. Physical needs
- Nutritional need
- Personal hygiene
- Improve sleep
- Protect from injuries to self and others.

IV. Recreational needs
V. Spiritual need
VI. Discharge plan

NURSING THE PATIENT WITH EXCITEMENT

INTRODUCTION

An excited patient presents accelerated psychomotor activities. He/she has an excessive, activity, especially as a defence against anxiety or as an expression of a manic state.

DEFINITION

The excited episode is characterised by predminately *increased motor changes.* For example, overactivity, irritability, demanding, prone to injuries; *Elated mood,* that is inflated self-esteem continuously happy and jovial, makes jokes, laughs at trivial matters, spends money extravagantly. *Increased thought:* For example, flight of ideas, pressure of speech.

ETIOLOGICAL FACTORS

— Genetic predisposition
— Neurophysiological factors
— Biochemical factors
— Psychological and interpersonal factors
— Severe stress
— Sociocultural factors.
(Refer Chapter VII, Unit XVIII.)

ASSOCIATED CONDITIONS

— The associated conditions in which excitement is presented are:
* Mood (affective) disorders
* Manic stage
* Schizophrena — catatonic excitement
* Anxiety disorders
* Organic disorders
* Organic mental disorders
* Psychoactive substance/drug abuse disorders.

PSYCHO-DYNAMICS

As in depression, the ego is affected and is not able to mediate the ID and Superego. ID predominates. The patient has dependency for love and affection. Though excited, the individual feels worthless and useless but denies these feelings as he is not able to tolerate them. Worthlessness is expressed with arrogance. He starts manipulating other people. Manipulation helps him to protect himself from failure. It also gives him a false sense of power and control. Elation and hyperactivity are an appeal for love. The family puts in pressure on the child to achieve high social and academic success. The child develops ambivalent feelings towards parents.

NURSING DIAGNOSIS

Increased physical activity (hyperactivity) change in nutritiona intake.
Inability to sleep
Change in weight
Increased sexual drive
Inappropriate dressing
Change in habits like use of alcohol and drugs
Refusal of medication
Increased irritability
Increased euphoria
Delusion of grandiosity/spending extravagantly
Expansive thoughts
Emotional liability
Argumentative
Decreased attention and concentration
Inflated self-concept
Impaired social functioning
Impaired communication
Impulsive in decision-making
Denial of problem
Related himself to God
or religious people.

TIPS FOR THE NURSE TO PROVIDE CARE TO HYPERACTIVE

Have a non-threatening approach
You should remain calm and firm
Provide support, recreation and appropriate diversion
Enforce limits
Restrain from getting involved in hilarity of the patient
Accept the patient here and now, avoid arguments
Cause of disturbed behaviour to locate, channelize activity
To see to physical, psychosocial needs of the patient
Immediate intervention to somatic complaints
Verbalize feelings, violent behaviour to be discouraged
Environment, calm, non-stimulating and safe.

NURSING CARE PLANS OF EXCITED PATIENT

NURSING NEEDS	GOALS	PLANNING	IMPLEMENTATION	EVALUATION
1	2	3	4	5
I. THERAPEUTIC NEEDS				
To help the patient to accept and take medicine.	STG To help the patient to take medicine regularly. LTG To enable the patient to: — take complete treatment — get the blood level checked, if required. — reduce a feeling of excitement and other symptoms.	* Plan giving medicine in time. Explain to the patient the need for taking medicine. * The patient refuses treatment because he enjoys elated feelings. * The patient has denial towards sickness, so discontinues medicine in between, plan explaining to relatives the continuity of treatment.	* Explain the need for treatment in short sentences. * Give medicine regularly to the patient. * Check side-effects of the medicine, record and report. * If the patient complains of earache or any injury, take him for a check-up. * Treat any wound of the patient because he neglects it and it may become infected. * Check the report of the lithium level, if the patient is on lithium carbonate. * Reduce salt in diet if the patient is getting lithium carbonate.	* Takes medicine as directed. * Expresses side-effects of the medicine. * Asks when the blood has to be sent for test.

1	2	3	4	5
II. PHYSICAL NEEDS				
To reduce physical activity and provide adequate sleep.	STG To help the patient to conserve his energy. Get less fatigued and exhausted. LTG To enable the patient to: — channelize energy — improve the sleep pattern.	* As these patients have boundless energy, they keep pacing up and down. Plan activities so that the patient can sit in between for some time. * Enforce on him a few rest hours on the bed. * Direct his activities.	* Allow the patient to tear a sheet and make some dusters for the ward. * Ask him to come to the duty room to take medicine (directing his activities) * Allow him to play throw ball so that his hostility is on inanimate things (channelizing energy). * See that play partner is not a depressive patient as his excitement will increase. Avoid competitive games. * Leave some magazine near the bedside. * Encourage him to complete activity which he has started. * Provide him with a calm environment. * Encourage naps in	* Sits in between, looks at a magazine and walks about. * Sits with another patient for 10 minutes.

1	2	3	4	5
			day-time. * Encourage him to sleep for six to eight hours.	
To improve diet and fluid intake.	STG To help the patient to improve his intake of food. LTG To enable the patient to: — give attention to his diet. — improve his weight. — improve his general health.	* Plan the foods which the patient can walk and eat as he/she feels that he/she does not have enough time to eat. * Concentration is poor and the patient cannot spend too much time on eating. * Due to exhaustion more food and fluids will be required.	* Give 'Finger Foods' the patient can hold, eat and walk * Put vegetable in a chapati roll and give to the patient. * Give an apple. * Peel off oranges and bananas and give to the patient. * Provide frequent and adequate meals. * Give plenty of water as these patients are on lithium carbonate. * Give no additional salt because of lithium therapy. * Give a high-protein, high-carbohydrate diet. * Serve food with minimum distraction in the environment. * Record weight.	* Improves in weight. The patient eats adequately while talking and walking. * Gradually sits and eats certain foods like rice and dal.

1	2	3	4	5
			* Maintain an intake/output chart.	
To protect the patient from injury to self and others.	STG To prevent homicide and suicide acts. LTG To enable the patient to: — avoid injury to himself. — avoid causing injury to others	* Plan less furniture in the room as the patient may injure him-self and will not bother about bleeding or an infected wound. * Due to hostility he/she may injure anyone, so check that a sharp instrument, glass or any other thing is not found near the patient.	* Maintain calm, supportive and structured environment. * Provide a non-stimulating environment. Avoid leaking taps, doors and fans making noise, for the patient may get irritated. * Avoid agruments in the ward. * Avoid competitive plays which may arouse hostility in the patient. * Check for injury, bruises or any infection. * Dress the wound even though the patient refuses.	* The patient checks himself before throwing a glass.
			* Limit his behaviour (if the patient went and shouted at the nurse/doctor) talk to him and tell him that today he can't	* Tells a relative of another patient: "I am sorry for throwing the cards while playing."

1	2	3	4	5
			watch T.V. because of his unacceptable behaviour) * Avoid keeping two excited patients in the same cubicle.	
To encourage appropriate dressing and grooming.	STG To help the patient to be accepted by others. LTG To enable the patient to: — dress according to weather and place. — develop a proper self-image. — come out of his elated symptoms. — improve judgement.	* Plan helping the patient to dress according to time, weather and place. * It is difficult to shave as the patient keeps moving. * He may wear bright clothes. A three-piece suit in hot summer. * Ladies may use red bright lipstick, bindi and flowers on head. * Sometimes the patient remains seminude.	* Help the patient to judge dressing according to weather. * The patient may come and say that "today my husband is coming to meet, Sister, I want to wear this red saree, red lipstick and some flowers. Explain to her that it is good to be happy, but in hospital these things are not appreciated. However, you can wear light lipstick, and a light-coloured saree. * Discourage too much of clothing in summer and inadequate clothing in winter.	* The patient gradually develops judgement that she needs to be clean and adequately dressed.

1	2	3	4	5
			* Enforce adequate clothing. Ignore their maladaptive behaviour towards inadequate clothing.	
To reduce verbal activity	STG To help him speak when it is required. LTG To enable the patient to: — allow others to speak. — prevent hoarseness of voice.	* Plan discussion in which the patient gets less opportunity to speak. * Explain to him the reason of pain in throat or hoarseness of voice. * The patient is verbally caustic, hostile, provocative or teasing. Prevent the patient from adopting this behaviour.	* Focus on a small topic for discussion. * Give a chance to others to talk. * Give him warm saline water for gargles. * If required, apply throat paint. * Encourage him to speak slowly and with pauses. * Give a low response to the patient's jokes and caustic remarks. * Discourage argument in the ward. * Set limits if the patient teases other patients. Tell him: "You will not be meeting that patient again."	* Gives chance to others to sepak. * Makes an attempt to listen to others.
Pursue to attend to personal hygiene	STG To develop a sense of well-	* During time of hyper-activity and	* Encourage the patient to attend	* Identifies the firmness in instruction.

1	2	3	4	5
	being. LTG To enable the patient to: — maintain personal hygiene. — develop concern about his belongings. — develop regular bowel habits.	grandiosity the patient might have given away own clothings and other belongings. Arrangement should be made for his clothing. * Help the patient to attend his activities independently. * The patient needs to be helped for regular bowel habits as he does not spend required time in these activities and has constipation.	to personal hygiene with minimum assistance. * Provide him with clothings and toilet articles because the patient might have given away his clothes due to his grandiosity. * Help the patient to select clothings according to weather. * Ensure that the patient attends to minimum care of brushing, bathing, changing clothes, combing in the morning. Be firm. * Encourage the patient to spend time in the toilet to develop regular bowel habits.	* Maintains personal hygiene.
III. PSYCHOSOCIAL NEEDS				
To improve judgement.	STG To protect him from personal loss of material and money. LTG To enable the patient to:	* Help the patient to learn the loss which he is suffering due to grandosity delusion like the loss	* Adopt a passive friendly attitude toward the patient. * Ignore bizarre behaviour.	* Listens with concentration. * Refrains himself from assaultive remarks and acts. * Respects privacy

1	2	3	4	5
	— improve his judgement ability — reduce delusion of grandiosity. — develop an insight into his behaviour. — prevent him from sexual assault on others. — reduce euphoric feelings.	of belongings and money. * Needs to be reinforced about his identity. * Set a limit on his behaviour because for lack of inhibitions there may be danger of a sexually assaultive behaviour. * Physical assault can be reduced by setting limits.	* Explain to relatives not to leave any cheque book with the patient. * Check articles daily. * Check that he does not give away small or big articles to anyone. * If the female patient in the ward complains of sexual approaches by a male patient, do not ignore. * Be firm with the patient to control his behaviour. * Use a firm and matter-of-fact approach. Otherwise the patient will involve the therapists in jokes, hilarity, caustic remarks. * Observe and limit impulsive behaviour. (If the patient is shouting in the ward, take him to bed and say that he is not incharge of the ward to shout at anyone).	of other patients.

1	2	3	4	5
To improve attention and concentration	STG To help the patient to attend to his activities completely. LTG To enable the patient to: — improve attention span and concentration. — develop a sense of satisfaction and worthiness.	* The patient needs to be helped to improve attention and concentration span so that irritability and dependency decreases. * Planning of activities which require individual performance.	* Give a simple and solitary task in the beginning such as making some cotton balls, reading two pages — writing about herself/himself. * Decrease stimuli and distraction during work such as putting on a good film on VCR. * Observe if the patient gets distracted to stimuli too frequently.	* Does not respond too frequently to multiple stimuli.
To improve communication	STG To help the patient to improve interpersonal relationship. LTG To enable the patient to: — feel accepted by others. — reduce a feeling of dependency. — develop an insight into his delusions.	* The patient does not communicate with others because of grandiosity. Plan environment in which the patient can communicate. * Other patient may avoid communication because of his caustic, hostile, provocative and teasing remarks.	* Accept the patient "here and now" with his present problem. * Use simple and brief sentences. * Avoid arguments. Give a calm reassurance by putting hand on his/her shoulders. * Help the patient identify the remarks which were appreciated by others. * Ignore his caustic	* Speaks slowly and clearly. * Does not use very strong words while talking to others.

1	2	3	4	5
			remarks. * "Laugh with" the patient sometimes but do no "laugh at him".	
To improve appropriate socialization.	STG To help the patient develop an appropriate social interaction. LTG To enable the patient to: — interact with others. — prevent social isolation. — develop a realistic self-concept.	* Plan interaction and socialization of the patient with other patients. These patients do not interact because of grandeur. * Prevent him/her from becoming a centre of attraction/talk. * Plan in helping-him/her to have a realistic concept about self.	* Encourage the patient to talk to others in clear words. * Help him speak slowly and clearly so that others can understand him. * Allow the patient some seclusion hours. It will provide him with time for realization. * Encourage the patient to give a chance to others to speak.	* Expresses now he feels nice in the ward because other patients also come and talk to him.
To enhance a realistic self-concept.	STG To help the patient to develop a realistic self-concept. LTG To enable the patient to: — reduce a feeling of helplessness — reduce unrealistic self-evaluation.	* Plan reducing grandiosity which actually is due to low self-esteem. * Provide activities in which dignity of the patient can be maintained. * Reinforce the positive efforts made by the patient.	* Address the patient by name * Allow the patient the freedom to choose activities e.g. bath, taking food. * Use a passive, friendly and matter-of-fact approach.	* Identifies the method of coping with the negative self-concept.

1	2	3	4	5
			* Reinforce the successful efforts made by the patient during group therapy such as accepting that he is not God when pointed out by other patients.	
IV. RECREATIONAL NEEDS				
	STG To help him channelize his energy in a productive way. LTG To enable the patient to: — divert his mind from delusions of grandiosity. — improve his attention and concentration.	* Plan activities in which the patient's energy can be used appropriately. * Plan activities so that the patient is able to socialize and check his negative behaviour.	* Too much encouragement to be avoided. * Give tasks which are simple and can be finished quickly like writing and drawing. * Provide rags for tearing during aggressive moments. * Allow working at an individual level in the beginning for lack of teams sport.	* Does some activity with concentration. * Demonstrates acceptable behaviour in the group.
V SPIRITUAL NEEDS				
	STG To help the patient to come out of an unrealistic world that he is God.	* Plan regular spiritual activities in which the patient participates with others.	* Encourage the patient to come to the prayer room daily. * Let him pray along	* The patient feels one among the group of members.

1	2	3	4	5
	LTG To enable the patient to: — learn the value of life. — improve the quality of life.		with others * Allow spiritual reading.	
VI DICHARGE PLAN				
	STG Help the patient to meet basic needs independently. LTG To enable the patient to: — develop a balance between his activities and rest. — have less recurrence of disease. — get and give support to family members.	* The patient can plan his daily activities and look after his needs independently. * The nurse along with the patient should work out a plan for his/her rest and activities. * The patient and relatives can be helped to work out the routine of the patient.	* Send the patient on trial visits to home two, three times before discharge. * Make an assessment of his behaviour after his visit to home. * Assess the self-care abilities of the patient. * Help the patient and relatives to identify the side-effects of drugs and recurrence of disease. * Encourage the patient and relatives for follow-up and continuing the medicine. * Help relatives to identify the patient coming out of excitement and going into depression (depressive dips).	* The patient reports his stay was enjoyable at home. * He felt better at home than in hospital. * Listens carefully to instructions regarding drugs and follow-up days.

TO RECALL

- **Definition of Excitement**
- **Etiological factors**
- **Associated conditions**
- **Psychodynamics**
- **Nursing diagnosis**
- **Nursing Care Plan**

I. Therapeutic Needs

II. Physical Needs

- **Reduce physical activities and provide adequate sleep.**
- **Improve diet and fluid intake.**
- **Protect the patient from injury to self and others**
- **Reduce verbal activity**
- **Pursue the patient to attend to personal hygiene**

III. Psychosocial Needs

- **Improve judgement**
- **Improve attention and concentration**
- **Improve communication**
- **Appropriate socialization**
- **Realistic self-concept**

IV. Recreational Needs

V. Spiritual Needs

VI. Discharge Plan

NURSING PATIENT WITH DEPRESSION

INTRODUCTION

Depression is a state associated with the affect (mood) of a person. It is a pathological mood disturbance characterized by feelings, attitudes and beliefs the person has about self and his environment. For example, pessimism, hopelessness, helplessness, low self-esteem and a guilt feeling. On a continum from normal to pathological depression varies from sadness to a depressive psychotic disease.

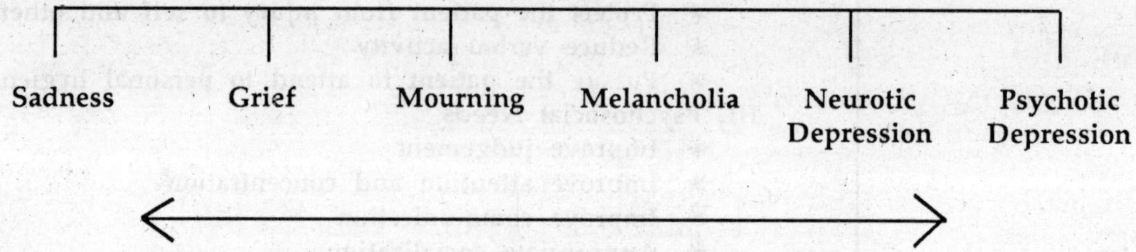

Fig. 27 : Continum from Normal to Pathological Depression.

DEFINITION

According to ICD- 10 (F 32), in a typical depressive episode of all three varieties, mild (F. 32.0), moderate (F. 32.1) and severe (F. 32.2 and F. 32.3), the individual usually suffers from a depressed mood, loss of interest and enjoyment, reduced energy leading to fatiguability and diminished activity. The other characteristic symptoms are:

a. reduced concentration and attention
b. reduced self-esteem and self-confidence
c. ideas of guilt and unworthiness
d. pessimistic views of the future
e. ideas or acts of self-harm or suicide
f. disturbed sleep
g. diminished appetite

ETIOLOGICAL FACTORS

* Genetic predisposition
* Neurophysiological factors
* Biochemical factors
* Psychological and interpersonal factors
* Severe stress
* Sociocultural factors
* *(Refer to Chapter VII, Unit XVIII)*

ASSOCIATED CONDITIONS WITH DEPRESSION

i. Anxiety disorders specifically separation anxiety
ii. Affective disorders — Depression caused in M.D.P. and involutional melancholia
iii. Schizophrenia presenting depressive symptoms
iv. Organic mental disorders — Dementia
v. Dysthymic disorder (depressive neurosis) and depression following OCN.
vi. Psychoative substance/drug abuse depression secondary to substance abuse.
vii. Depression associated with physical illness, chronic disease, surgery such as mastectomy, amputation, hysterectomy.
viii. Depression associated with other conditions such as divorce, death, side-effects of drugs, premenstrual period, postpartum psychosis.

TYPE OF DEPRESSION

Typical depressive episodes are: mild depressive episode, moderate depressive episode, severe depressive episode, including stupor.
(Refer to Chapter, VII Unit XVIII).

PSYCHODYNAMICS

Depressive reactions usually originate with an experience of loss. Loss may be material or personal. This leads to anger in the patients. Instead of directing anger towards others, the individual turns anger inwards. They are also excessively dependent on love, affection and encouragement given by others. Too much of dependency on others leads them to disappointment. The more they demand, the more others reject them. These people become hostile and angry towards those who reject them. Then they feel guilty because of hostility and develop a self-punishing attitude. These patients present (a) chronic hunger for affection, (b) a chronic guilt, (c) a need for control, (d) low self-esteem (e) a feeling of helplessness and powerlessness

DIFFERENCE IN ENDOGENCOUS AND EXOGENOUS

CRITERIA	ENDOGENOUS DEPRESSION	EXOGENOUS DEPRESSION
Synonomous Terms	Also called biological or psychotic depression.	Also called reactive or neurotic depression.
Genesis	Resulting from biological and personality deficit factors. Environment triggers it of, otherwise environment	Resulting from external and environmental stimulus. Change in environment will change the intensity of

CRITERIA	ENDOGENOUS DEPRESSION	EXOGENOUS DEPRESSION
	does not play a significant role.	depression
Intensity	Severity is marked. The client shows marked motor retardation or agitation. Not able to meet family, social and occupational commitments.	Less marked. The client is able to manage all types of commitments fairly well.
Physique	Typically pyknic/ mesomorphic in physique.	No typical body physique.
Premorbid Personality	Personality deficit such as cyclothymic personality presenting mood swings; can cope with a stressful situation when well.	Anxiety-prone reaction to envirnomental stress leads to a depressive episode.
Precipitating Factors	Absence of any specific factor.	Identification factors such as loss of person or money.
Social Class	Poor, lower and working class.	Middle or upper class.
Sex	Women especially at childbirth, menopausal phase, also in old age.	Men in most cultures.
Physiological Process	Physiological process slows down, muscles sag, posture slumps, face appears sad, walk is slow and dragging.	Physiological changes are less marked and change according to external factors. (happy environment will also bring change in the client)
Mood	The individual often cries, difficulty in sleeping, loss of appetite, thinking and concentration is decreased, does not change according to envirnoment.	Mood patchy, happy and sad. Changes according to environmental alteration.

CRITERIA	ENDOGENOUS DEPRESSION	EXOGENOUS DEPRESSION
Physical Care	Loses interest in physical care. May become constipated, dirty and sick.	The client is able to attend to his physical needs.
Sleep Pattern	Late insomnia. Early morning awakening. Sleeps in time, gets up at 3 or 4 AM (attempts/commits suicide in these quiet hours).	Early insomnia not able to get sleep. Once asleep, gets up in the morning only.
Diurnal Change	Feels lowest/depressed in the morning, may improve during the day.	Less depressed in the morning, may become more depressed as the day progresses.
Change in Thought and Perception	Severe delusional ideation, usually somatic, the patient says he lacks appetite because he has no stomach and bowels have turned into snakes. Mouth is a cave with no exit, depression may lead to stupor. Hallucination present, expresses suicidal thoughts.	Presents anxiety, restlessness and attention-seeking mechanisms.
Loss of Libido	Marked decrease in libido. No sexual desire at all.	Not usual. It may increase for seeking comfort or relief from anxiety.
Response to Treatment	Responds well to ECT and anti-depressant drugs.	Responds well to anti-depressants and psychotherapy.

Fig. 28 : Table Explaining Difference between Endogenous (Psychotic) and Exogenous (Neurotic) Depression.

NURSING DIAGNOSIS

The most common nursing diagnoses of depression for planning nursing care are:

* Suicidial ideation and attempts
* Decreased activity
* Increased weight loss
* Altered affect; apathy, ambivalence
* Loss of interest
* Reduced attention and concentration
* Impaired communication
* Impaired socialization
* Reduced self-esteem and self-concept
* Increased ideas of guilt and unworthiness
* Decreased sleep and appetite
* Self-care deficit (personal hygiene — bath, unkept, care of clothes and hair; diet intake)

NURSING CARE PLAN OF DEPRESSED PATIENT

NURSING NEEDS	GOALS	PLAN	IMPLEMENTATION	EVALUATION
1	2	3	4	5
I. THERAPEUTIC NEEDS				
Administering medicines and other treatment.	STG Reduce suicidal ideation. Prevent the patient going into stupor. LTG To help the patient to show decrease in depressive symptoms.	* Plan giving medicines as prescribed by the psychiatrist. * If electro-convulsive-therapy (ECT) is required, make preparation for the patient and relatives. * Plan for constant observation of the patient.	* Check the type of anti-depressants to be given. * Ensure the patient takes the medicines. * Give medicine at the right time (keep 5R in mind) * Observe for side-effects specially EPS *(Refer to Chapter VII, Unit XV)* * Prepare the patient and relatives for ECT *(Refer to Chapter, VII, Unit XVI).* * Make observation after drugs and ECT. * Ensure individual and group psychotherapy. * Constant observation of the patient	* Sits up in the bed. * Verbalize suicidal thoughts and plan.

1	2	3	4	5
			(one-to-one observation).	
II. PHYSICAL NEEDS				
To prevent suicidal ideation and attempt.	STG To prevent the patient from attempting to commit suicide. LTG To help the patient to: — find pleasure and meaning in life. — provide mental catharsis — prevent the patient from attempting to commit suicide. — reduce a feeling of ambivalence to live or die.	* Provide protection to the patient. * Plan a safe environment. * Plan observation for 24 hours. * Make an assessment of the method the patient has planned for attempting to commit suicide.	* Don't leave the patient alone. * Check for sharp instruments, glasses, necktie, rope or any such things by which the patient can strangulate. * Observe for "passive suicide" —the patient may starve or fall asleep in the bath tub/sink. * Close observation specially when the patient is coming out of depression, because he/she may have the energy and opportunity to kill himself/herself. * Check if he is collecting some drugs. * Check in the bathroom and toilet, as the patient might have	* Discusses his suicidal ideation with the nurse. * Explains the method adopted by him for attempting to commit suicide earlier. *

1	2	3	4	5
			planned to commit suicide, accompany him/her to the bathroom. * Don't allow patient to put bolt on the door of bathroom or toilet. * Encourage the patient to talk about his/her suicidal plan and method (check lethality). * Explain to the relative to inform him successful or happy events of the family. * Help the patient to gain an insight into the seriousness of the problem. * Help him identify new ways of coping with life situations (discussing the problems with friends and relatives). * Talk about an ambivalence feel-	

1	2	3	4	5
			ing the patient has. * Explain him that at certain moments the will to die overpowers but there are good things about living, specially when he is a wanted person by some people.	
To improve nutrition intake.	STG To help the patient to maintain body requirement To help him relief from' constipation. LTG To help the patient to: — take an adequate diet. — develop interest in eating. — improve weight — maintain physical health.	* The patient needs to be encouraged by the nurse and relatives to eat nutritional and adequate food to prevent from passive suicide. * The intake of food is less because of the intensity of depression, the patient should be allowed to talk about depressive thoughts. * Increase in weight will increase the patient's self-concept that he is improving. * Plan a schedule of diet to provide	* Provide food in a small quantity and at a time but frequently. * Ask the choice of food and serve in an attractive manner (would you like to have a boiled egg or omelete). * Serve food when everyone is eating. * Be with the patient when he is eating food. * Talk about his success and good behaviour while the patient is eating. * Pursue the patient	* The quantity of food intake improves. * Expresses happpiness when meals of his choice are served. * Grandual increase in weight.

1	2	3	4	5
		him relief from constipation.	to eat a full meal. * Give plenty of fluids and roughage, green leafy, vegetables, salad. * Plan out with the patient his diet for the next day. * Record the patient's weight. * Inform the patient about weight gain. * In case of stupor the patient needs to be tube-fed.	
To persue the patient to maintain personal hygiene	STG To help the patient keep clean, for a sense of well—being. LTG To help the patient to: — develop a sense of well-being. — take interest in his personal hygiene. — improve his appearance — improve his self-concept. — feel accepted by others.	* The patient does not show interest in his cleanliness due to depressive thoughts. * The patients has ideas of worthlessness, hopelessness which can be reduced by encouraging him to maintain his personal hygiene and feel accepted by others. * Plan that the patient wears clean and ironed	* Pursue the patient to brush his teeth in the morning. * Ensure that he takes his bath regularly. * In case of men, see that he shaves and takes care of his hair. * Explain to the patient to apply glycerine on his lips and women can use a light-coloured lipstick. * Explain to him to keep his nails	* Takes initiative in self-care. * Feels accepted by others. * The nurse may say,"You look clean and fresh today." * Starts his routine activity and feels nice. "Sister , today I have taken my bath and worn this dress which my wife brought." * Takes pride in his appearance.

1	2	3	4	5
		clothes. * Plan his skin care. * Plan to help him regulate his bowels and bladder habits.	clean. * Check that the patient has changed into clean and pressed clothes. * Encourage fluids to prevent cracking of skin and constipation. * Tell the patient to sit in the toilet for sometime for paristalaltic stimulation. * Encourage the patient to go out of the bed after maintaining his personal hygiene. * Explain to other team members to appreciate his cleanliness.	
To balance activity, rest and sleep.	STG To help the patient improve his sleep pattern. LTG To help the patient to: — develop a regular pattern of sleep. — get adequate hours of rest. — feel active during	* Plan day-time activities according to the patient's occupation. * Rest is significant as fatigue will reinforce depression. * The nurse can plan simple new activi-	* Pursue the patient to do activities during day time. * Encourage the patient to come to the activity room. * Encourage him to have a bath before going to bed. * Provide a hot glass	* Gets an adequate amount of rest and sleep.

1	2	3	4	5
	the day time.	ties with new achievable goals. * The patient expresses his inability or inadequacy in performing even small activities like bath, eating.	of milk. * Provide a clean and comfortable bed. * Allow the relative to stay with him. * Provide a calm environment with minimum noise and disturbance in the ward. Explain to the patient that activities will help him/her feel better. * Explain that day-time activity will lead to some amount of fatigue, thereby good sleep at night.	
II. PSYCHOSOCIAL NEEDS				
To reduce a feeling of dependency and helplessness	STG To help the patient to develop a feeling of self-sufficiency. LTG To help the patient to: — develop a positive self-concept. — reduce a feeling of helplessness. — improve his sefl—	* The nurse must plan with the patient activities which he' can perform independently. * Family members should be explained to take the patient's suggestion on any family	* Allow the patient to make a decision when he wants to go for a bath. It gives him freedom to decide. * Encourage him to eat, comb his hair, shave without any assistance. * Provide activities	* The patient feels confident of doing his activities. * Says confidently, "Now I can take care of myself."

1	2	3	4	5
	concept.	decision.	according to the interest and capability of the patient. * Show respect by calling the patient by name. * Listen to the patient carefully if he is making any self-depreciatory remarks (such as I am good for nothing).	
To improve self-concept.	STG To help the patient improve his self-image. LTG To help the patient to: — feel confident in the group. — reduce a feeling of worthlessness. — feel that he is important and wanted.	* Planning of activities which help in raising his self-concept. * Help the patient to identify his positive points/assets. * Help the patient to identify daily gains and provide positive reinforcement. * Avoid oppportunities in which the	* Provide brief explanations of activities. * Encourage him to do those activities of which he is confident. * Inform the patient the progress he has made and encourage him. For example, "Everybody appreciated the way you distributed breakfast in the ward." * Discuss with the patient how things have	* Walks with confidence in the ward. * Takes initiative to socialize. * Finds out what all is going on at home or work place.

1	2	3	4	5
		patient may take an inappropriate decision.	changed because now he is not so depressed. * Explain to relatives not to put him in difficult decision-making situations.	
'To improve communication	STG To help the patient develop self-confidence. To develop confidence in others. LTG To help the patient: — develop trust in others. — express his anger in a non-destructive manner. — reduce his emotional flatness/ apathetic attitude.	* Planning of a non-threatening environment. * Provide an opportunity to verbalize his emotionall and painful experience. * Plan teaching certain communication skills. * Encourage the patient to develop relationship with people with whom a positive conversation takes place. Avoid letting him talk to elated pateints. The patient may feel more discouraged. * Help him verbalize the meaning of his gestures.	* Talk to the patient. * Use an active friendly approach. * Listen to the patient actively by responding such as by nodding and by using such words as hum, hai, continue. * Encourage him to talk. * Explain his emotional flatness to a particular situation. * Explain his emotional flatness to a particular situation. "Not responding to the patient's relative who is very happy because his son	* Talks clearly. * Likes to talk to some people about his problems. * Expresses happiness on seeing the relatives of another patient.

1	2	3	4	5
			stood first in the class." * Be brief in conversation. * Relate an incident where others also make mistakes. * Calmly accept the patient's angry response. * Help him know that expression of his anger did not harm anyone. * Encourage him for talking to relatives in an effective manner. "I am missing children, why did'nt you bring them even once?" * Observe non-verbal gestures. The patient may say that he is happy but looks sad. Tell him the difference in what he is saying and feeling.	
To improve socialization	STG To Help the patient develop self-confidence to	* Plan encouragement in socialization as these	* Accept the patient with whatever feelings he has	* The patient says that he does not feel very lonely

	2	3	4	5
	help him learn the importance of socialization LTG To help the patient: — improve the quality of life. — prevent self-absorption. — Enjoy a meaningful relatioship. — improve his self-concept. — reduce social isolation.	patients are self-absorbed. * They are not interested in developing a relationship. * Help the patient feel confident to interact with others. * Adopt a non-rejecting attitude. * Social isolation needs to be reduced.	come to the hospital. * Remind him of his worthiness. The patient says, "Everybody in my family is worried about my sickness." * Help the patient gradually to socialize with others. * Discourage socialization with manic patients because it may reinforce self-condemning ideas. * Create a socially interesting situation. For example, call all the patient and tell themto spend time in your patient's cubicle. * Gradually help him to move out of the bed and interact with others.	now. * Takes initiative in interacting with others.
To reduce a feeling of guilt and apathy.	STG To help the patient verbalize	* Discuss with the patient what guilt	* Help the patient verbalize his guilt	* The patients may express "Oh, so

1	2	3	4	5
	a feeling of guilt. LTG To help the patient : — overcome a feeling of guilt. — develop a realistic approach to life. — reduce his apathetic feelings.	feelings will be removed by depressive acts or suicide ideas. * Plan activities in which the patient describes what he is going through. * Encourage him to learn that mistakes are made and one can always improve.	feeling. * Make an assessment of his guilt feeling and relationship with depression. * Encourage him to talk about an alternative solution to his guilt feeling. * Help him identify the secondary gains due to depression such as not going for work. * Encourage him to attend group therapy. * Allow other patients to talk about their experience. * Allow him to clean his surroundings, wash his own dirty clothes.	these types of difficulties are faced by many people."
III. RECREATIONAL NEEDS				
	STG To help the patient become more active. To help the patient divert himself from self-absorp-	* Plan recreational activities which the patient likes. * The patient gradually should be encouraged to	* Find out interests of the patient. * Help the patient do activities of his choice first with his relatives or	* Enjoys the activities in the wards. * Helps in organizing Independence Day activities in the ward.

1	2	3	4	5
	tion. LTG To help the patient: — improve the quality of life. — find pleasure in life. — develop a sense of recovery.	initiate the activities in the day-care room. * Plan activities in which he feels successful and satisfied.	nurse. * Encourage him to go to another patient for playing cards or ludo. * Allow him to sit outside where other patients are playing badminton or table tennis. * Encourage him to play badminton.	* Feels confident and says: "Sister, I also help in my office at functions."
V. SPIRITUAL NEEDS				
	STG To help the patient enjoy his routine life. LTG To help the patient: — find meaning in his life. — develop a sense of satisfaction. — enjoy the quality of life.	* Plan out regular spiritual activities. May be praying, reading of some religious book or meditation.	* Encourage the patient to go to the prayer room. * Help him read the religious book of his choice. * Divert his mind from self-absorption and a feeling of worthlessness by encouraging him to discuss yoga and meditation. * Encourage the patient to make a confession.	* The patient enjoys his routine. * Participates in the morning prayer and yoga.
VI. DISCHARGE PLAN				
To reduce depressive	STG To avoid read-	* Plan a free and	* Encourage the	* The patient looks

1	2	3	4	5
feelings.	mission. To help the patient adjust to his family and work place. LTG To help the patient: — overcome the depressive episodes. — adjust in his job. — develop a sense of adequacy and being accepted. — participate in family activities. — find a meaning in his life, with no suicidal ideas.	frank discussion with the patient and family members. * Work out a discharge plan with the patient and his relatives. * Help family members identify the change in the behaviour of the patient. * Plan encouraging the patient to develop a support system from other than relatives.	patient to talk about his anxieties after discharge. * Help the patient express the difficulties at his job prior to sickness. * Allow relatives to participate in discussion. * Help the patient identify key members in his support system. * Re-establish relationship with these key members. * Educate family members and the patient on the continuity of medicine and follow-up. * Discuss plans of helping at home after discharge.	forward to discharge from the hospital.

TO RECALL

- Definition of depression
- Etiological factors
- Associated conditions with depression
- Types of depression
- Psychodynamics
- Difference between Endogenous and reactive depression
- Nursing diagnosis
- Nursing care plan

I. Therapeutic Needs

II. Physical Needs
- Prevention of suicide
- Improve nutrition
- Maintenance of personal hygiene
- Encourage adequate rest and sleep

III. Psychosocial Needs
- Reduce feelings of dependency and helplessness
- Improve self-concept
- Improve communication
- Improve socialization
- Reduce a feeling of guilt and apathy

IV. Recreational Needs

V. Spiritual Needs

VI. Discharge Plan

NURSING PATIENT WITH WITHDRAWN BEHAVIOUR

INTRODUCTION

Withdrawn behaviour is common to many psychiatric disorders. It is a defensive reaction consisting of retreat from social contact and involvement or from threatening situations. The patient avoids an opportunity to interact with others.

DEFINITION

Withdrawn means removed from immediate contact or easy approach. Isolated, socially detached and unresponsive (Webster Dictionary).

Withdrawn behaviour is an attempt in which the patient tries to avoid social interaction. Usual pattern of withdrawn behaviour is slow onset, developed over a periood of months or years. Friends and relatives observe the decrease in normal interest. Mood or affect is flat and inappropriate, blunting of emotions. Speech is unintelligible as the patient does not care whether he is understood or not. Not interested in communicating. Talks to self. Thinking is disturbed. The patient has persecutory delusions. Has delusion of grandeur, thinks that he can direct everyone. Hallucination, auditory, olfactory, tactile and gustatory present. Judgement is poor.

So the withdrawn behaviour may be physical like in *Stupor*. It can be verbal in which the patient does not talk to anyone and remains *Mute*.

ASSOCIATED CONDITIONS

According to DSM-III-R, withdrawn behaviour may be presented in conditions such as schizophrenia, mood disorders (depression), organic mental disorders, delusional disorders, avoidant personality disorders.

Other conditions can be physical handicap, mental disharmony, aging and physical illness, specially with odours like colostomy, open wound, ulcers due to cancer.

PSYCHODYNAMICS

In these individuals the ego functioning is impaired. Ego is not able to mediate between self and external reality. When a person is not able to cope up with external reality he/she regresses to an early development stage. Then the Id predominates. The individual tries to isolate himself from others. He is not able to think at the adult level. He has a problem in thinking and judgement also.

NURSING DIAGNOSIS

- Non-compliance to treatment due to poor insight.
- Impaired communication.
- Altered perception.
- Disturbed thought; delusions, self-preoccupation and narcissism, suspicious, feeling of guilt.
- Impaired socialization.
- Low self-concept.
- Self-care deficit; personal hygiene, diet, clothings, impacted stool.
- Protection from self-harm.
- Decreased activity/activity intolerance

NURSING CARE PLAN OF WITHDRAWN BEHAVIOUR PATIENT

NURSING NEEDS	GOALS	PLAN	IMPLEMENTATION	EVALUATION
1	2	3	4	5
I. THERAPEUTIC NEEDS				
Compliance to treatment	STG To help the patient to develop a feeling of improvement. LTG To help the patient to: — get rid of a feeling of guilt and self-destructive behaviour — decrease a feeling of worthlessness.	* The patient needs to be given anti-depressants/antipsychotic drugs as prescribed. * Some patients are given ECT. Relatives need to be explained.	* Help the patient accept the treatment. * Be firm that the patient swallows the medicines. * Prepare the patient for ECT, if required. * Observe for any untoward effects of drugs and ECT. * Record and report any side-effects.	* The patient takes the medicine regularly. Guilt feeling is reduced. * Becomes more responsive.
II. PHYSICAL NEEDS				
Help the patient to maintain personal hygiene.	STG Help the patient to remain clean. Help him in improving appearance. LGT To help the patient to: — attend to his personal hygiene — have a sense of well-being — maintain personal hygiene for aesthetic sense.	* Withdrawn behaviour leads the patient to neglect personal hygiene like bath, mouth care, mouth may smell and a crust will be formed on lips, eyes dirty with discharge. Men do not shave. Hair is unkept and there may be pediculosis in	* Use an active friendly approach. * Assist in maintaining personal hygiene. * Pursue the patient to get up from the bed. * Take him/her to the bathroom to brush teeth, take bath, wash hair and change dress	* The patient feels fresh and clean. * Sits up in the bed for some time.

1	2	3	4	5
		hair. * The patient avoids changing clothes because of a feeling of uselessness or having no energy to change. * The patient does not bother about his/her appearance.	daily. Provide the patient with his/her own clothings. * If the patient has pediculosis, give treatment. * Ensure that the patient combs his/her hair. * Give some glycerine to apply on lips. * Encourage the patient to maintain personal hygiene daily. * In case of females help the patient to maintain perineal care/menstrual hygiene.	
Help the patient for regular evacuation of bowels and bladder.	STG To help the patient develop regular bowel habits. LTG To help the patient to: — prevent himself from complications of impacted stool or urinary infection.	* Withdrawn patient is slow and sluggish in all activities. * He/she avoids going for defecation and urination which may lead to impacted stool or urinary infection.	* Encourage the patient to get up from bed and take three or four rounds of the ward. * Insist on going to the toilet for urination and defecation. * If constipated, provide plenty of fluid, roughage in	* The patient develops regular bowel habits.

1	2	3	4	5
			diet and green leafy vegetables. * If the stool is impacted, 'Glove Finger' removal needs to be done. * Maintain an intake-output chart.	
Improve in take of food and fluids.	STG To privde adequate nutrition. LTG To help the patient to: — develop interest in eating. — promote physical health.	* The patient does not have interest in eating or physically feels very weak (tired) to eat, so neglects eating or takes more time to finish up one meal. At times the patient needs to be fed. * The patient wants to punish himself by not eating because of a guilt feeling.	* Serve to the patient food of his choice. * Give small and frequent meals. * Give liquids and semi-solids in the beginning in which the patient does not require much of mastication such as custard, curd and rice. * Serve food in an attractive manner. * Allow the patient to eat slowly, do not hurry through. * Sit with the patient when he/she is eating, discuss pleasant topics. * Give fluids like water, milk, juice in between.	* Starts eating food on his own. * Increase in food intake.

1	2	3	4	5
			* If the patient-feels too weak to eat, feed him/her with a spoon. * Rarely tube feeding is required. * Maintain an intake/output chart.	
Improve activities and sleep	STG To involve the patient in activities. To have good sleep at night. LTG To help the patient to: — regain energy. — identify positive assets.	* A withdrawn patient has decreased activities because he/she lacks energy (feels). Guilt predominates and thinks it is better not to live. * Keeps lying in the bed. Even finds it difficult to turn the position. Takes very long to get up from the bed. * Feels exhausted even while playing cards or sitting in the bed. * The patient keeps lying without activities and cannot sleep at night.	* Develop therapeutic inter-personal relationship. * Accept the patient but be firm in approach. * Ask the patient to get up and sit in the bed. * Provide a simple concrete activity like clean his/her bed, side locker. * Fold his/her clothes, comb hair. * The patient may take time, ask her/him to do activity in less time the next day. * Pat him/her when the patient finishes activity early. * Walk with the patient in the	* The patient feels less exhausted.

1	2	3	4	5
			cubicle/ward. * Limit nap during day time. * Provide a calm and secure environment, so that the patient sleeps well.	* Sleeps throughout night.
Protect self or others from injury	STG To prevent the patient from self-injury. LTG To help the patient: — not to harm others and self.	* The patient may attack self or others due to hallucination or delusion. * Provide a safe environment.	* Provide a safe environment * Discourage condemning remarks by others (He cannot even take food). * Observe the patient for his behaviour such as hostility. * Remove articles by which he can harm himself or others.	* The patient feels he is wanted. * Discusses feelings of self-injury.
III. PSYCHOSOCIAL NEEDS				
Improve communication.	STG To help the patient develop communication. LTG To help the patient to: — develop self-confidence. — communicate with others.	* A withdrawn patient also withdraws from verbal communication and becomes mute or non-communicative. * It may be due to negativism, denial	* Share the patient's silence by sitting near him/her. * Silence of nurse Conveys to the patient that silence is not "bad". * Be calm and tolerant.	* Starts talking in a low pitch initially.

1	2	3	4	5
	— improve social interaction.	of existence, fearful of others' reaction. Using means of control. * Dependency on the nurse, non-communication are like one-sided relatedness that is from the therapist side.	* Presence of the nurse may encourage the patient to talk. * Do not probe, interrogate the patient. * Do not get impatient. * If the patient opens his/her eyes and looks at you after one week, it shows the patient has accepted you and wants your presence. * Appreciate the nonverbal communication such as waiting for the nurse, preparing the place for interaction. * Concentrate on mumbling of the patient and a low-pitch talk. * Establish a positive relationship.	
Improve self-concept and socialization.	STG To help the patient socialize. LTG To help the patient :	* The patient feels ucomfortable in a social setting. Accept his behav-	* Stay with the patient in silence. * Encourage the patient to social-	* Sits with others. * Participates in activities with confidence.

1	2	3	4	5
	— reduce social isolation. — reduce a feeling of unworthiness.	iour. Gradualy enlarge his/her socialization. * Allow the patient to interact with people who will accept him/her. * Prevent this patient from becoming comfortable with loneliness. This will decrease his/her self-concept.	ize/interact frequently. * Limit the number of persons with whom he interacts. * Gradually increase the number * Discourage the patient from spending long hours in his room by self. * Start a topic in which he can participate. * Discourage an excited patient to talk to a severely withdrawn patient. * Encourage the patient for his positive performance.	* Responds to questions * Initiates conversation.
Help to decrease hallucination.	STG To help reduce misperception LTG To help the patient: — have a realistic perception.	* The patient develops social isolation and becomes autistic. Hallucination replaces his/her interaction with others, specially auditory hallucination.	* Help the patient to talk about his anxiety. * Encourage the patient to come and inform the nurse about his hallucination. * Talk about other	* The patient talks about his anxiety and association with voices he hears. * States that he does not hear any more voices. * Interaction im-

1	2	3	4	5
		* Development of relationship will help in reducing hallucination.	things but not hallucination. * Dismiss the patient's hallucination as "oh, these voices!" * Ensure that someone is available in whom he/she has trust.	proves.
Help in improving thinking and memory.	STG To help in taking an immediate decision. — To reduce delusion of the patient. LTG To help the patient: — improve in his thinking. — reduce delusions.	* Planning needs to be done to stimulate thinkings as the withdrawn patient has poverty of ideas and difficulty in taking decisions. * Marked delusional thinking interferes with abstract thinking. * The patient's regression needs to be reduced. Because of neologism, echolalia and rumination thinking does not make progress. * The patient needs to be helped to improve his thinking and memory.	* Give a magazine or book to read. * Do not force the patient to make decisions intially. * Gradually, provide him with a simple situation like "would you like to brush your teeth now ?" * Be alert to listen to the delusional thought and identify its relationship with withdrawn behaviour. * Ignore the delusion, Tell others also to do the same. * Divert the delusional thought	* Take initiative in making a decision. * Less preoccupied with his thoughts. * Tries to maintain self-care.

1	2	3	4	5
			into some simple activity (helping the nurse in counting blankets). * Check for improved recent and remote memory. * Reorient the patient to time, place and people.	
To reduce withdrawn behaviour.	STG To help the patient develop trust in others. To help him/her to interact with others. LTG To help the patient to: — improve his/her self-confidence. — identify his worth.	* Try to identify the causes of withdrawn behaviour and help the patient learn his positive points. * Explore situations in which his/her withdrawn behaviour can be reduced.	* Allow the patient to talk how he/she developed the withdrawn behaviour. * Encourage the patient to verbalize his/her feelings by which he can bring a change in his behaviour. * Encourage him/her to talk about his/her guilt feelings. * Allow him to wash his dirty clothes, clean the dirty locker. * Explain to him the importance of his participation in family matters. * Help him assess his positive points,	* The patient identifies new ways of handling his/her problems.

1	2	3	4	5
			like how sincere worker he had been in his office, contribution made in children's education, family crisis. * Encourage the patient to react to others' happiness and sorrow. * Allow the patient to express hostility.	
IV. RECREATIONAL NEEDS				
	STG To help him divert his/her mind from delusions, guilt feeling and feeling of worthlessness. LTG To help the patient to: — develop interest in activities	* The patient is unable to initiate activites due to withdrawn behaviour. * Feels he is useless, worthless and helpless to do any activity. * Help the patient to choose recreational activities of his choice.	* Ask for the hobbies of the patient. * Encourage him/her to do one activity of choice. * Take the patient to the day-care room. * Encourage him to play with other patients.	* Starts enjoying some of the activities in the ward.
V. SPIRITUAL NEEDS				
	STG To develop a meaning in life. LTG To help the patient to:	* Planning needs to be done to promote optimistic feelings in the	* Encourage the patient to participate in religious activities if he	* The patient gets relief after confessing to the nurse his/her guil

1	2	3	4	5
	— reduce a feeling of despair, worthlessness. — enjoy life. — promote a positive self-concept.	patient. Help the patient see life realistically with an improved self-image.	wants. * Discuss the positive things which are likely to occur in his life in future. * Take the patient out to see the beautiful things in the environment. * Provide an opportunity for confession if the patient so desires.	feeling.
VI. DISCHARGE PLAN				
	STG To help the patient to attend to self-care. Take medicine regularly. LTG To help the patient to: — find a support system among friends and family members. — initiate social interaction.	* The patient should be encouraged to discuss his discharge activities. Explain to relatives the slow progress made by the patient. * Discourage them to do activities for the patient, if required.	* Encourage the patient to talk about his discharge plan. Send him home on parole. * Observe his expression of happiness or sadness on discharge. * Encourage the patient to verbalize his/her feeling. * Discuss with the patient and relatives together the self-care activities which the patient should perform himself. * Encourage his compliance to treatment and follow-up.	* The patient expresses the feeling that he is better and wants to go home.

TO RECALL

- * Definition of withdrawn behaviour
  Associated conditions
    Psychodynamics
    Nursing diagnosis
    Nursing care plan
      I Therapeutic needs
      II Physical needs
        * Maintain personal hygiene
        * Encourage regular bowel and bladder habits.
        * Improve intake of food and fluid
        * Protect self and others from injury
      III Psychosocial needs
        * Improve communication
        * Improve self-concept and socialization
        * Decrease hallucination
        * Improve thinking
        * Reduce withdrawn behaviour
      IV Recreational need
      V Spiritual need
      VI Discharge need plan

NURSING PATIENT WITH SUICIDAL IDEATION

INTRODUCTION

Suicide is an act or instance of taking one's own life voluntarily. In psychiatric nursing, suicide threats and gestures are taken as an emergency. It may be a symptom of depression schizophrenic withdrawal, turning of hostility inward to self, an attempt to make others feel guilty and means to release unbearable pain.

MYTHS ABOUT SUICIDE

a. It is felt that the suicide threat is just a bid for attention and should not be taken seriously.
b. Suicide/thoughts should not be discussed.
c. Only psychotics commit suicide.
d. Persons from good families do not attempt to commit suicide.
e. A failed suicide attempt should be treated as manipulative behaviour

(Refer to Chapter VII, Unit XX)

EPIDEMIOLOGY

The variables which can be considered to assess the epidemiology of suicide are:

a. Social
b. Demorgaphic
c. Clinical
d. Self-destructive personality/people

(Refer to Unit XX)

ASSOCIATED CONDITIONS

Related DSM III-R Conditions

— Bipolar disorders
— Major depressions schizophrenia
— Delusional (Paranoid) disorders
— Psychoactive substance - use disorder
— Dysthymic

Other conditions may be physical deformity due to accident, chronic illness i.e. the patient on heamodilaysis terminal state, aging and a crisis situation like appearing in a court case, debts, unemployment, marital disharmony and separation.

ETIOLOGY

Shives L-R has described the causative or motives for attempting to commit suicide.

1. *A progressive failure to adapt*—the individual no longer is able to adapt to stressers.
2. *Feeling of alienation or isolation* — especially in teenagers. Isolation may occur gradually. It can be self-imposed or due to lack of assertiveness.

3. ***Feelings of anger and hostility towards a significant person*** — Son may commit suicide to let father feel very bad for his continuous scolding. It can be anger towards guilt which the client may use by self-killing.
4. ***A reunion wish or fantasy*** — reunion with a friend who dies in an accident.
5. ***To end a feeling of hopelessness and helplessness***— The client may feel that everything what he wanted to achieve has been done, now there is nothing to be done in his life, so he commits suicide.
6. ***A cry for help.***
7. ***An attempt to live with death from a feeling of frustration, ambivalence***— life (Eros) and death (Thanatos) exist in every individual. A person has an ambivalent feeling of living and dying. For example, a stuntman, a rash driver.
8. ***An attempt to save face*** — due to business failure or debt.
9. ***Terminal or chronic illness.***
10. ***Impaired thought process*** (delusions)

SUICIDE

Suicide is sometimes based on an individual's ties in society.

a. *Altruistic Suicide* — A term used by Durkheim for what he described as suicide associated with excessive integration with a group. For example, suicide by old people who believe they are a burden to their families.

b. *Egoistic Suicide* — A type of suicide that is the result of the individual's feelings of extreme alienation from others and from society in general. For example, an extremely sincere and honest worker in a corrupt setting.

c. *Anomic Suicide* — A term introduced by Durkheim to identifiy a type of suicide caused by the disorientation of the individual after an unfavourable change in a financial or social situation due to loss of money in business. The subject believes his previous life style is no longer possible.

d. *Samsonic Suicide* or *Suicide of Revenge* — to spite others or experiencing as being unfriendly. If the husband is unfaithful to his wife, she may attempt to commit suicide to take revenge from him.

PSYCHODYNAMICS

A person attempting to commit suicide has a feeling of isolation, hopelessness and helplessness. Is depressed markedly. Avoids social interaction. Expresses a desire fo kill himself because of worthlessness or a guilt feeling. The associated conditions of attempting to commit suicide are schizophrenia, depression and anxiety. *(Refer to Unit XX)*

NURSING DIAGNOSIS

* Marked depression — guilt feeling, self-accusation, dejection.
* Self-directed injury (statement of self-destructive wishes/plans)
* Disturbed sleep pattern.
* Passive suicide by getting sunk in a wash basin, bath tub, starvation, Confused decision—making abilities.
* Impaired communication.
* Complaining of physical symptoms, fatigue, low energy level.
* Altered nutrition intake and physical appearance.
* Low self-esteem.
* Decreased interest in personal, social interpersonal, spiritual, financial activities.

NURSING CARE PLAN OF PATIENT WITH SUICIDAL IDEATION

NURSING NEEDS	GOALS	PLAN	IMPLEMENTATION	EVALUATION
1	2	3	4	5
I. THERAPEUTIC NEEDS				
	STG To prevent suicide LGT To help the patient : — recover from depression and associated symptoms. — overcome a feeling of guilt and suicidal ideation.	* The patient will have marked depression with a feeling of worthlessness and helplessness. * Guilt feelings enhance the suicidal ideation. The patient needs to be given antidepressants and ECT. * Nursing care should be planned when the patient is on these therapies.	* Provide a comfortable environment. * Allow relatives to stay with the patient. * Administer antidepressants. * Observe, record and report side-effects. * Do MSE to assess the mode of committing suicide and its lethality. * Help the patient go through ECT. * Constant observation of the patient. * Enter in all records that the patient has a suicidal ideation.	* Depressive ideas and suicidal ideation decreases.
II. PHYSICAL NEEDS				
Safe Environment	STG To help the patient feel secure LTG To help the patient:	* Because of high anxiety the patient will have self-directed violence	* Ensure adequate staffing in the ward. * One-to-one obser-	* The patient identifies that he is being cared and observed.

1	2	3	4	5
	— overcome a feeling of depression.	and hostility. * He/she may keep collecting drugs or articles by which he/she can attempt to commit a successful suicide. * Careful observation of the patient during vulnerable time, that is 3 AM to 4 AM, when everyone in the ward is fast asleep. * Avoid sending the patient alone any where. * Removal of objects which the patient may use for self - harm.	vation— one nurse constantly should observe the patient. * Remove any sharp instrument, articles of glass, ropes, string of pyjama, petticoat, neckties from the room. * Avoid long sheets the patient may use for hanging. * Food should be served in paper plates, the patient may use glass plates for harming himself. * Accompany the patient to the bathroom and toilet. * Don't leave electrical connections open. * Lock medicines and instruments in the ward. * Check the patient's belongings. * Ensure that the patient swallows medicines.	

1	2	3	4	5
			* Check the patient at night when he is awake and alone. * Maintain close observation during change of shift,meal time, Sunday when few staff members are on duty. * Provide room near the nurses' station.	
Personal Hygiene	STG To help the patient develop a sense of well-being. LTG To help the patient: — maintain cleanliness. — feel accepted by others. — enhance self-esteem.	* Depression and a feeling of hoplessness cause loss of interest in personal hygiene too. * The patient does not maintain cleanliness, has constipation, and feels helpless and fatigued to do any activity. * Wants to punish	* Develop a therapeutic relationship. * Encourage the patient to maintain oral hygiene. * Encourage for regular bowel habits. Pursue him/her to take bath and comb hair. * Enforce him/her to change clothes. * Help him go and take a round of the ward. * Help the patient to verbalise why he does not want to attend to his physical needs.	* The patient maintains personal hygiene.

1	2	3	4	5
		himself.	* Help him identify his worth father says Ramesh you are looking nice today, I am happy).	
Improve Intake of Food.	STG Help the patient improve his intake of diet. LTG To help the patient: — develop a feeling that he needs to survive. — maintain physical health.	* Because of low self-esteem and ideas of guilt the patient wants to try "passive suicide" by not eating. * Encourage the patient to talk why he does not want to take his meals.	* Encourage the patient to verbalize his food habits. * Help him identify the reasons of not taking food and association with disinterest in life. * Develop a warm and trusting relationship. * Help the patient identify the positive aspects of living and taking food. * Serve food in an attractive manner. * Provide small and frequent meals. * Record intake and output. * Record weight of the patient	* The patient develops interest in eating.

II. PSYCHOSOCIAL NEEDS

1	2	3	4	5
	STG To help the	* The patient starts	* Encourage the	* Starts discussing

1	2	3	4	5
Trusting Relationship	patient develop confidence. LTG To help the patient : — identify his/her worth. — improve his/her self-concept.	developing a feeling of lack of trusting relationship and support system from family members and friends. * Develops a feeling of isolation and worthlessness.	patient to talk. * Listen patiently. * Keep to the appointments * Provide privacy while interacting. * Reinforce positive achievements of the patient. * Encourage relatives to visit the patient. * Convey a hopeful attitude towards recovery of the patient.	his feeling of disgust and despair with his nurse.
Reduce Suicidal Ideation.	STG To assess the lethality. LTG To help the patient: — verbalize his suicidal plan. — prevent self-harm. — become others-centred rather than self-centred.	* Encourage the patient to talk about his anger, guilt or hostility. * Help him identify situations which may arouse hostility. * Encourage him to express these feelings which are normal instead of diverting them to self-destruction.	* Encourage the patient to talk about his suicidal plan. * Check the lethality of the method used. * Check whether the articles needed to carry out his suicidal plan are available. (Gun, hanging rope, pills). * Alert relatives and the ward staff. * Ensure that the patient does not have any harmful	* Explain the alternative like "I think I will take a loan from my bank and start business again. All is not over."

1	2	3	4	5
			articles. * Help the patient list alternatives to suicide. * Encourage him to identify consequences of suicide on family members.	
Improve self-esteem	STG To decrease a feeling of worthlessness. LTG To help the patient: — identify his strength. — prevent failures.	* Because of depression and associated symptoms the patient has a very low self-concept. * Continuous failures lead to more negative self-concept. * The nurse and relatives need to reinforce strength of the patient and his contribution to the family.	* Call the patient by name. * Give positive strokes (compliance to medication). * Give him an activity which he can complete. * Show it to others. * Help him identify his positive points and achievements in life.	* Talks with confidence.
Improve communication.	STG To help the patient overcome his feeling of guilt and self-punishment. LTG To help the patient: — use his communi-	* These patients are self-absorbed in planning suicide they avoid talking. * Communication will help the patient talk about	* Use active friendly approach. * Encourage the patient to talk to others. * Respond with warmth. * Discourage lone-	* The patient initiates conversation in the day-care room.

1	2	3	4	5
	cation skills. — find a meanig in life. — overcome his feeling of guilt and depression.	his guilt feeling and may get a feedback about the pleasures of life. * Discouragement of attempt suicide from many will enhance a feeling his worth.	liness to prevent suicidal ideation. * Encourage other patients to go and talk to him. * Motivate the patient to go to a nearby patient. * Use various communication techniques such as restating, clarifying, pinpointing and reflecting.	
Improve socialization	STG To help the patient to interact with his family members. To help him develop a feeling of belongingness. LTG To help the Patient to intract with others.	* The patient has social isolation because of depressive symptoms and low self-esteem. Encourage him/her to fall back on family support.	* Don't leave the patient alone. * Place some other patients also in his cubicle to prevent any suicidal attempt. * Gradually encourage him to get up from his bed and talk to others. * Help the patient socialize from a smaller to larger group. * Encourage the patient to participate in group activities.	* Shows happiness in playing with some patients.

1	2	3	4	5
Improve coping abilities.	STG To help the patient identify his coping abilities. LTG To help the patient: — use a problem-solving approach. — promote a feeling of worth. — decrease dependent behaviour.	* Due to depression the patient feels incapable of handling problems and gives in due to a feeling of incapability. * Feels more depressed and worthless and thinks of attempting to commit suicide. * Encourage him to use a problem-solving approach and decision-making ability.	* Encourage the patient to talk about his problems. * Help him find out a solution to the problem other than suicidal ideation. * Encourage the patient to make simple decisions initially. * Explain to relatives to discuss family issues and take the patient's suggestion. * Help the patient identify his worth and decision-making abilities.	* Identifies his coping abilities * Takes decisions for family members and himself with confidence.
IV. RECREATIONAL NEED				
	STG To divert the patient's mind. LTG To help the patient: — do his routine activities. — enjoy life.	* The patient needs to be encouraged to explore his hobbies and restart one by one. * In the beginning encourage him to do activities on his own, gradually help him to socialize with others and play.	* Help the patient to identify his favourite hobby or game. * Provide enough time to the patient. * Encourage him for outdoor activities. * Help him/her enjoy success and	* Looks forward to the recreation time. * Expresses " thank God, I came to hospital."

1	2	3	4	5
			accept defeat without getting much disturbed.	
V. SPIRITUAL ACTIVITIES	STG To reduce pre-occupation with self-harm. LTG To help the patient: — develop positive aspects of life. — find value of life. — identify the idea of death and religious belief.	* Help the patient explore his belief and self-harm and reasons for living, that is reinforcement of positive aspects and achievement of life. * Help the patient live in the present. * Relate ideas of death and religious belief.	* Ask the patient why he wants to die. * Ask him what are the things he would like to do if he lives. * Encourage reading religious books. * Discuss the attitude towards life in religious books. * Help him make a list of his qualities. * Show him the list and his worth.	* The patient gets solace and verbalizes with determination "never I shall think of suicide, oh God".
VI. DISCHARGE PLAN	STG To help the patient get help if he has a suicidal ideation. LTG To help the patient: — identify support system — attend a follow-up clinic.	* Family members should be helped to keep observing the patient. * Allow the patient to talk to relatives in case he/she has suicidal ideas. * Contact the therapist even at	* Ensure family support to the patient. * Discuss with relatives in front of the patient. * Provide an opportunity to relatives to discuss the fear "if the patient	* The patient and relatives feel secure. * Attends the follow-up clinic regularly.

1	2	3	4	5
	— develop ready contact with the therapist in case of suicidal ideas.	midnight if he has suicidal ideas.	attempts". * Ask the patient to discuss his support system in case of suicidal ideas. * Give the telephone number of the therapist. * Allow relatives and the patient to talk any time. Help will be extended on telephone also (Hot Line counselling). * Link the patient with a social network. * Educate the patient and relatives to attend the follow-up clinic and ensure compliance to treatment.	

TO RECALL

- ✳ Introduction and definition of suicide
- ✳ Myths about suicide
- ✳ Epidemiology
- ✳ Associated conditions
- ✳ Etiology
- ✳ Psychodynamic
- ✳ Nursing Diagnosis
- ✳ Nursing Care Plan

I. Therapeutic needs.

II. Physical needs
- — Safe environment
- — personal hygiene
- — improved intake of food

III. Psychosocial needs
- — Trusting relationship
- — Reduce suicidal ideation
- — Improve self-esteem
- — Improve communication
- — Improve socialization
- — Improve coping abilities

IV. Recreational needs

V. Spiritual needs

VI. Dicharge plan

NURSING THE PATIENT WITH ANXIETY

INTRODUCTION

During the period of stress everyone goes through anxiety. An individual is able to cope up with the associated symptoms of anxiety. But when the individual is not able to do so and starts developing marked symptoms, he/she requires help. Sometimes this basic factor of anxiety may turn into other neurotic disorders.

DEFINITION

Anxiety is a pervasive feeling of dread, apprehension and impending disaster. It is different from FEAR. Fear is a response to a clear and present danger. For example, fear of dark, fear of a dog. Anxiety is a response to an undefined or unknown threat which may be due to unconscious conflict or insecurity (like undergoing surgery). The psychological and physiological changes occur in fear as well as in anxiety.

TYPES OF ANXIETY DISORDERS

According to ICD-10 (F 41), anxiety is classified as decribed below:

(I) PANIC DISORDERS

It is also called episodic paroxysmal anxiety. The individual has recurrent attacks of severe anxiety. These attacks are not restricted to any particular situation or circumstance and are unpredictable. The person has an onset of palpitations, chest pain, choking sensation, dizziness and a feeling of unreality (Depersonalization). A fear of dying, losing control or going mad may also be present. The attack lasts for minutes or a little longer. Panic attack is often followed by a fear of having another attack.

(II) GENERALIZED ANXIETY DISORDERS

The essential feature is anxiety. It is generalized and persistent but not necessarily due to environmental circumstances. It is also called a 'Free Floating' anxiety. Common symptoms are nervousness, trembling, muscular tension, sweating, lightheadedness, palpitation, dizziness and epigastric discomfort. "Like a feeling that someone in the family is going to be very ill." Generalised anxiety is a common disorder in women than men.

On a continuum, anxiety can vary from mild to panic.

ANXIETY

Mild+ | Moderate++ | Severe+++ | Panic+++++

Fig. 29 : Explaining Anxiety Continuum.

ASSOCIATED CONDITION OF ANXIETY

1. Anxiety disorders.
2. Schizophrenia.
3. Delusional (Paranoid) disorders.
4. Psychophysiological conditions
   — Crisis
   — Phobia
   — Obesity
   — Physical disorders
5. Dissociative disorders.

ETIOLOGICAL FACTORS

I. Biological factors
II. Psychological factors
   — Maladaptive learning
   — Blocked personal growth
   — Pathogenic interpersonal relationship
   — Stress and decompensation
III. Sociocultural Factors.

(Refer to Unit-XIX).

PSYCHODYNAMICS

Anxiety is basically due to a conflict, a conflict between ID and Superego where ego is not able to mediate effectively. Failure to this anxiety occurs. Faulty parental modelling. When parents become anxious about any stressful situations, their expectation from the child also leads to stress on the child, leading to anxiety. An individual's learnt coping abilities will also determine how anxious the person is to handle stressful situations. Fear of losing something or the parent also may arouse anxiety.

NURSING DIAGNOSIS

* Exaggerated fear
* Changed physiological status
* Impaired communication
* Decreased orientation
* Lowered self-esteem
* Altered socialization
* Ineffective coping abilities
* Disturbed sleep pattern
* Disturbed eating pattern
* Increased activity
* Dehydration
* Decreased family support
* Self-care deficit.

FORMS OF ANXIETY

CHANGES	MILD	MODERATE	SEVERE	PANIC
Physiological changes	Increased heart rate, respiration, BP and gastric mobility (diarrhoea). Skin cold and clamy, pupils slightly dilated. Decreased salivation.	All the symptoms increase. Mild anxiety. There may be urinary urgency.	Symptoms are marked, decreased hearing, dilated pupils, decreased perception to pain or injury.	Physiological changes are severe.
Attention and concentration	Increased alertness, concentration poor, appears confident.	Misperception of stimuli, concentration very poor. Paces up and down, may irritate others.	Decreased and distorted perception.	Attention and concentration highly affected.
Speech	Volume and rate is appropriate to what a person is communicating.	Frequent changes of topic, joking, repetitive questioning. Speech volume and rate increase.	Uses words like "it is impossible for me." Demands help.	Not clear. May talk with action.
Activity	Increased	Body position changes frequently, restless, unable to meet routine social and vocational demands.	Gross motor tremors, facial grimaces, purposeless activity such as pacing up and down, wringing hands.	May scream and run about or may stick to something.
Appetite	Decreased due to a slowed digestive process.	Poor, or they eat very fast without chewing properly.	Marked loss of appetite.	No appetite.
Muscle Tone	Slightly tightened	Tense all the time	Tense and rigid muscles. Degrees of anxiety with associated symptoms	Very poor motor coordination.

Fig. 30 : Desciption of mild, moderate, severe and panic form of anxiety.

NURSING CARE PLAN OF PATIENT WITH ANXIETY

NURSING NEEDS	GOALS	PLAN	IMPLEMENTATION	EVALUATION
1	2	3	4	5
I. THERAPEUTIC NEEDS				
	STG To prevent the patient from going into shock. LTG To help the patient to: — overcome anxiety — prevent systemic complications.	* Physiological changes can lead the patient to shock. * The nurse must try to maintain the B.P. of the patient. Restore warmth of the body, reduce dehydration by providing liquids.	* Observe and record the vital signs of the patient. * Record the blood pressure of the patient. * Give chewing gum to improve salivation. * Administer anti-anxiety drugs, if prescribed. * Observe for the side-effects of drugs. * Give liquids to drink. * Massage the patient's feet and hands to improve peripheral circulation. * Cover to provide warmth.	Due to anti-anxiety durgs the B.P. , Pulse respiration stabilizes.
II. PHYSICAL NEEDS				
Improve sleep pattern.	STG To reduce physical exhaustion	* Due to increased actvitiy and apprehension the	* Reassure the patient. * Provide a comfort-	Feels fresh on getting up.

1	2	3	4	5
	LTG To help the patient to: — have adequate sleep hours. — feel less exhausted.	patient does not sleep adequately. He/she looks and feels exhausted. Encourage the patient to sleep for a longer duration.	able environment * Allow relatives to stay. * Switch on the bedside light. * Hold the patient's hand. * Slowly massage the head/back. * Provide a hot glass of milk. * Encourage the patient to sleep for six to eight hours. * Encourage afternoon naps.	
Decreased activity/ restlessness	STG To reduce exhaustion to the patient. LTG To help the patient to: — find the relationship between anxiety and increased activity. — reduce the purposeless activity.	* Plan the activities in which the patient is discouraged to walk too much. The covert anxiety (not expressed) may lead to increased activities, help the patient to identify.	* Calm and serene attitude of the nurse. * Detect covert anxiety (presence of a particular relative or situation or message). * Observe the increased activity. * Encourage the patient to verbalize relationship between the visit of a relative and increased activity and restlessness. (Are you feeling uncomfortable	The patient becomes less restless. Activity is decreased.

1	2	3	4	5
			because of your relative's visit ?)	
Improve hydration.	STG To maintain fluid and electrolyte balance, LTG To help the patient to: — recover from a dehydration phase — cope with a stressful situation.	* The patient has marked diarrhoea and may be vomiting. Intake of fluids is very poor. Lips become dry and cracked. Skin also becomes loose due to dehydration, provide adequate fluids	* Observe and record vital signs of the patient. * Provide liquids in a small amount but frequently. * Give chewing gum/chicklet to chew to improve salivation. * Apply glycerine on lips. * Give antidiarrhoeal drugs, if prescribed. * Maintain an intake/output chart.	The patient looks hydrated skin turgor improves.
Improve appetite & weight.	STG To increase intake of food. LTG To help the patient to: — improve diet intake. — improve in physical health.	* Due to anxiety the appetite is poor or the patient eats too fast without chewing. * Very few patients eat too much and show increase in weight. Because of a poor diet the patient looks cachexic.	* Observe the amount of intake of diet. * Encourage small and frequent meals. * Explain to the patient to chew and eat food. * Help him to develop interest in eating. * Provide foods of his/her choice.	Enjoys eating food. Shows increase in weight.

1	2	3	4	5
			* Record wight. * If the patient is eating too much, reduce the intake of high CHO (carbohydrate foods).	
Prevent from injury.	STG To protect the patient from self injury. LTG To help the patient to: — protect himself/others from injury and accidents.	* The patient is very restless due to anxiety, paces up and down hurriedly, may cause injury to self and by neglect or by mistake injure other persons. * Provide a safe environment.	* Provide a safe environment with less equipment. * Cut fruit and give him. * Pour milk/tea from the flask and give it to the patient. * Ensure that the floor is not slippery.	Bumps less.
III. PSYCHOSOCIAL NEEDS				
Reduce anxiety.	STG To help the patient to overcome anxiety. LTG To help the patient to: — use coping mechanisms. — reduce complications.	* Plan care to decrease symptoms of anxiety. * Identify the source of anxiety like threat to self-security or others, inability to gain respect from others, actual or impending interference with basic needs like food, sleep.	* Adopt a reassuring and friendly attitude. * Encourage the patient to talk (mental catharsis). * Listen actively (by responding, nodding your head). * Remain with the patient (feels secure.). * Use simple but firm sentences.	The patient feels relieved and anxiety is reduced.

1	2	3	4	5
		* Being left alone increases anxiety.	* Observe the patient's covert (hidden) anxiety. * Allow the patient to talk about the cause of anxiety. * Repeat the question for the patient, if required.	
Improve perception	STG To help the patient to be oriented to time, place and person. LTG To help the patient to: — develop accurate perception — improve attention and concentration.	* Plan activities in which the patient's attention and concentration are improved. Misperception is due to high anxiety and decreased attention and concentration.	* Orient him to ward/unit and staff. * Encourage the patient to sit down and do some activity. * Give a painting and ask the patient to identify the figure and the colures used. * Motivate the patient to complete activity which he has started. * Observe for any distraction the patient has. * Ask the patient whether he hears any sounds.	Has less misperception. Can sit and do his work with concentration.
Improve Communication	STG To reduce	* Too many hurried	* Provide support	Speech is clear.

1	2	3	4	5
	speech pressure and communicate clearly. LTG To help the patient to: — use his communication abilities — overcome anxiety	thoughts come at a time due to anxiety and the patient wants to convey to every-one. So speaks fast, conveys wrong, incomplete messages. * At times it may be incoherent.	and reassurance to the patient. * Environment should be calm. * Talk to the patient slowly with pause. * Help him to convey slowly the message. * Use communication techniques of reflecting, pinpointing, clarifying, restating and summarizing. * Help the patient to identify clarity in his/her talk.	
Improve coping abilities	STG To identify and overcome a stressful situation leading to anxiety. LTG To help the patient to: — be able to manage a stressful situation in future without an anxiety episode.	* The patient has a lot of coping abilities, help him to identify and use them. * Re-educate him to use these abilities in future also to overcome stress.	* Encourage the patient to talk about coping mechanism used by him/her in the past. * Help him/her identify the successful approach. * Ask him/her the alternative to meet the stress. * Help him identify that he has coping abilities (Tea was	Identifies a solution to the problem. Feels comfortable.

1	2	3	4	5
			not brought by 8 o'clock. He requested one of the relatives to get tea for him from the canteen).	
Improve Socialization	STG To reduce irritability to others. LTG To help the patient to: — regain his/her socialization abilities.	* Due to anxiety the patient has a purposeless activity and speech (purposeful for him) which may irritate others and they may avoid him/her. The patient starts feeling lonely and more anxious.	* Explain to family members that the phase of symptoms is temporary. * Encourage relatives to support his/her appropriate behaviour. * Help him not to disturb others. * Accept the patient with his symptoms. * Help him talk clearly. * Encourage the patient to participate in activities like day care, occupational therapy. * Control irritation at the patient's behaviour.	Enjoys socialization.
Improve Family support	STG To feel secure and have less anxiety.	* Help the patient to identify who all can support him.	* Encourage the patient to talk about the support	The patient feels secure in the presence of family members.

1	2	3	4	5
	LTG To help the patient to: — identify the available family support. — feel secure during stress.	He needs to identify and develop the support system. * Explain family members to initiate their role during stress.	system in the family. * Help him/her identify and develop relationship. * Encourage family members to provide security (social) to the patient. * Ensure that it is a temporary phase. * Listen to the relatives (Anxious patients make relatives anxious).	
IV. RECREATIONAL ACTIVITIES				
	STG To divert from an anxiety situation. LTG To help the patient to: — find pleasure in life. — Divert his mind.	* The patient is too preoccupied with stress and anxiety. His/her mind can be diverted by providing activities of choice. * Feeling of normalcy will be strengthened.	* Ask the patient about his hobbies. * Encourage him/her to go to the day-room. * Provide material if he likes to do painting, writing or drawing.	The patient initiates his hobbies.
V. SPIRITUAL NEED				
	STG To restart his/her spiritual activity.	* During the phase of anxiety the patient neglects his/	* Help the patient identify his spiritual activities.	The patient restarts his spiritual activities and shows happiness.

1	2	3	4	5
	LTG To help the patient to: — find meaning in life. — get peace and thereby decrease in anxiety.	her spiritual activities. Remind and encourage the patient to restart these activities.	* Enourage him/her to start his morning prayer and meditation/yoga/pooja. * Provide him with an opportunity to go to the prayer room.	
VI. DISCHARGE PLAN				
	STG To help the patient to cope with stress. LTG To help the patient to: — identify what triggered off anxiety. — identify his coping abilities problems faced by the patient/family due to inappropriate coping mechanisms.	* Help the patient identify the real cause of anxiety, his abilities to manage it. Also manage stress to the family caused by physiological problems. * Help him to identify the mechanisms to cope in future.	* Allow the patient to talk about his recovery. * Help him identify his role in recovery. * Help him to identify the available family support. * Re-educate his coping abilities. * Help him identify the coping mechanisms depending on stress in future.	The patient identifies his coping abilities.

TO RECALL

- ✻ Definition of Anxiety Disorders
- ✻ Types of Anxiety Disorders
- ✻ Table describing degrees of anxiety disorders — Mild, Moderate, Severe, Panic
- ✻ Etiological Factors
- ✻ Associated Conditions
- ✻ Psychodynamics
- ✻ Nursing Diagnosis
- ✻ Nursing Care Plan

I. Therapeutic Needs

II. Physical Needs
- ✻ Improve Sleep pattern
- ✻ Decrease Activity restlessness
- ✻ Improve hydration
- ✻ Improve appetite and weight

III. Psychosocial Needs
- ✻ Reduce anxiety
- ✻ Improve perception
- ✻ Improve communication
- ✻ Improve coping abilities
- ✻ Improve socialization
- ✻ Improve family support

IV. Recreational Activities

V. Spiritual Needs

VI. Discharge Plan

NURSING PATIENT WITH OBSESSIVE COMPULSIVE DISORDER

INTRODUCTION

Obsessive compulsive disorder is a neurotic disorder in which obsession and compulsion are a significant source of distress and interfere with an individual's ability to function. *Obsessions* are persistent, recurrent ideas and impulses (ideas of doubts, thoughts of committing violence). Though these thoughts appear senseless to an individual, they cannot be ignored or suppressed by him/her. *Compulsions* are repetitive, stereotype acts (hand washing, counting, checking, touching) which must be performed by an individual to relieve tension even though they are recognized senseless by the individual.

DEFINITION

According to ICD - 10 (F 42) obsessive compulsive disorder has an essential feature of recurrent obsessional thoughts or compulsive acts.

Obsessional *thoughts* are *ideas, images* or *impulses* that enter the individual's mind again and again in a stereotype form. They are distressing because they are violent or obscene or senseless and the sufferer often tries unsuccessfully to resist them. An example for obsessional thought or rumination: a woman may suffer because of repeated thought that she may ultimately kill the child whom she loves so much.

Compulsive acts or rituals are stereotype *behaviour* repeated again and again. They are not enjoyable by an individual. This behaviour is recognized by an individual as pointless and purposeless. Repeated attempts are made by the individual himself to resist in the beginning. The patient has anxiety due to obsessional symptoms. Obsessive compulsive thought has a positive relationship with depression.

Obsessive compulsive disorder is common in men and women. Its onset is usually in childhood or early adult life.

ETIOLOGY

I. Biological factors.

II. Psychological factors.
- — Maladaptive learning.
- — Blocked personal growth.
- — Pathogenic interpersonal relationship.
- — Stress and decompensation.

III. Sociocultural factors.

(Refer Unit XIX).

ASSOCIATED CONDITIONS

— Anxiety disorders
— Schizophrenia
— Phobic disorders
— Obsessive compulsive personality
— Psychoactive substance abuse
— Alcoholism
— Eating disorders— Anorexia Nervosa, Bulimia Nervosa
— Obesity.

PSYCHO-DYNAMICS

The individual is fixated at the anal stage of psychosexual development. The child develops pleasure in controlling his feacal matter. Tries to be neat and tidy and comes upto the expectation of parents in toilet training. Works properly, does not wet the bed. He/she is always tyring to please parents or significant people. Psychodynamically, the characteristic defenses used in obsessive compulsive behaviour are regression, isolation, undoing and reaction formation.

REGRESSION: The person goes back to the earlier stages of development, manipulation of genitalia, masturbation.

ISOLATION: It is an ego defense in which the patient withdraws himself socially. Due to obsessive thoughts the individual has increased anxiety but he/she is not able to attach the emotional intensity which had been gone through. So the patient isolates himself.

UNDOING: The patient is always worried about the acts he/she has been performing, gets anxious to overcome them. For example, to undo his act of masturbation the patient repeatedly washes hands.

REACTION FORMATION : The patient has a reaction formation of undoing his acts by repeatedly washing hands. But underlying these is a feeling of performing acts which he/she feels are 'dirty'.

NURSING DIAGNOSIS

* Increased anxiety
* Decreased coping ability with compulsion
* Acceptance attitude of the nurse
* Inspired judgement— Ritualistic acts.
* Decreased communication
* Lower self-esteem
* Self-care deficits— bathing, eating, activity, loss of weight
* Disturbed sleep pattern
* Need for behaviour modification.

NURSING CARE PLANS FOR PATIENT WITH OBSESSIVE COMPULSIVE DISORDER

NURSING NEEDS 1	GOALS 2	PLAN 3	IMPLEMENTATION 4	EVALUATION 3
I. THERAPEUTIC NEED				
	STG To help the patient reduce anxiety. LTG To help the patient to: — reduce his obsessional acts — prevent him from exhaustion.	* To reduce anxiety or guilt the patient performs acts repeatedly. He will get physically exhausted and preoccupation will lead to no other activities. So it should be reduced by drugs and behaviour modification.	* Recognize the cause of anxiety. * Administer antianxiety or antidepressant drugs as prescribed. * Observe record and report the side-effects. * Participate and continue giving psychotherapy such as assertiveness and cognitive psychotherapy; for example, positive reinforcement, response shaping. *(Refer to Chapter VI Unit XVI)*	Anxiety and associated symptoms are reduced.
II. PHYSICAL NEED				
Encourage Personal Hygiene	STG To reduce the feeling of dirt. LTG To help the patient to:	* The patient has a feeling of dirt around him and washes hands/	* Observe for anxiety-arousing situations. * Provide a clean	Attends to his toilet needs. Takes bath regularly.

1	2	3	4	5
	— maintain personal hygiene — reduce ritualistic acts.	takes bath/ washes clothes frequently (one of these acts). * Usually he doesn't perform other activities due to preoccupation with ritualistic acts. * Don't hurry through the activities which increase anxiety in the patient.	toilet and bathroom to the patient. * The patient maintains personal hygiene but avoids going to dirty bathrooms and toilets (according to him/her). * Allow the patient to continue with his ritualistic behaviour initially. * Encourage him to maintain personal hygiene specially bath, hair wash and evacuation of bowels and bladder at his own pace.	
Care of skin	STG To protect the patient from dryness of skin. LTG To help the patient to: — control his/her urge to wash hands. — prevent his skin from cracking and dryness.	* The patient may keep washing clothes/hands repeatedly. Scrubs them so much that it causes injury. Marked dryness of the skin due to repeated wash.	* Provide a good quality soap to the patient. * In winter provide warm water. * Encourage the patient to use cold cream, or vasaline and wear gloves. * Gradually set a limit on the number of times the	Reduces frequency of washing hands. Skin of hands looks healthy.

1	2	3	4	5
			patient washes hands in one hour. * Don't punish the patient. It would arouse more anxiety. * When he has less anxiety explain to the patient the effects of his ritualistic acts on his skin.	
Improve appetite and weight.	STG To help the patient improve his intake of diet. LTG To help the patient to: — improve his general health. — protect him from infections.	* The patient is so preoccupied in his obsessed thought and acts that he is not able to eat.* * Thinks that his hands will get dirty. * People who have cooked food may not be clean. There may be so many germs in their hands.	* Serve food in the patient's own utensils. * Help the patient to wash hands. * Encourage him to use fork and spoon if he feels his hands will get dirty. * Initially, allow food from home. * Record his weight.	The patient starts eating. Shows improvement in weight.
Improve sleep pattern.	STG To provide adequate rest hours to the patient. LTG To help the patient to: — control ritualistic	* The patient's preoccupation to ritualistic behaviour and obsessive thought disturbs him/her at night also and he/she	* Assess the patient's anxiety because of his ritualistic act. * Encourage him to do thorough washing before	The patient feels comfortable at night.

1	2	3	4	5
	behaviour at night. — get adequate sleep at night.	has distubed sleep. * Allow the patient to attend to his ritualistic behaviour at night before sleeping.	going to bed. * Administer antianxiety drugs, if prescribed. * Encourage him to repeat the act only in the morning after getting up.	
III. PSYCHOSOCIAL NEEDS				
Psychotherapeutic environment.	STG To provide a secure social environment. LTG To help the patient to: — decrease anxiety. — reduce his social isolation.	* A calm environment will decrease the patient's anxiety, thereby decreasing stress on his/her ritualistic act.	* Provide a calm, comfortable and neat environment. * Don't hurry through the instructions. * Use a relaxed approach with the patient. * Give positive reinforcement to his non-compulsive behaviour. * Encourage the patient to set limits himself for his behaviour. * Initially, set limits if the patient feels it difficult. For example, from 7 AM to 8 AM you have washed your hands 10 times. As	Controls his ritualistic behaviour.

1	2	3	4	5
			a result, the skin of your hands must be very dry. * Set limits but provide adequate time for his rituals. * Divert his mind to activities which required concentration like reading a story book or religious book for other patients. Don't provide new activities.	
Help in coping with obsessive compulsive behaviour	STG To reduce anxiety of the patient. LTG To help the patient: — learn new ways of coping with anxiety. — overcome compulsive acts.	* The patient needs to be helped to find new ways of coping with anxiety. * Initially, don't attack or belittle the patient for his ritualistic acts. * Gradually, limit the behaviour when it starts affecting his health.	* Be warm and sympathetic in approach. * Accept compulsive acts of the patient initially. * Avoid arguing. * Allow the patient to complete his compulsive act. * Help him/her realise that his/her act is time-consuming. * Assist him/her in new ways of problem-solving. * Help him/her to	The patient controls his ritualistic behaviour.

1	2	3	4	5
			identify how other actitivies like eating, changing clothes, spending time with family members are getting affected because of ritualistic acts. * Limit the ritualistic acts (reduce rigidity) * Remind the patient that in the past one hour he/she has not gone to wash hands. * Help the patient to decrease the need for perfection. * Gradually increase the duration of ritualistic acts. * Do not punish him for his symptoms. * Use cognitive and assertiveness training therapy. * Teach relaxation approach. * Behaviour modification can be made by modelling, reaction pre-	

1	2	3	4	5
			vention (*Refer to Unit XVI*). * Verbal control on the frequency of ritualistic acts.	
Help in improving communication.	STG To help the patient develop effective relationship LTG To help the patient to — reduce obsessional stickiness. — Divert the patient's mind from ritualistic acts.	* The patient is preoccupied with his ruminating thoughts and compulsive acts. He/she does not find time to develop relationship with other patients. * Feels that others are not as clean as he is, though the underlying feeling of guilt is present. * The nurse needs to plan to reduce his/her anxiety. * Dependence-	* Provide a trusting environment. * Disover the source of anxiety. Talk about other symptoms, (rigidity, frustration, ambivalence). * Encourage the patient to talk about his anxiety. * Encourage him to talk to a few people at a time and can carry on his ritualistic acts too. * Gradually encourage him to talk to more people. * Enhance self-confidence by reinforcing non-compliance to ritualistic behaviour. * Help the patient to accept treatment. * Encourage the patient to cooper-	The patient starts accepting the therapist. The patient initiates relationship with others.

1	2	3	4	5
		independence conflict should be reduced.	ate and put in efforts to bring about change in his behaviour. * Help the patient to identify the cause of conflict with the therapist.	
To enhance self-concept and socialization.	STG To increase the feeling of competence and adequacy. LTG To help the patient to : — re-establish social interaction. — decrease the feeling of social isolation.	* The patient's anxiety is marked to finish up ritualistic acts. Because of his need for independence rigidity, he avoids social relations. * Socially isolated, he starts practising his ritualistic acts more.	* Provide information to the patient when anxiety is at a low level. * Call the patient by name. * Help the patient's relatives to participate in his treatment. * Encourage the patient to participate in ward activities. * Encourage him to interact with others'. * Laugh and use humour. * Help him/her to accept compliments. * Help the patient identify pleasure in social interaction and adopting	The patient feels comfortable with others. Identifies less use of ritualistic behaviour.

1	2	3	4	5
			flexibility in his rigid behaviour. * Protect him from criticism or ridicule by others. * Ensuring that other patients are not kept waiting because of him by reducing the frequency of his ritualistic act.	
Help in Reducing Anxiety.	STG To decreae compulsive behaviour. LTG To help the patient to : — Express his hostility — Cope with negativistic feeling.	* The patient's increased anxiety leads him to compulsive acts. * The hostile feeling makes him more anxious and negativist. Even when pointed out, he does not accept that his ritual acts are baseless.	* Observe the intensity of anxiety. * Identify the anxiety-prone situation. * Provide a clean and comfortable environment. * Allow the patient to express his hostile feeling in a non-destructive manner (Speaks loudly). * Discourage his resisted compulsive behaviour.	Feels comfortable with decreased ritualistic acts.
IV. RECREATIONAL ACTIVITIES				
	STG To divert the patient's attention from ritualistic	* The patient's ritualistic acts can be diverted by pro-	* Observe activities in which the patient's rituals	The patient enjoys the recreational activities. Identifies the reduced

1	2	3	4	5
	acts. LTG To help the patient to: — prevent the need for compulsive act. — use his orderly qualities in a constructive manner.	viding activities in which he/she can use perfection skills. * Identify a situation in which the patient's anxiety gets reduced, * Group therapy may be encouraged.	are decreased (presence of an influential person like Dotor,Nurse, Relative). * Encourage him to do activities of his choice. * Ask the patient to draw columns in the register. * Help him to maintain attendence record in the day-care room.	need of his ritualistic act.
V. SPIRITUAL NEEDS				
	STG To help the patient identify the value of life. LTG To help the patient to: — gain strength (moral) — enhance self-confidence.	* The patient is too indulged in his behaviour. Neglects his spiritual activities like other activities. * Encourage him to attend to his spiritual activities.	* Ask the patient about his spiritual interests. * Provide him with facilities. * Ask relatives to get the religious book which he/she is used to read. * Encourage the patient to do meditation.	Reduces his obsessive compulsive behaviour.
VI. DISCHARGE PLAN				
	STG To help the patient not to use ritualistic acts. LTG To help the	* Help the patient to talk about his various coping abilities which he	* Help the patient learn to identify an anxiety situation. * Encourage him to	The patient feels comfortable without ritualistic acts.

1	2	3	4	5
	patient to: — cope with anxiety without a compulsive act. — find a support system among friends and relatives.	used in the past to overcome stressful situations. — To help him identify the use of compulsive acts and their effect on daily activities.	use new ways of problem solving. (catharsis writing, discussing). * Encourage him to use various coping skills like talking to family members and friends.	

TO RECALL

- Definition of Obsessive Compulsive Disorder
- Etiology
- Associated Conditions
- Psychodynamics
- Nursing Diagnosis
- Nursing care plan
  - Therapeutic Needs
  - Physical Needs
    - Encourage Personal Hygiene
    - Care of Skin
    - Improve appetite and weight
    - Improve the sleep pattern
  - Psychosocial Needs
    - Psychotherapeutic Environment
    - Help in coping with Obsessive Compulsive Behaviour
    - Improving Communication
    - Enhance Self-concept and Socialization
    - Reduce anxiety
- Recreational Needs
- Spiritual Needs
- Discharge Plan

NURSING PATIENT WITH CONVERSION DISORDER (HYSTERICAL NEUROSIS — CONVERSION TYPE)

INTRODUCTION

In ICD 10 (F 44) conversion disorders have been previously described as 'conversion hysteria'. DSM-III-R describes conversion disorders (or hysterical neurosis conversion type) under somatoform disorders (300. 11). In this text, DSM-III-R classification will be discussed (i.e. conversion disorders) under somatoform disorders.

DEFINITION OF SOMATOFORM DISORDERS

The patient has repeated presentation of physical symptoms with a persistent request for medical investigation inspite of repeated negative findings and reassurance by the doctor that symptoms have no physical basis. The patient converts his psychological symptoms into body symptoms such as palpitation, pain in abdomen instead of insecurity.

CLASSIFICATION OF SOMATOFORM DISORDERS

DSM-III-R classifies it as:

a — Body dysmorphic disorders
b — Conversion disorders (or hysterical neurosis, conversion type).
c — Hypochondriasis
d — Somatization disorders
e — Somatoform pain disorders
f — Undifferentiated somatoform disorders

(A) BODY DYSMORPHIC DISORDERS

These patients are preoccupied with imagined defects in appearance, specially facial problems. They go to a dermatologist or a plastic surgeon with complaints of face. It may start from adolscence and persist for several years.

(B) HYPOCHONDRIASIS

In hypochondriasis, the patient has an exaggerated concern over his bodily health. Feels ill without any actual medical basis or pathology.

(C) SOMATOFORM PAIN DISORDER (PSYCHALGIA)

In this the patient complains of severe prolonged pain without any organic pathology, starts from adolscence and continues in adult age.

(D) CONVERSION DISORDERS

Conversions disorder, hysterical type, is a somatoform disorder.

DEFINITION

Conversion disorder, hysterical type, is a somatoform disorder in which repressed inner conflicts are unconsciously converted or transformed into physical symptoms that have no organic basis, eg. paralysis, blindness, loss of sensation, seizures or fits. Conversion symptoms are used for *primary gain,* i.e. the patient gets relief from anxiety by not going through the threatening situation; for example, not going for an interview. *Secondary gain* is by sympathy and attention from others. "Oh, poor Mahesh, he could not go for an interview, though he had prepared himself so well.' Secondary gain can be freedom from responsibility or economic compensation also.

SIGNS AND SYMPTOMS

BEHAVIOURAL CHARACTERISTICS :— These patients have a subtle behaviour self-dramatization, exihibitionism, narcissism, emotionalism, manipulativeness, suggestible and child-like behaviour.

MOTOR SYMPTOMS :— Tremors, convulsion, mutism but the patient can cough, aphonia but the patient can whisper, astasia abasis the patient can control his leg movement while sitting or lying but cannot control and walk properly and has muscular weakness.

SENSORY SYMPTOMS :— Analgesia or diminished ability to feel pain, anasthesia, hypothesia (partial loss of sensitivity), hyperesthesia (excessive sensitivity), paraesthesia (exceptional sensation of tingling)

VISCERAL SYMPTOMS :— A feeling of lump in throat (Globus hystericus), nausea, vomiting and a choking sensation. Anorexia nervosa, the patient has *'la belle* indifference' to symptoms i.e. unconcerned about symptoms. Sometimes malingering is confused with a conversion disorder. In malingering, a conscious effort is made to exhibit the symptoms of illness for some type of gain. For example, complaining pain in chest and back due to a car accident to get financial gain from an agency.

PSYCHODYNAMICS

In these patients the conflict has been respressed. This arouses anxiety, which is converted into physical symptoms. There is a desire to escape or flee from stress. Conversion reaction grows out of guilt and necessity of self-punishment. Sometimes the patient wants to punish others for their harsh behaviour by having a conversion reaction. Attention seeking mechanism is issued by prolonging complaints of physical illness even after recovery.

NURSING DIAGNOSIS

* Impaired interpersonal relationship.
* Increased attention - seeking mechanism (demands reassurance and praise, sexually seductive)
* Impulsive behaviour
* Maladaptive learning
* Low self-esteem
* Communication difficulties
* Decreased socialization
* Increased concern of physical symptoms
* Inappropriate exaggeration of emotions, over-expression of emotions, superficial or shallow emotions, demonstration of anger.
* Self–centred approach
* Alteration in speech.

NURSING CARE PLAN FOR PATIENT WITH CONVERSION DISORDER

NURSING NEEDS 1	GOALS 2	PLAN 3	IMPLEMENTATION 4	EVALUATION 5
I. THERAPEUTIC NEEDS				
	STG To reduce symptoms of the patient. LTG To help the patient to: — develop an insight into his problems — cope with the stress without converting it into physical symptoms.	* These patients are not admitted, but treated through out-patients because they are highly suggestible. They adopt symptoms of other patients too. * Some patients who have a health problem due to conversion reaction are hospitalized. These patients, outdoor as well as indoor, are given intensive psychotherapy like reality therapy, uncoverng ventilation, modification, re-education, hypnotherapy.	* Provide a comfortable environment. * Neglect the physical symptoms but not the patient. * Help team member to do the same. * Develop a therapeutic relationship. * Help in carrying out hypnotherapy, abbreaction. * Make observation and record seizures or fits.	The patient demands less attention of therapists.

1	2	3	4	5
II. PHYSICAL NEEDS				
Supervise the physical needs.	STG To help the patient to remain clean. LTG To help the patient to: — identify that he can maintain self—care.	* The patient does not have any self-care deficits. However, sometimes he/she does not maintain personal hygiene for seeking attention. * May feel like vomiting before/after meal.	* Supervise personal hygiene of all the patients. * Be firm but sympathetic towards the patient's behaviour (Patient — Sister, I could not wash my hair. I feel tired. Nurse — Ignored the word "tiredness" and tell the patient to wash tomorrow). * Ignore if the patient vomits before meal. It will be alright after eating. Should be the answer. * Avoid keeping a kidney tray or emesis tray near the bedside for vomiting.	Attends to physical care without persuastion.
III. PSYCHOSOCIAL NEEDS				
Discourage maladaptive Learning.	STG To help the patient avoid using maladaptive learning. LTG To help the patient to :	* During the childhood the patient might have seen mother/father reacting to stress with anger or	* Encourage the patient to talk about situations in which he uses a maladaptive behaviour.	Demonstrates modification in behaviour.

1	2	3	4	5
	— re-educate himself about appropriate behaviour.	throwing things. The patient adopts this learning and is excused by saying, 'Like father'.	* Help him relate the maladaptive behaviour with situations. * Help him identify the appropriateness of behaviour. * Encourage him/her to explore new ways to solve problems (planning before hand what dress to wear for a party and getting it ready also).	
Decrease Manipulative behaviour.	STG To help the patient to be less dependent. LTG To help the patient to: — identify his/her own poteníalities. — use new ways of coping with a situation himself/herself.	* Manipulative behaviour helps these patients to attain a 'primary gain' or plea for help like having a severe headache on the arrival of a guest at home. She may not have to attend to guest (primary gain). * Help the patient to decrease manipulative behaviour by psyhchotherapy. * Help the patient	* Help the patient identify the relationship of manipulative behaviour and situation. * Encourage him/her to verbalize. * Encourage the patient to identify the frequency of these types of behaviour. * Help her to express the response of her husband and children during behaviour. * Teach the patient	Identifies that without using manipulative behaviour also attention is gained.

1	2	3	4	5
		to reduce use of manipulative behaviour.	effective ways of handling a problem. * Limit the manipulative behaviour (The patient starts having belching in the presence of her husband.) * Use role playing or psychodrama. * List situations in which the patient has used manipulative behaviour.	
Decrease attention-seeking mechanisms.	STG To reduce the feeling of inadequacy. LTG To help the patient to: — cope with stress. — reduce physical symptoms.	* The patient demonstrates physical symptoms of headache, crying, belching, pain in arm,paralysis and anger on others. * Help the patient to control symptoms and use an appropriate defense mechanism to fight the situation rather than getting away from it (flight). The patient tries to attain a secondary gain.	* Develop a therapeutic relationship. * Listen to the patient. * Give attention to the patient. * Avoid attention-seeking mechanisms. * Be firm but sympathetic. * Evaluate physical symptoms. * Verbalize his symptoms to focus the restlessness (During the visitors' hour the	Demonstrates less of physical symptoms.

1	2	3	4	5
			patient's wife reached late. He started with severe headache.) * Help him make an independent decision. * Re-educate the patient about his physical strength and coping-up ability. * Help the patient verbalize his problem rather than converting in bodily symptoms.	
Decrease concern about physical symptoms	STG To reduce attention to physical symptoms. LGT To help the patient to: — divert his mind from physical symptoms. — use an appropriate mechanism to overcome stress.	* Use of physical symptoms by the patient is to get attention and affection. He/she exploits these symptoms for lack of affection and insecurity, wants to be independent but because of low self-esteem can't take up independent roles. * Help the patient to identify his positive aspects.	* Ignore physical symptoms but not the patient. * Provide attention and affection when the patient is not complaining physical symptoms. * Help the patient identify physical symptoms and its relationship with situations. * Encourage him/her to talk about other ways by	Attends more to others' needs than being self-centred.

1	2	3	4	5
		* The patient demonstrates *'La bell'* indifference' to symptoms.	which he/she can overcome stress. * Provide a situation in making a decision (the husband informs the patient that the child is not well. The patient says: "Don't come tomorrow, be with the child at home.") * Re-educating use of physical symptoms is avoidance of a psychological stress. * Help the patient identify his physical symptoms and effect on health.	
Appropriate use of Emotions.	STG To help the patient develop ability for appropriate use of emotions. LTG To help the patient to: — avoid overconcern about situations. — be concerned about others.	* The patient shows over-concern about himself. * Feels very happy or sad of a situation which may not demand so much concern. * Educate the patient on the appropriate use of emotions. As the	* Help the patient identify a situation. Relationship of the patient to that situation. * Help the patient to react appropriately (A relative of the patient is crying because of delayed recovery. The patient starts	Reacts appropriately.

1	2	3	4	5
		patient is highly suggestible, re-education will help.	crying also). * Help the patient identify his role and emotional attachment to the patient and the relative.(crying patient)	
Enhance Self-Esteem.	STG To help the patient overcome fear of rejection. LTG To help the patient overcome a feeling of inferiority and dependency.	* The patient has need for approval and praise. * Due to a feeling of inadequacy and low self-esteem he becomes more and more dependent. * Help him identify his achievements which will enhance his self-concept.	* Call the patient by name. * Develop a trusting relationship * Give tasks which the patient can complete like knitting, stitching, painting, drawing. * Help the patient to see the outcome. * Provide supportive psychotherapy * Discuss his success and achievements in the past. * Discourage the use of physical symptoms to get away from situations. * Help him/her to identify his/her ability by which he	Does not use physical symptoms on arrival of relatives.

1	2	3	4	5
			she can cope with situations.	
Improve Communication.	STG To help the patient communicate clearly. LTG To help the patient identify his/her communication ability.	* Communication is not severely affected but while talking, the patient talks according to what suits him/her and gaps filled up can be identified. Use various communication techniques.	* Use firm and sympathetic approach. * Encourage the patient to talk clearly. * Use communication techniques such as relfecting, pinpointing and summarizing. * Help the patient to know gaps while talking (I get headache if someone gets angry at someone. I get more sometimes, instead of saying I get more when my husband gets angry).	Identifies the communication gaps.
Improve Socialization	STG To Help the patient divert his/her mind. LTG To help the patient to: — enhance his self-concept, — enjoy socialization.	* The patient tries to socialize but whenever she/he wants to avoid, converts in physical symptoms. Help the patient identify the occur-	* Encourage the patient to attend to all social events. * Help the patient identify the typical social situation and occurrence of symptoms. * Encourage the pa-	* The patient socializes without the use of physical symptoms.

1	2	3	4	5
		rence of physical symptoms in specific social situations.	tient talk about the reaction of others. * Help the patient to understand that appropriate socialization will improve his self-concept.	
IV RECREATIONAL NEEDS				
	STG To divert the patient from physical symptoms. LTG To help the patient to: — use time effectively — use his/her ability appropriately.	* The patient needs to be helped to get busy in some activities, idle time will lead to preoccupation with his/her symptoms.	* Encourage the patient to work on his area of interest like gardening, reading books. * Help him identify the appropriate use of time so as to reduce physical symptoms. * Encourage the patient to go to a dayroom. * Ignore his physical symptoms.	Demonstrates no physical symptom during recreational activity.
V SPIRITUAL NEED				
	STG To help the patient to attend to his routine activities. LTG To help the patient to: — get satisfaction in life	* The patient needs to be encouraged to attend to his/her spiritual activities. He/she will feel more comfortable and derive strength	* Help the patient to practise his/her religious rituals. * Encourage him to discuss his feeling of recovery after religious activities.	The patient finds pleasure in life.

1	2	3	4	5
	— be others centred rather than seld-centred.	after meditation or yoga.	* Encourage him to join social work during leisure time.	
VI DISCHARGE PLAN				
	STG To help the patient to decrease the use of physical symptoms. LTG To help the patient to: — identify his/her recovering abilities. — assess his enhanced self-concept.	* The patient should not use physical symptoms. Should find pleasure in life. As no medication is required the patient can attend psychotherapy, if suggested by a therapist.	* Help the patient identify his potentials. * Encourage the patient to discuss handling of a stress situation without use of physical symptoms. * Counsel the relatives to be sympathetic but firm. Not to give in to physical symptoms. * Encourage relatives to give attention and affection whenever the patient does not show physical symptoms. * Discourage dependency.	Identifies all situations are not that difficult as he/she thinks. No physical symptoms present.

TO RECALL

- — Definition of Somatoform Disorders.
- — Classification of Somatoform Disorders
  - — Body dysmorphic disorders
  - — Hypochandriasis
  - — Somatoform pain disorders
  - — Undifferentiated somatoform disorders
  - — Conversion disorders (Hysterical Neurosis) Conver sion-type.
- — Conversion Disorders
  - — Definition
  - — Signs and Symptoms
    - ✱ Behaviour characteristics
    - ✱ Motor symptoms
    - ✱ Sensory symptoms
    - ✱ Visceral symptoms
  - — Psychodynamic
  - — Nursing Diagnosis
  - — Nursing Care Plan
    - I. Therapeutic Needs
    - II. Physical Needs
    - III. Psychosocial Needs
      - ✱ Decrease attention-seeking mechanisms
      - ✱ Decrease concern about physical symptoms
      - ✱ Appropriate use of emotions
      - ✱ Decrease maladaptive behaviour
      - ✱ Decrease manipulative behaviour
      - ✱ Enhance self-esteem
      - ✱ Improve communication
      - ✱ Improve socialization.
    - IV. Recreational Needs
    - V. Spiritual Needs
    - VI. Discharge Plan.

APPLICATION TO NURSING

Reading of the unit on 'Nursing Care Plans for Patients with Mental Disorders' will enable the nursing students to develop a concept in helping the client/patient in various mental disorders. This specifically will help the learners to plan nursing care for patients with schizophrenia, delusional/paranoid disorders, excitement, depressions, withdrawn behaviour, suicidal ideation, anxiety, obsessive compulsive neurosis and conversion reaction. (Somatoform disorders)

The learners will be able to make a nursing diagnosis and plan nursing care based on the psychodynamics of the disorder.

BETTER STUDY SECTION UNIT XXII

1. VOCABULARY (Refer Dictionary)

Alienation	Jovial
Altered	Lethality
Blunted	Milieu
Channelize	Modification
Choking	Narcissism
Compliance	Persuade
Deficit	Realistically
Disharmony	Reflecting
Dizziness	Relevantly
Episode	Shallow
Exhaustive	Suggestible
Extravagantly	Trustworthy
Fantasies	Verbalize
Guilt	
Impulses	
Incongruence	
Insidious	
Interchangeably	

2. ASSIGNMENT

Identify the nursing needs of the patient with the following conditions during your clinical posting in a psychiatric O.P.D./Unit

— Delusional Disorders
— Excitement
— Depression
— Withdrawn Behaviour
— Anxiety
— Suicidal Ideation
— Obsessive Compulsive Neurosis
— Conversion Disorders.

3. STUDY QUESTIONS

* Write the difference between Endogenous and Reactive Depression.
* Develop a nursing care plan on each of the conditions you have read in this unit and discuss with your teachers.

4. READING REFERENCES.

Beek, Rawltins and Williams. *Mental Health Psychiatric Nursing — A Holistic Life Cycle Approach* (2nd ed) . The C.V. Mosby Company, Toronto (1988).

Kalkman M.L. & Davis A.J. New Dimensions in *Mental Health Psychiatric Nursing* (4th ed), McGraw Hill Book Company, New York (1974);

Shives L.R. *Basic Concepts of Psychiatric-Mental Health Nursing* (2nd ed), J.B. Lippincott Company, Philadelphia (1990);

Taylor C.M., *Essentials of Psychiatric Nursing* (11th ed), The C.V. Mosby Company, London (1982).

Kaplan Harold and Sadeock B.J., *Comprehensive Textbook of Psychiarty* (5th ed), Williams and Wilkins, London (1989);

Kapoor, Bimla, *A Textbook of Psychiatric Nursing,* Kumar Publishing House, Delhi (1992).

Knesil, C.R. & Wilson, H.S, *Psychoatric Nursing.* Addison-Wesley Publishing Company, Mento Parle, California (1979).

Lego S. *The American Handbook of Psychiatric Nursing,* J.B. Lippincott Company, Philadelphia (1984).

Johnson's B.S. *Adaptation and Growth — Psychiatric Mental Health Nursing* (200 ed), J.B. Lippincott Company, Philadelphia (1989).

UNIT XXIII
NURSING CARE PLANS FOR SPECIAL PROBLEMS IN MENTAL HEALTH NURSING

UNIT OUTLINE

Nursing Patient with Organic Mental Disorders
* Introduction
* Causes
* Nursing Diagnosis
* Nursing Care Plan.

Nursing Patient with Alcoholic Problem
* Definition
* Causes
* Withdrawal Symptoms
* Psychodynamics
* Nursing Diagnosis
* Nursing Care Plan.

Nursing Patient with Drug/Substance abuse
* Definition
* Psychodynamics
* Commonly Abused Substance/Drugs
* Nursing Diagnosis
* Nursing Care Plan.

Nursing Client Who is Mentally Retarded (MR)
* Definition
* Epidemiology
* Causes of Mentally Retarded
* Difference in Mental Retardation and Mental Illness
* Myths about Mental Retardation
* Degrees of Mental Retardation
* Nursing Diagnosis
* Nursing Care Plan.

Application to Nursing

Better Study Section

INTENDED LEARNING BEHAVIOUR

After reading this unit, you will be able to:

a) Explain the types of organic mental disorders.
b) Develop skill in nursing patient with mental disorders.
c) List the causes of alcoholism.
d) Identify the withdrawal symptoms.
e) Plan the nursing intervention of patient with alcoholic disorders.
f) Enumerate the types of substance/drugs clients may abuse.
g) Develop skill in identifying withdrawal symptoms.
h) Plan and implement nursing intervention.
i) List the causes of mental retardation.
j) Differentiate between mental retardation and mental illness.
k) Identify the degrees of mental retardation.
l) Plan nursing intervention.

NURSING PATIENT WITH ORGANIC MENTAL DISORDERS

INTRODUCTION

Organic mental disorders, acute or chronic, involve impairment of brain tissue functions due to such factors as head injury, toxic conditions, encephalitis, systemic infections, brain tumor or cerebral arteriosclerosis. The resulting symptoms include mild-to-severe impairment of memory, orientation, judgement, general intellectual functioning and emotional impairment.

Organic mental disorders are described in *Chapter VII, Unit XVIII.*

CAUSES OF ORGANIC BRAIN DISORDERS

— Head Trauma
— Fever specially common in children
— Metabolic, toxic and other causes
— Dementia may occur in any age but it is more common in elderly persons *(Refer Chapter VII, Unit XVIII).*

NURSING DIAGNOSIS

* Alteration in thought process
  — inability to recognize
  — confused and disoriented
  — impaired judgement (paranoia)
  — loss of memory for recent events
  — misplacement of things
  — loss of things.
* Impaired attention and concentration.
* Self-care deficit due to loss of independent functioning, bath ing, eating, bowel and bladder incontinuence.
* Social isolation may lead to depression, agitation.
* Prone to injuries due to sensory deficits.

NURSING CARE PLAN FOR PATIENT WITH ORGANIC MENTAL DISORDER

NURSING NEEDS 1	GOALS 2	PLANNING 3	IMPLEMENTATION 4	EVALUATION 5
I THERAPEUTIC NEEDS				
	STG To reduce any type of infection. LTG To enable the patient to : — recover from any infection. — help him develop a sense of security that he is being cared for.	* Any type of illness or complaints may be treated symptomatically.	* Give medicine as prescribed. * Help the patient to express any of his physical complaints. * Give an assurance that medicine will be provided in time. * Involve relatives in giving the patient medication in time.	* The patient confirms whether complete treatment is given.
II PHYSICAL NEEDS				
Prevent from injuries.	STG To help the patient to avoid repeated injuries. LTG To help the patient to : — feel confident that the environment is safe. — avoid a sense of insecurity.	* Plan a safe and less congested environment. * Plan to keep a fewer number of articles which are not injurious to the patient.	* Provide just adequate furniture in the room. * Check tha. no wires, tubes or other things are spread in the room. * Electricity connection should be covered. * Provide the same	* Moves about in the room with confidence.

1	2	3	4	5
			physical set-up so that the patient gets used to it. * The patient should be informed of any change brought about in the room. * Provide a bell. * Switch for light and fan should be near the bedside. * Provide adequate light in the room. * Maintain a pleasant and quiet environment.	
Encourage and help in personal hygiene.	STG To help the patient feel fresh LTG To help the patient to: — develop a sense of well-being. — develop the habit of cleanliness — prevent from infection. — feel accepted.	* Set up a routine for the patient to attend to his personal hygiene. * Plan out some activities and help him maintain his regular bowel and bladder habits.	* Help the patient to brush his/her teeth, and take bath. * If the patient can't clean his back the nurse can help in doing so. * Give massage at the back to prevent bedsores and change the patient's position frequently. * Observe skin for any injuries, bruises, abrasions.	

1	2	3	4	5
			* If the client has incontinence, change the dress and put Eau De Cologne deodorant to prevent odour. * If the patient is constipated, provide a laxative with doctor's prescription. * Provide all things near the client, it will help him carry on activities easily. * Avoid doing things for the client, however step-by-step directions can be given. * Don't be in a hurry. * The client may repeat some activities such as cleaning of some area, allow it but gradually enforce limits. * Encourage the client to comb hair.	* The patient brushes his/her teeth, takes bath, combs hair. Tries to be self-sufficient.

1	2	3	4	5
			* In the case of male tell him to shave. In case of muscle incoordination, he would need partial help in shaving. * In winter provide adequate clothing; the patient may not ask for it and may die of cold.	
Attend to Nutritional needs	STG To build general health of the patient. LTG To enable the patient to : — take regular meals. — build up his/her general health.	* The patient may take small and frequent meals for fear of incontinence. * As chewing ability is also decreased, soft, easily digestable food may be planned.	* Ask the patient's likes and dislikes. * Provide soft and frequent meals. * Sometimes the foods can be churned in the mixer and given to the patient. * Don't scold the patient if he has messed up while eating. * Allow the patient to eat at his/her own pace, don't hurry. * Provide roughage, and green leafy vegetables in diet to relieve constipation.	* The patient enjoys soft meals.

1	2	3	4	5
Improve sleep pattern.	STG To reduce loneliness and depression at night. LTG To enable the patient to : — feel fresh in day time. — participate in day activities — get less fatigued.	* Planning of a sleep schedule for the night. * A calm and quiet environment.	* Discourage the patient to sleep in day time. * Keep him/her busy in activities * Encourage for a lukewarm bath in winter and tap water bath in summer at night. * Keep the environment calm and quiet. * Give good back massage. * Allow the patient to read a magazine if she/he likes. * Leave the light on if the patient is having hallucination. * Put up bedside rails.	* Sleeps for longer hours at night.
III. PSYCHOSOCIAL NEEDS				
Promote socialization.	STG To reduce a feeling of social isolation. LTG To enable the patient to : — develop a sense of belongingness — enhance self-concept.	* The patient feels alien among his own people. * He/she likes to participate in activities and give suggestions. * Plan and provide an attitude of con-	* Call the patient by name. * Tell relatives to come and sit next to the patient. * Encourage him/her to participate in activities. * Actively listen to	* Feels satisfied talking to others.

1	2	3	4	5
	— feel that he/she is accepted/wanted.	cern and helpfulness. * The patient starts feeling lonely and through socialization it can be reduced.	the patient's past experience/ memories. * Help the patient realise why significant people in the family can't give enough time now as before. * Listen to him/her with respect and regard. * Encourage visit by children of the family.	
Promote communication	STG To help the patient to enhance his/her self-concept. LTG To enable the patient to : — develop a sense of satisfaction of interacting with others. — feel being accepted by others.	* Gradually these patients become non-communicative, thinking others do not have time for them. This sense can be reduced by spending time with the patient. * Communication also gets decreased because of impairment of brain and sensory deficits. So clear, brief and selective communication needs to be done.	* Approach in a slow, calm manner. * Observe for non-verbal communication (N. Do you want water, Mukesh ? P-remains quiet N-offers water, P-drinks) * Face the patient. * Talk gently; loud tones create threat and irritability for the patient. * Give a simple and clear message. * Encourage the pa-	* Expresses happiness that he/she is able to convey his/her message clearly.

1	2	3	4	5
			tient to talk. * Listen to him/her with respect and regard. * Repeat instructions, if required.	
Reduce Disorientation	STG To help the patient feel comfortable and less confused. LTG To enable the patient to : — help in regular activities. — feel secure and less restless	* Due to disorientation the patient is confused, so reorientation is required. * Patient and clear communication helps the patient to understand the meaning of the message being conveyed.	* Orient the patient to time, place and person with the help of a wall clock, calendar in the ward and the physical set-up * Call the patient by name. * Repeat the routine activity of the patient. * Avoid argument * Speak slowly, clearly and in simple sentences. * Convey warmth and concern. * Touch the patient to provide a sense of security. * Respond to the patient's questions. * Encourage him/her to speak clearly and not to mumble words.	* The patient looks less confused. * Feels comfortable in the setting

1	2	3	4	5
			* Create a comfortable environment without stress or hurry.	
Help to adjust with perceptual changes.	STG To help the patient reduce anxiety. LTG To enable the patient to : — adjust to perceptual deprivation — improve in his sensation. — reduce irritability.	* Due to misperception these patients are very anxious. * Specially the patient is not able to recognize direction and place even though sorroundings are familiar. * Help in reducing confusion. * Help in coping with frustrating situations. The patient may get frightened due to hallucination and relatives may also be disturbed.	* Reorient the place * Allow the patient to touch everything and feel the familiarity. * Allow the patient to smell the old perfume which he/she is used to. * Prevent the patient from burns. * Lack of sensitivity to heat may cause burns, prevent it. * Be available to the patient whenever he needs help. * Speak clearly, as the patient may concentrate due to suspiciousness but can't hear due to sensory misperception. * Give sedation, if prescribed. * Help the patient and relatives understand that change is due to disease.	* The patient feels less restless.

1	2	3	4	5
Help to adjust in alteration in memory & attention.	STG To help the patient improve his attention span. LTG To enable the patient to : — adjust to memory changes (transient or permanent).	* The patient gets irritated because he/she is not able to recall immediate and recent events, but remote memory is intact. * Feels inadequate in front of relatives and friends.	* Help the patient and relatives understand that change is due to disease. * Help relatives not to get irritated if the patient is not able to inform them about a telephonic message or what the doctor told him/her. He may not be able to recall. However, he may be able to tell what the doctor told him at the time of admission. * Switch on old songs, music or show old photographs to stimulate memory. * Provide activities of his/her choice so that the patient can attend and complete them. * Encourage the patient for any work that he/she has completed. * Provide an oppor-	* The patient shows concentration and efficiency on the work which he had been doing. * Feels comfortable with old things and says : "I feel bad when I can't remember the recent things."

1	2	3	4	5
			tunity to do the tasks which he had been doing for many years.	
Limit Inappropriate behaviour.	STG To help the patient to enjoy support from others. LTG To enable the patient to: — feel comfortable with others. — reduce pressure on family members. — feel that he/she is wanted.	* The patient is not able to decide whether to go to a social gathering at home or not. * Tendency to misplace things, finds them, loses them again. * Help him not to be defensive about any mistakes. * The patient demands attention.	* Identify support of family members. * Encourage the patient and relatives to be tolerant. * Help him control his anger and irritability. * Help the patient find out a misplaced thing as early as possible to reduce anxiety. Encourage him to keep things in a place where he can remember. * Encourage the patient to participate in a family decision. * If the patient has made a mistake, explain him that he does not need to be sensitive about it. But he should be careful	* Tries to control his anger and irritability.

1	2	3	4	5
			in future. * Don't overprotect them.	
IV. RECREATIONAL NEEDS				
	STG To reduce social isolation. LTG To enable the patient to: — spend time productively — enjoy life — feel useful for family members.	* Help in diverting the patient's mind. * Simple recreational activities may be provided: hobbies of his/her choice in which some productive outcome is possible.	* Tell children to go and play with the patient simple games like cards, ludo. * Provide knitting which the patient enjoys. * Male patient may like to cover the books of children. * Read a story for children. * Likes to watch T.V. programmes of choice. * Encourage the patient to interact and socialize with his own group.	* The patient enjoys life and feels that she/he is useful for family members.
V. SPIRITUAL NEEDS				
	STG To help the patient to follow his/her routine. LTG To enable the patient to: — maintain his/her routine activity — reduce distress	* These patients are ritualistic in their religious activity, help them to maintain it. * Trips to religious places may be reduced and they	* Allow the patient to attend her/his regular prayers. * Don't get irritated with extra time spent by the patient. * Gradually help	* The patient says: "Now I am not able to pray for long because I get tired."

and despair.	should be helped to adjust to it.	him reduce time in case it is affecting his diet intake. * Provide religious books video/ audio cassettes.	

VI. DISCHARGE PLAN

STG To help the patient to be self-sufficient. LTG To enable the patient to: — cope with the change due to sickness. — be self-sufficient.	* Planning of discharge also depends on the family support. The nurse needs to make an assessment. * Discussion with family members and the patient on his independent and dependent roles. * To develop realistic goals towards the patient's recovery.	* Encourage relatives to talk about the problems they have to face at home. * Allow the patient and his relatives to discuss the plan of care at home. * Explain to relatives and the patient what probable physical and social adjustments they need to make. * Educate the patient and relatives for after-care help from various agencies.	* Relatives and the patient get prepared to adjust in a home situation. * Stable vital signs. Reduced tremors and change in associated symptoms.

TO RECALL

* Definition of Organic Mental Disorders.
* Causes
* Nursing Diagnosis.
* Nursing Care Plan.
  - I. Therapeutic Needs
  - II. Physical Needs
    - — Prevention from injuries.
    - — Encourage and help in personal hygiene.
    - — Nutritional needs.
    - — Improve sleep pattern.
  - III. Psychosocial Needs
    - — Promote socialization.
    - — Promote communication.
    - — Reduce disorientation.
    - — Help to adjust with perceptual changes
    - — Help to adjust in alteration in memory and attention.
    - — Limit inappropriate behaviour. (inappropriate)
  - IV. Recreational Needs.
  - V. Spiritual Needs.
  - VI. Discharge Plan.

NURSING PATIENT WITH ALCOHOLIC PROBLEM

INTRODUCTION

Addiction to alcohol and drugs has become a problem for the individual, family and community. With a large number of people taking to alcoholism due to psychological and socio-cultural factors, the health problems have also become alarming. Alcoholic Anonymous describes alcoholism as a physical condition associated with mental obsession. It is considered to have physical, psychological, sociological and alcoholic parts of sickness.

DEFINITION

Alcoholism is defined as chronic dependence characterized by compulsive drinking of alcohol to such a degree that it produces mental disturbance, interferes with social and economic functioning. Major signs of addiction are increasing consumption, sneaking and gulping drinks, morning drinking, excessive drinking when alone, confusion and tremors, uninhibited behaviour and severe withdrawal symptoms.

CAUSES

Interpersonal factors
Socioeconomic factors
Cultural and ethnic factors
Pharmocological factors
Ecological factors

(Refer Chapter VII Unit XX)

WITHDRAWAL SYMPTOMS

Withdrawal symptoms include sleeplessness, sweating, poor appetite, tremors, convulsions, hallucinations and even death.

PSYCHO-DYNAMICS

The personality make-up of these people is a weak ego and superego. The individual remains fixated at the oral stage of development. He uses it as a primary method of relieving stress and frustration. He has low self-esteem and poor impulse control. There may be the presence of a negative role model at home in which father may take to alcohol in stressful situations.

NURSING DIAGNOSIS

* Non-compliance of treatment.
* Impaired physical care.
* Decreased intake of food and fluids and weight loss.
* Increased tremors of hands and legs.
* Highly violent — suicide/homicide.
* Disturbed sleep pattern.
* Decreased energy.

* Impaired judgement: may jump out of the window in delirium.
* Increased anxiety.
* Depression.
* Use of defense mechanisms; denial, projection and rationalization.
* Manipulative behaviour.
* Low self-esteem due to dependency.
* Perceptual changes, hallucination, bizarre thinking.
* Systemic changes — B.P., Pulse, Seizures, Gastro-intenstinal.
  — disturbances, Neurological changes.
* Marked withdrawal symptoms.

NURSING CARE PLAN FOR PATIENT WITH ALCOHOLIC PROBLEM

NURSING NEEDS 1	GOALS 2	PLAN 3	IMPLEMENTATION 4	EVALUATION 5
I THERAPEUTIC NEEDS				
Compliance to treatment.	STG To help the patient to take medicine regularly. LTG To help the patient to: — control his symptoms like delirium tremors. — reduce anxiety and depression. — reduce other associated symptoms like hallucination, rigidity, confusion, disorientation. — Prevent complications.	* The patient will have a denial for taking medicine. Plan giving him medicine regularly and in time. * Explain the patient that medicine will help reduce symptoms associated with alcoholism.	* Encourage the patient to take medicine as prescribed. * Administer sedatives as prescribed and observe for reduced discomfort. * If the patient is found to be in an acute state of intoxication, attend to medical care and maintain a vital sign chart.	* Stable vital signs. * Reduced tremors and change in associated symptoms.
II PHYSICAL NEEDS				
Provide adequate nutrition and maintain weight.	STG To help the patient to take an adequate and nutritional diet. To take adequate fluids. LTG To help the	* The patient refuses to take a diet and develops vitamin deficiency. * The patient looks dehydrated and	* Encourage the patient to take adequate diet. Force eating, if he/she refuses. * Add vitamins in the diet or treat-	* Starts eating meals. * Shows gain in weight.

1	2	3	4	5
	patient to: — improve his/her general health — prevent malnutrition due to use of alcohol.	malnourished. * Plan an adequate diet and fluid intake. * The patient may lose fluids due to vomiting caused by alcohol intake, assess ability of self-feeding, * Nausea, vomiting or diarrhoea may be present due to withdrawal.	ment, specially thiamine. * Give plenty of fluids. * Ensure that the patient takes a full meal. * Maintain his weight record. * Record intake and output. * Help the patient to feed if tremors are marked. * Give small and frequent feeds. * Maintain electrolyte balance.	
Improve Sleep Pattern.	STG To improve duration of sleep. LTG To help the patient to: — have adequate hours of quality sleep. — develop a sense of recovery.	* The patient has a disturbed sleep pattern because of agitation. * The patient gets a few hours of sleep. * He/ she may not be able to sleep because of frightening visual hallucinations such as insects, animals.	* Provide a calm and soothing envirnoment. * Be with the patient. Don't leave him alone. * Observe the patient for any interruption of sleep. * Give a hot glass of milk. * Rub the back to make the patient comfortable. * Switch on soft	* The patient has long hours of sleep.

1	2	3	4	5
			music and allow the patient to read a book. * Leave the lights on. * If hypontics are prescribed administer the dose.	
Protect self and others from injury.	STG To protect the patient from commiting suicide due to depression. To prevent his homicide acts due to violent behaviour. LTG To help the patient control his impulsive behaviour.	* The patient may jump out of window due to disorientation or hallucination. * Lack of alcohol intake may lead to irritation and violent behaviour. * The patient may attack others due to delusional (paranoid) disorder. Provide a safe environment. The patient may fall due to imbalance or lack of muscle coordination.	* Assess his depressive feelings. * Reorientation to the patient of time, place and people around. * Provide care by the same nursing personnel. * Do not discuss the patient near bedside. * Observe the violent behaviour of the patient. * Use restraints as a last resort.	* Does not attack anyone.
Maintenance of health of the patient.	STG To help the patient improve holistically. Reduce and control symptoms like	* Maintaining physical health of the patient, specially B.P., pulse, respiration.	* Constant observation and recording of vital signs and neurological status.	* The patient shows improvement in his health.

1	2	3	4	5
	B.P. Neurological symptoms. LTG To help the patient to: — reduce complications. — recover completely with less sequlae.	* Identify stages of withdrawal symptoms. * If the patient presents seizures, care should be taken to protect him from any injury.	* Make note of withdrawal symptoms and give nursing care accordingly. * If the patient has seizures (convulsions), provide a padded bed, give care prior, during and after seizures. * Assess for physical complaints. * If the patient is too peaceful during the withdrawal stage, look for possession of alcohol.	
To maintain personal hygiene.	STG To help the patient to develop a sense of well-being. LTG To help the patient to: — maintain personal hygiene — be self-sufficient.	* The patient needs to be encouraged to maintain personal hygiene,as he/she is disturbed because of his/her withdrawal symptoms. * Is preoccupied in obtaining alcohol.	* Pursue the patient to maintain personal hygiene. * Ensure that he/she changes clothes daily. * If the patient is confused, assist him in his personal hygiene.	* The patient feels fresh and looks neat and clean.
III. PSYCHOSOCIAL NEEDS				
To help the patient withdraw from use of alcohol.	STG To help the patient identify the problems	* The patient needs constant observation during the	* Encourage the patient to talk about his drink-	* The patient shows symptoms of detoxification.

1	2	3	4	5
	associated with the use of alcohol. LTG To help the patient to: — lead a normal life. — prevent himself from complications, specially tremors, neurological change, malnutrition, death.	withdrawal phase. * Explain to the patient to assess his physical health during the use of alcohol and without it after withdrawal symptoms are reduced. * Help the patient to find pleasure in life without the use for alcohol.	ing pattern. * Find out his/her plan of stopping intake of alcohol. * Encourage the patient to change his social group. * Observe vital signs of the patient.	
To help in reducing anxiety and depression.	STG To help the patient reduce restlessness. LTG To help the patient to: — be able to manage without the use of alcohol. — develop confidence that symptoms will be reduced.	* The patient is worried about getting alcohol, otherwise he thinks that symptoms will be unbearable. * Depression may also be due to relatives' pressure in stopping the use of alcohol.	* Accept the patient with his problem. * Give care to the patient during withdrawal symptoms. * Provide support of relatives by letting them to be with the patient. * Be firm with relatives and the patient if he/she keeps asking for alcohol. * Be non-judgemental. Avoid saying it was bad for you to take alcohol.	* The patient is less restless.

1	2	3	4	5
			* Restrain your biased feeling toward the alcoholic. Observe for suicidal ideation, may attempt suicide due to depression.	
Help reducing hallucination.	STG To protect the patient from injury to self. LTG To help the patient to: — learn that hallucinations are transient. (temporary) — have peaceful sleep. — prevent reuse of alcohol.	* Marked hallucination leads to discomfort. The patient keeps seeing insects, animals or frightening, distorted faces during the chronic stage. * The patient needs to be reassured that hallucination will decrease during treatment. * During hallucination he may jump out of the window and die.	* Encourage the patient to talk about his hallucination. * Don't leave the patient alone. * Explain to relatives and the patient that once he/she recovers these symptoms will disappear. * Protect the patient from self-injury.	* The patient has very less hallucinations.
Limit Manipulative Behaviour.	STG To stop use of alcohol. LTG To help the patient to: — identify his manipulative behaviour.	* Withdrawal symptoms become difficult to tolerate, so the patient starts begging relatives for alcohol.	* Explain to relatives not to feel emotionally disturbed at the patient's withdrawal symptoms.	* The patient uses less of manipulative behaviour. * Relatives do not get alcohol even though the withdrawal symptoms

1	2	3	4	5
	— bear the withdrawal symptoms. — use less of defense mechanisms.	* Relatives need to be educated to support in recovery of the patient. * The patient may rationalize that if a little bit of alcohol is given, he will never take in his life again.	* Ensure the patient and relatives safety in the hospital. * Explain to the patient the emotional manipulation he/she is trying with relatives. * Instruct relatives and ward employees not to get alcohol for the patient. * Check for possession for alcohol if the patient is not showing withdrawal symptoms.	are intolerable.
Enhance Self-Esteem.	STG To help the patient to feel comfortable with others. LTG To help the patient to: — learn that he is important.	* The patient feels that society may not accept and may condemn him as an alcoholic. * Relatives and his own children have shown lack of concern during the alcoholic stage. * Inadequacy feel-	* Call the patient by name. * Explain to relatives and the patient that symptoms are temporary. * Allow relatives and children to visit the patient frequently and discuss family issues. * Discourage rela-	* The patient identifies that he is more comfortable. * Identifies that he is being accepted by larger groups.

1	2	3	4	5
	— can interact with everyone.	ing due to physiological changes like tremors. * Should be encouraged to take up his roles gradually.	tives to make derogatory remarks, "It is only because of your bad habit everybody has come to know." * Explain to relatives that the patient's habit has taken into illness. * Help the patient in doing his/her activities. * Encourage him/her to socialize. * Help family members to develop confidence in the patient.	
Help the patient to socialize.	STG To develop a sense of support. LTG To help the patient to: — enjoy socialization without the use of alcohol. — identify his capability of interacting with others. — enhance his/her self-concept.	* These patients only socialize with their 'alcoholic groups'. * The patient feels that others may condemn him because he is alcoholic.	* Help the patient to try out new relations. * Encourage interaction with other patients. * Encourage the patient to spend time in day-room.	* Feels that he/she can socialize without the use of alcohol.
IV. RECREATIONAL NEEDS				
	STG To divert the patient's mind	* Socialization with others will im-	* Help the patient to identify his hobbies.	* The patient takes initiative on get-

1	2	3	4	5
	from withdrawal symptoms. LTG To help the patient to: — find pleasure in life without the use of alcohol. — feel confident.	prove his self-concept. * The patient had been always pre-occupied with getting alcohol and did not spend enough time on his/her hobbies.	* Allow the patient to do painting if she/he wants to. * Provide him with recreational articles like making paper meshe articles. * Avoid articles which can cause injury due to muscle incoordination.	ting articles of his choice from home to spend his time.
V. SPIRITUAL NEEDS				
	STG To regain an insight into life. LTG To help the patient to: — have hope and gain pleasure in life without the use of alcohol.	* Help the patient to attend to his spiritual needs.	* Encourage the patient to attend to his daily prayers. * Attend to yoga which he was practising before.	* Enjoys life, looks relaxed.
VI. DISCHARGE PLAN				
•	STG Not to reuse alcohol. LTG To help the patient to: — attend to alcoholic anonymous groups. — Attend a follow-up clinic.	* Help family members to support, protect and care at home. * Encourage the patient to change his social group. * Spend time on his occupational activities and with family.	* Encourage the patient to attend the follow-up clinic. * In case of a crisis encourage him to attend alcoholic anonymous groups. * Help him to go back to his job.	* The patient starts with his routine work at job and home.

TO RECALL

- Definition
- Causes
- Withdrawal Symptoms
- Psychodynamics
- Nursing Diagnosis
- Nursing Care Plan
  - I Therapeutic Needs — Compliance to treatment
  - II Physical Needs
    - Provide adequate nutrition and maintenance of weight
    - Improve sleep pattern
    - Protect self and others from injury
    - Maintenance of health
    - Maintenance of personal hygiene.
  - III Psychosocial Needs
    - Withdrwal from alcohol
    - Reduce anxiety and depression
    - Reduce hallucination
    - Limit manipulative behaviour
    - Enhance self-esteem
    - Help the patient socialize
  - IV Recreational Needs
  - V Spiritual Needs
  - VI Discharge Plan

NURSING PATIENT WITH DRUG/SUBSTANCE ABUSE

INTRODUCTION

Drug addiction/substance abuse is a social problem worldwide. It is a problem of the individual, family and society. The non-medical use of dependence-producing drugs involves dynamic interaction between three major factors:

a. the properties of the durg taken and the manner of use
b. the characteristics of the users; and
c. the nature of the immediate and larger socio-cultural environment in which the durg use occurs.

DEFINITION

Drug addicts or "Junkies', as they are called by peers, take in drugs for a number of reasons, such as to relax, to forget problems, to be social at parties. Some use drugs because it is fun, or drugs help them feel better when they are under stress. Use of the drugs is due to peer pressure also.

Drug abuse/substance abuse is a term applied to pathological use of drugs or alcohol with impairment in social and occupational functioning (e.g. failure to meet family obligations, erratic or criminal behaviour, missing work or school) and a minimal duration of disturbance of at least one month.

ETIOLOGY OR CAUSES

i. Interpersonal and psychosocial factors
ii. Socioeconomic factors
iii. Cultural and ethnic factors
iv. Pharmocological factors
v. Ecological factors

(Refer Chapter VII,Unit XX)

PSYCHO-DYNAMICS

These people have difficulty in having relationship with family members. Psychoanalytically, they are described as regressed and fixed at the oral stage of psychosexual development. Families in which the parents are self- centred and are preoccupied with success and prestige may lead their children to drug addiction. These children may face personal insecurity, show rebellious attitude towards authority and try to escape from a difficult situation. Critical behaviour due to self-doubt and absence of strong and efficient ego.

COMMONLY ABUSED SUBSTANCES/ DRUGS

The drugs which are commonly abused can be classified as:

i. Narcotics
ii. Sedative and depressants.
iii. Stimulants
iv. Psychodelics and hallucinogens

v. Minor tranquillizers

(Refer Chapter VII,Unit XX)

NURSING DIAGNOSIS

* Increased anxiety due to nonavailability of drugs, lack of money, fear of police, poor performance at home and job.
* Altered sleep pattern.
* Impaired social interaction.
* Disturbed self-esteem.
* Poor intake of diet.
* Impaired communication.
* Manipulative behaviour.
* Decreased coping abilities of withdrawal symptoms.

These clients are brought to the hospital by police, or forcibly by relatives. Very rarely they come on their own for treatment of stopping the use of drugs. Nursing care will depend upon which stage the patient has come. However, the common approach by the nurse is discussed in the following text.

NURSING CARE PLAN FOR PATIENT WITH DURG/SUBSTANCE ABUSE

NURSING NEEDS	GOALS	PLAN	IMPLEMENTATION	EVALUATION
1	2	3	4	5
I THERAPEUTIC NEEDS				
	STG To help the client to cope up with withdrawal symptoms. LTG To help the client to: — avoid taking drugs again.	* The nurse needs to participate in caring for the patient during detoxification. Specially helping the patient to develop an insight into the problems associated while on drugs.	* Develop trusting relationship. * Identify the types of withdrawal symptoms the patient is presenting. * Help the client to cope up with symptoms. * If any alternative drug is prescribed give it to the client. * Explain the relative not to feel emotionally upset and give the drug. * Check if the client is possessing or getting a drug in the ward through some source.	* The patient tries to cope with withdrawal symptoms.
II PSYCHOSICAL NEEDS				
Help in decreasing anxiety.	STG To decrease restlessness. LTG To help the client to:	* The client is anxious to get the next dose. Tries to look for a safe	* Develop trusting relationship. * Accept the client 'here and now'	* Shows decreased restlessness because of treatment and support from

1	2	3	4	5
	— overcome anxiety. — find family support.	place for taking the drug because of police fear. * Goes back to the addict group for lack of emotional support from the family.	with his/her problem. * Don't belittle him in front of others as a 'drug addict'. * Assess his/her anxiety. * Encourage him to verbalize the reason of anxiety. * Check if the client is possessing money. * Observe with whom the client is interacting and what is the motive. * Encourage family members to provide support. * Check if he spends too much time outside the ward or in the toilet/ bathroom.	family members.
Reducing Maladaptive Behaviour.	STG To help the client to be accepted by others. LTG To help the client to: — change his habits — stop stealing — reduce aggressiveness	* The client, on not getting money, starts stealing, selling household things. * May beat up children, wife or other members of the family.	* Develop therapeutic relationship. * Encourage the client to express his views on obtaining the drug. * Ask him about the difficulties the	* The client controls his/her maladaptive behaviour.

1	2	3	4	5
		* The family members should be explained not to give in to the client's impulsive behaviour.	family members face for lack of money. * Encourage him/her to decide a solution to the problem of shortage of money. * Explain relatives not to get worried about threats of the client to leave home. * Limit his/her maladaptive behaviour by letting him realise it.	
Reducing manipulative behaviour.	STG To help the client not to take drugs again. LTG To help the client to: — realise that he/she is using manipulative behaviour. — cope with withdrawal symptoms.	* The client will be restless and emotionally blackmail the relatives that he/she will die, get him/her the dose. Hospital nurses and doctors don't understand these. * Help relatives not to give in to the client's demand.	* Explain to relatives that the client is safe in hospital without the use of drugs. * Explain to them not to get emotionally upset because of withdrawal symptoms. * Be present with the client. * Ignore his symptoms, but keep giving care. * Encourage fluids	* The client tries to cope with withdrawal symptoms.

1	2	3	4	5
			to prevent dehydration (I.V. fluids, if required). * Encourage him to take a good bath and change clothes. * Ensure clients that these symptoms are due to withdrawal of drugs and symptoms are temporary.	
Improve communication.	STG To help the client to express his feelings. LTG To help the client to: — reduce preoccupation of procuring drugs. — develop self-confidence.	* The client feels confident to talk only in the peer group. He/she has a feeling that others may reject him as an addict. * Does not interact because of low self-concept.	* Help the client to talk about his difficulty. * Ensure the presence of a relative. * Give a feeling that he/she is being cared for by being present near the client. * Help him to identify his strength like writing ability, good worker prior to the use of drugs. * Allow relatives and friends to visit him/her. * Encourage him/her to talk to others.	* The client identifies his/her behaviour prior to the use of drugs.

1	2	3	4	5
			* Be non-judgemental (Don't irritate your relative any more).	
Improve Socialization and self-concept.	STG To help the client to socialize. LTG To help the client to: — find pleasure in socialization. — develop self-confidence.	* The client does not socialize with others except his peer group (drug addicts). He/she may socialize from where he can take money. * Self-concept is decreased because of social neglect.	* Develop an active friendly attitude. * Help the client to socialize with people other than drug addicts. * Encourage him to join rehabilitation groups. * Provide him with activities in which he shows excellent performance. * Encourage relatives to take his suggestions. * Don't force them to interact only with mentally ill patients in the ward.	* The client intiates socialization.
III PHYSICAL NEEDS				
Help to cope with withdrawal symptoms.	STG To help the client to get relief from nausea, vomiting and other symptoms. LTG To help the client to:	* As the withdrawal symptoms are marked the client is not able to tolerate the detoxification. Observation needs to be	* Observe the intensity of withdrawal symptoms. * Administer stat medication. * Record vital signs and symptoms.	* The client feels secure.

1	2	3	4	5
	— tolerate withdrawal symptoms. — ensure him a safe medical environment.	done constantly. * Create an environment in which the client and relatives feel medically safe and secure.	* Give plenty of fluids to reduce dehydration. * Change clothes of the client if stinking due to excessive prespiration. * Provide a plan for the client's relatives. * Hold the client's hand during episodes of pain. * Be with the client.	* Tries to tolerate withdrawal symptoms.
To improve sleep pattern.	STG To help the client to have good night sleep. LTG To help the client to: — develop a regular sleep pattern. — feel less need of drugs.	* Stimulants lead to decreased sleep in drug users, with the result the client keeps thinking of continuity of drugs. * Feels fatigued and irritable for lack of sleep. Hallucination may also interfere.	* Encourage the patient to sleep for six to eight hours minimum at night. * Provide a secure environment. * Leave the floor lights on. * Allow a relative to sleep near the client. * Give back massage at night. * A hot glass of milk will induce sleep. * Allow the client to read some story books of his/her choice.	* Sleeps for six to seven hours, gradually shows increase in the duration of sleep

1	2	3	4	5
To improve food intake.	STG To help the client take an adequate and nutritious diet. LTG To help the client to: — eat regularly. — prevent malnutrition.	* The client may not feel like eating due to the effect of drugs. May eat very little. Starts losing weight, becomes malnourished.	* Provide small and frequent meals. * Serve food of his/her choice. * Maintain weight record. * Show the patient change in his/her weight.	* Takes food on his own.
To prevent injury and infection.	STG To help the client to protect himself from injury. LTG To help the client to: — prevent infection, local and systemic.	* Taking of oral and inhalant drugs leads to injury to mucous membrane. * Repeated use of injection with infected needles leads to local and systemic infection. * Malnutrition also leads to reduced immunity.	* Check for localized trauma due to repeated injections. * Evaluate the vein thrombosis. * Care for any infection. * Don't put the patient with other clients who are having infection. * Give medicine as prescribed for systemic infection.	* The client feels that he is being cared for.
IV RECREATIONAL ACTIVITIES				
	STG To divert attention of the client from drugs. LTG To help the client to: — channelize frustration in productive work.	* For many months or years the client has been only busy to be on 'street' either to get a drug or to use it. * Provide him with	* Plan activities for the client. * Encourage all the clients to come in the open space, take exercise and yoga. * Tell him to help	* The client says if there is so much to do in the ward, at home I can help in many things.

1	2	3	4	5
	— reduce lethargy. — improve zest for life.	activities of his interest. * Help him know that life has more meaning than just having drugs. * Help him know that change in his behaviour will bring changes in relatives.	in cleaning his locker. * Encourage him to distribute diet in the ward. * Tell him to take out articles for the occupational therapy room. * Prepare the T.V. room for all the clients to sit down. * Put on music and allow clients to burn out their energy. * Prepare for group therapy for clients on deadiction.	
V SPIRITUAL NEEDS				
	STG To help the client divert his mind from procuring drugs. LTG To help the client to: — develop an insight into his behaviour. — take an opportunity of getting fully recovered. — be socially productive again.	* The client needs to be explained the other methods which he can use to cope with frustration and failure. * Reduce the feeling of helplessness.	* Encourage him to come to the prayer and yoga room. * Attend to spiritual talks. * Provide an opportunity for confession. * Give reward for activities and accomplishment. * Encourage him to talk positively about himself.	* Interacts with others discusses pleasurable moments of life.

1	2	3	4	5
VI DISCHARGE PLAN				
	STG To help the client not to restart the use of drugs. LTG To help the client to: — identify the painful withdrawal symptoms. — change the support system. — stop taking drugs.	* 'Old habits die hard' is applicable for these clients. * Intensive follow-up of activity, related groups, recreational group and reaction of the client. Friends and relatives need to be helped. * The client can look for a change of social support instead of depending on his "drug pals".	* Encourage verbal catharsis. * Remind repeated admissions. * Educate when the symptoms are painful. * Encourage him to join a drug deaddiction group. * Explain family members to take the client to a deaddiction group. * Identify the friends and family supports. * Search for room of the client if he is too quiet, passive, not hungry and sleeps unusually long hours.	* Takes another friend to hospital for deaddiction. * Comes for follow-up.

TO RECALL

- ✱ Definition
- ✱ Etiology/Causes
- ✱ Psychodynamics
- ✱ Commonly abused substances/drugs

Nursing diagnosis

- ✱ Nursing Care Plan
  - I. Therapeutic Needs
  - II. Psychosocial Needs
    - ✱ Decrease in anxiety
    - ✱ Reducing maladapative behaviour
    - ✱ Reducing manipulative behaviour
    - ✱ Improve communication
    - ✱ Improve socialization and self-concept
  - III. Physical Needs
    - ✱ Help cope with withdrawal symptoms
    - ✱ To improve the sleep pattern
    - ✱ To improve food intake
    - ✱ To prevent injury and infection
  - IV. Recreational Activities
  - V. Spiritual Needs
  - VI. Discharge Plan

NURSING CLIENT WHO IS MENTALLY RETARDED

INTRODUCTION

Persons with retardation or slowness in their mental growth and capacities are called "Mentally Handicapped" or "Mentally Retarded". They are also referred to as "slow developers, "slow learners" or "less intelligent".

DEFINITION

Mental Retardation is a disorder characterised by significantly subaverage general intellectual function, an I.Q. of 70 or below, with impairment in adaptive behaviour (including thinking, learning, social and occupational adjustment) and manifested during the development period (below age of 18). Abbreviation used for mental retardation is MR (Longman Dictionary).

ICD-10 defined — Mental retardation is a condition of arrested or incomplete development of the mind, which is especially characterized by impairment of skills manifested during development period that contribute to cognitive (knowledge) language, motor and social abilities.

EPIDEMIOLOGY

Frequency :— No all-India survey has been undertaken to determine the exact number of the mentally retarded in our country. However, more than 20 million people are mentally retarded in India. About three of every 100 people belong to this category. And one of these will not be able to care for himself. So he/she becomes totally dependent on others, while others will be partially handicapped.

Incidence :— Incidence of MR seems to increase sharply at the age of five with the number of cases identified at the age of 15.

CAUSE OF MENTAL RETARDATION

The cause of MR can be explained under the following heading:

GENETIC FACTORS

Chromosomal defects. For example, mongolism, Down's syndrome.

CAUSES RELATED TO PREGNANCY AND CHILDBIRTH

Prenatal :— Lack of an adequate nutritional diet to mother, viral infection in the first trimester (3 months) of pregnancy such as pertusis, mumps, rubella infection, RH incompatability, premature birth.

Natal — During birth — birth trauma, mechanical injury to the child's brain while helping in delivery. Asphyxia, difficult labour, anoxia leading to MR, 25 to 30% of feeble-mindedness occurs due to mismanaged childbirth.

Post-natal :— After birth if the infant had bacterial encephalitis, meningitis which is the most common cause of mental feebleness, post-natal cerebral trauma, convulsive disorders.

Infection — Congenital Rubella, influenza to mother, congenital syphilis.
Trauma/head injury.
Malnutrition — In the first two years of development leads to Mental Retardation.
Disorders or Metabolism — Phenylketouria Hypothyriodism.
Intoxication — Biliurubin encephalopathy, lead poisoning, postvaccinal encephalitis.
Sociocultural — Prolonged isolation during the developmental period leads to sensory and social deprivation, cultural familial retardation in which the child feels it difficult to interact with others.
Untreated epileptic fits.

DIFFERENCE IN MR AND MENTAL ILLNESS

Mental illness is a disease which can be cured. Mental retardation is developmental disorders in which there is impaired ability. So MR is not a disease. It cannot be cured. However, the associated conditions like deafness, poor vision and emotional disturbances can be treated. So the handicap can be reduced.

MYTHS ABOUT MR

Certain myths about MR are given below:

1. ***There is nothing like mental retardation.*** It is wrong. It is probably more difficult to accept and visualize MR than physical illness. Blindness, defect in limbs can be seen but MR cannot be seen unless the child starts growing and finds difficulty in learning problem solving, adjusting socially and I.Q. is below 70.
2. ***Mental retardation is always hereditary.*** It is wrong. Hereditary factors contribute but a list of other causes is included in this unit which leads to MR.
3. ***Mental retardation is not common.*** It is wrong. As described in epidemiology, MR is 3% in the general population.
4. ***Mental retardation can be cured by tonic,*** vitamins and marriage. It is wrong. No tonics can increase mental abilities. Marriage rather may cause adjustment and legal problems.
5. ***All mentally retarded are alike.*** It is wrong. Mental retardation varies from mild, moderate, severe to profound. Assessment by proper I.Q. will help in assessing the potentials of these clients.
6. ***Mentally retarded cannot be educated or trained.*** It is wrong. Depending upon the degree of mental retardation, education and training can be given.

DEGREES OF MENTAL RETARDATION

ICD-10 (F 70 to 72) has classified MR as:
— Mild mental retardation.
— Moderate mental retardation.
— Severe mental retardation.
— Profound mental retardation.

DEGREE	IQ LEVEL	DEFICIT	COPING ABILITIES
Mild	50 — 69	Difficult in academic school work, problem in reading and writing. Difficulty in complex ideas and drawing generalization, can learn motor skills better than verbal skills Education upto the 6th grade.	Fully independent in self-care. Development of domestic skills, behaviour, social and emotional adjustment is like a normal person. As many as 80 per cent can fully adjust, **"educable"**.
Moderate	35 — 49	* Progress in school work limited. * Education upto 2nd grade * Intelligence level similar. to 4 to 7 years old child. * Unaware of needs. * Requires supervision during self-care. * Can learn few basic skills.	* Requires supervision during work. * Can be placed under a sheltered workshop but for unskilled work like counting 10 buttons and putting in one box. **'Trainable'.**
Severe	20 — 34	Marked degree of motor impairment associated with deficit. Minimal speech.	* Requires complete supervision for self-care. * May learn to perform very simple working, picking up something and putting nearby in a bundle.
Profound	20 & below	Can't comply with request or instructions. Immobile, incontinent, rudimentory form of non-verbal communication like("gggggg"). No ability to care their basic needs	* Custodial care. Can't do anything on their own.

Fig. 31 : Table describing Degree of MR, IQ Level, Deficit Coping Abilities.

Behaviour modification of a mentally retarded person can be made by operant conditioning and token economy at least in some of the self-care areas like eating, bathing, toileting, dressing.

NURSING DIAGNOSIS

Nursing diagnosis in this text is discussed of moderate and severely retarded persons.

Preventive Approach	— Assessing the degree of mental retardation. Early detection, genetic counselling. — Antenatal care, postnatal care.
Psychosocial Deficit	— Parents. — Acceptance by society. — Developmental changes. — Sexual abuse. — Decreased attention and concentration. — Helping in fostering group behaviour. — Speech and communication.
Physical Deficit	— Bathing, brushing, dressing, toileting, eating, health care.
Recreational and Occupational Activities	— Group activity. — Visits outside. — Sheltered workshop.
Rehabilitation	— Home. — Rehabilitation Home. — Half-way homes. — Day-care home. — Vocational training programme.

NURSING CARE PLAN FOR PATIENT WITH MENTAL RETARDATION

NURSING NEEDS 1	GOAL 2	PLAN 3	IMPLEMENTATION 4	EVALUATION 5
I. PREVENTION OF MENTAL RETARDATION				
	STG To help in reducing the number of people with MR. LTG To care for already existing MR persons.	* If there is a family history of MR, the couple should be educated about the probable chances. * During the antenatal period help mother to improve diet and prevent from infection. * Help her to go through easy labour and prevent any trauma to the child. * Postnatal care — prevent infection to mother and her child. Help her to check for milestones of the infant.	* Give genetic counselling to the couple if there is history of MR in the family. * Prevent the mother from having any type of infection. * Encourage abortion if the mother had Rubella infection. * Discourage taking of drugs for abortion. * Enrol the mother for a regular antenatal check-up. * Educate the couple for delivery in a good hospital with adequate facilities. * Protect the infant	* The couple ensures regular check-up. * Brings the infant to a well—baby clinic regularly.

1	2	3	4	5
			from any type of infection. * Teach the mother not expose to X-Rays unnecessarily. * Explain to the mother to check-whether the child holds the head erect at six months, sits without support at nine months, stands and walks by 18 months and talks at 24 months. * Put up exhibitions in an antenatal clinic and community health centre on prevention of MR.	
II. ASSESSMENT OF DEGREE OF MR				
	STG To help parents know if the child is MR. LTG To help parents: — learn the degree of MR. — plan for the help of the child.	* Educate parents if the milestones of the child are not normal, get him/her tested in a child guidance clinic. Parents need help not to go to many places as the result will	* Encourage parents to bring the child to a well baby clinic regularly. * Check for the milestones and teach the mother also. * Ensure any	* Parents start accepting that something is wrong with their child.

1	2	3	4	5
		be the same. * Help them to bear the shock of "WHY MY CHILD" is having Mental Retardation.	physiological handicap before informing or creating doubt in parents about MR specially deafness (partial) * Inform parents about good child guidance centres. * Help handling anxiety of parents. * Ensure the presence of both the parents for diagnosis.	
III PSYCHOSOCIAL SUPPORT				
Acceptance of Child with Mental Retardation.	STG To help parents to accept the deficit of client. LTG To help parents to treat the child as other children in the family.	* Parents find it difficult to accept. * Proper investigation and reports should be explained to them. * Develop an empathetic attitude towards parents. Parents start looking for a place where they can leave the child and pay monthly expenditure.	* Encourage parents to talk about the report. * Listen patiently and with supportive attitude. * Educate parents that home environment is safe psychologically and physically for the child. * Encourage mother to clarify her doubts at each stage of child development.	* Parents starts coping with the development of the client.

1	2	3	4	5
			* Explain to parents to accept the child and society will also accept. * Explain that they don't have to be ashamed of having a MR child at home.	
Help parents in Developmental Changes.	STG To help parents to accept the growth of their child. LTG To help parents to: — meet needs of the growing child. — protect the child from sexual assault.	* These children have good physical growth, boys are physically strong an can hurt anyone. Girls grow physically well. * Boys may not have judgement and sexually assault their own sisters. * Females can also be exploited sexually. This causes apprehension in parents.	* Prepare parents to accept the physical growth of the child. * Train and care for a female child during her menstruation. * Do not leave a young girl alone at home with a male MR client. * Control and punish the impulsive behaviour of the child. * Do not over protect.	* Takes care of himself/herself during growth.
Help in Communication.	STG To help the client express what he/she needs. LTG To help the client to:	* These children have poor communication ability. * In severe cases it is at a very ru-	* Help parents to use simple names and ask the client to repeat Dad,. Mom, names of toys, dolls.	* The child learns few words and then formulates a sentence "Give water, milk".

1	2	3	4	5
	— learn to formulate a sentence. — enjoy talking to others.	dimentary level. So gradually help the client to learn the words.	* Call by name people at home. * Give reward when the client tries to call a correct name.	
Improve Attention and Concentration.	STG To help the client to familiarize and learn about things in his nearby environment. LTG To help the client to : — gradually increase the attention span. — improve concentration.	* Parents need to be explained that the client may improve in concentration gradually. He/she should be given activities of a similar kind. This takes time.	* Explain to parents to give one activity at a time like taking out water with a mug from one bucket till it is empty. * Encourage the client to repeat these activities.	* Gradually the client concentrates for a longer duration.
Help in Fostering Group Behaviour.	STG To feel part of the group. LTG To help the client feel that everybody can do some activity. — To give encouragement to the parents.	* Parents need to be explained that the group will motivate the child to learn some activities. * Parents also will feel that they are not the only one having a child with Mental Retardation.	* Allow the child to attend to group activities. * Help the child to learn behaviour which is accepted in the group such as not throwing things here and there. * Be quiet when guests have come.	* The childtries to maintain behaviour in the group.
Help Coping with Physical Stimulation	STG To assess the sensory abilities of	* Stimulation of senses that is eye,	* Put the bed near the window so	* The client starts responding to

1	2	3	4	5
of Senses.	the child. LTG To stimulate the senses of the child. — To train the child to become self-sufficient.	ear, skin and nose. They will also help the client to start identifying things.	that the client can see a variety of things. * Use bright colours. * Name the colour repeatedly. * Allow the child to listen to music & sound of utensils. * Put the child over a blanket, smooth cloth, rough cloth. * Bring certain foods; flowers, scents near the nose. * Show a picture of dog repeatedly, then show the real dog and say 'DOG'.	some stimulants.
IV PHYSICAL NEEDS				
Train the Child for Personal Hygiene; Care of Teeth and Skin.	STG To help the child to keep teeth and skin clean. LTG To help the client to learn self-care. — try to become partially dependent.	* The child is to be taught by modelling and demonstration. * Teaching with patience, and simplicity.	* Take a brush and hold it in your hand. * Tell the child to hold it in a similar manner. * Put paste on your brush and the child's brush. * Take near your mouth.	* The child may make many attempts to hold the brush but demonstrates the skill after a few months.

1	2	3	4	5
	— protect mouth and skin from infection.		* Make the child repeat it. * Open your mouth, put teeth together and brush. * Step-by-step see the child repeats. * Take the child to the bathroom. * Demonstrate bathing procedure step-by-step like brushing. * Repeat activities for several days/ weeks. * Show happiness at each positive act of the child.	
Helping in Dressing.	STG To help the child to adequately dress. LTG To help the child to: — develop skill in buttoning and unbuttoning. — remain in clean clothes.	* This is a long procedure. The nurse therapist has to be patient with the child. It is difficult to button and unbutton the dress. To remove and wear the dress is also difficult for children with Mental Retardation.	* Demonstrate buttoning and ubuttoning of the shirt without wearing it. * Explain to the parents to give clothes with big holes and buttons. No back bottons, use press buttons. * Provide clothes with zips. * Demonstrate repeated opening	* Shows new clothes to sister and brother. Feels happy.

1	2	3	4	5
			and closing of the zip. * Get bright-coloured clothes for the child with a picture on them. * Give these to the child and tell him these belong to him/her.	
Helping in Toilet Training.	STG To help the child not to bed-wet. LTG To help the client to: — develop regular habits. — enjoy passing urine and stool in the toilet.	* Ask for cooperation of family members. * Help them not to feel shy in demonstrating to the child.	* Ask children to pass urine in the toilet in front of the M.R. child. * Tell the child to repeat the same act. * Demonstrate to the child how to sit in the toilet. * Ask him to demonstrate. * Show washing after passing stool. * Allow the child to repeat. * Reward the child with the favourite toy/game or car ride.	* The child finds pleasure in getting up in a dry bed.
Training in Eating.	STG To help the child to enjoy eating like other	* It may be difficult initially for the child for lack of	* Take a slice of bread and hold it in your fingers.	* Gradually the child starts taking other semisolid

1	2	3	4	5
	children. LTG To help the client to: — Become less dependent on others.	muscle coordination. But repeated demonstration and return demonstration will help him/her to eat on his/her own.	* Tell the child to do the same. * Help in putting the bread slice in his/her fingers. * Open your mouth and bite a small piece. * Now ask the child to repeat the same. * Chew slowly. * Ask the child to chew. * Swallow it in front of the child. * Ask the child to do the same. * Provide the child with his own utensils.	foods also.
Health Care.	STG To prevent the child from any infection. LTG To protect the client : — from any accidents such as burns, cuts. — from infections.	* Teach parents that these children are prone to accidents and infections. If the child has hearing and visual defects, explain to parents to get hearing aids or spectacles.	* Explain to parents not to overprotect the child. * Teach what is hot by letting him feel it once. * Avoid keeping gun, knife, scissors in the open. * Treat infection if the child develops it. * Teach relatives the use of hearing aids or spectacles.	* The child grows with less of deformities.

1	2	3	4	5
V. RECREATIONAL ACTIVITIES				
	STG To help the child join the group in play. LTG To help the child to: — develop abilities to be in the group. — attain pleasure. — learn activities through recreation.	* Help parents to develop a schedule of activities for children. * Allow the Mental Retardation child to play with other children.	* Provide simple craft activity like folding paper in two. * Playing with mud and making small toys. * Colouring a toy with one or two colours. * Providing the child to paint what he/she likes.	* The child gets pleasure claps and laughs.
VI. REHABILITATION OF CHILDREN				
	STG To help the child to be occupied. LTG To help the child to: — learn productive activities. — be occupied. — become more indenpendent.	* Help parents to identify the interests of the child. * Locate the nearby facilities like a factory where simple work can be performed by the child.	* Allow the child to do small activities at home. * Help parents to send the child to a day-care centre, half-way homes. * The child should be put in a sheltered workshop where he can be supervised constantly by someone.	* Parents feel relief that the child is learning something. * The child gets ready and wants to go.

TO RECALL

— Definition
— Epidemiology
— Causes of MR
— Difference between MR and Mental illness
— Myths about MR
— Degrees of Mental Retardation
— Nursing Diagnosis
— Nursing Care Plan

I. Prevention of Mental Retardation.
II. Assessment of Degree of MR.
III. Psychosocial Support
   * Acceptance of child with MR.
   * Help parents in developmental changes.
   * Help in communication.
   * Improve attention and concentration.
   * Help in fostering group behaviour.
   * Help Coping with Physical stimulation of senses.
IV. Physical Needs
   * Train the child for personal hygiene.
   * Helping in dressing.
   * Helping in toilet training and eating
V Recreational activities rehabilitation of children.
VI. Rehabilitation.

APPLICATION TO NURSING

Reading of the Unit on Nursing Care Plans for Special Problems in Mental Health Nursing will help the student to plan nursing intervention based on psychodonamics and nursing diagnosis in organic brain disorders, alcoholic disorders, drug abuse and mental retardation.

Reading of *Unit XXII* and Unit *XXIII* will enable the student to plan nursing intervention based on the nursing process for disorders other than described in these units.

BETTER STUDY SECTION OF UNIT XXIII

1. **VOCABULARY** (Refer Dictionary)

Arteriosclerosis	Impaired
Ecological	Impulse
Gulping	Interruption
Handicapped	Prestige
Holistically	Vocational
	Soothing

2. **ASSIGNMENT**
   a) List the withdrawal symptoms of the client who is addicted to drugs.
   b) Prepare a tabular presentation of the degree of Mental Retardation

3. **STUDY QUESTION**
   a) List the deficit of a child with mental retardation while working in Pediatric/psychiatric O.P.D.
   b) Prepare a discharge and rehabilitation plan for a client with drug abuse.

4. **READING REFERENCES.**

Shives L. R. ***Basic Concepts of Psychiatric Mental health Nursing*** (2nd Edition) J. B. Lippincott company, Philadelphia (1990).

Longman ***Dictionary of Psychology and Psychiatry*** Longmen. NewYork and London (1984).

Walker J.I. ***Essentials of clinical Psychiatry*** I.B. Lippincott company London (1985).

COMPREHENSIVE TEST OF CHAPTER VIII

1. List four steps of Nursing Process.
   (i)
   (ii)
   (iii)
   (iv)

2. Assessment of needs includes three aspects:
   (i)
   (ii)
   (iii)

3. Planning consists of the following aspects:
   (i)
   (ii)
   (iii)
   (iv)

4. List the types of nursing actions:
   (i)
   (ii)

5. A list of mental disorders is given in column B and statements of psychodynamics in column A. Place an appropriate alphabet from column B in the space given along with statement in column. A.

Column A	Column B
i.— The patient uses projection as a major defense mechanism.	a. Anxiety b. OCN
ii.— The patient develops a feeling of isolation, hopelessness and helplessness.	c. Depression d. Excitement
iii.— The patient represses conflict that arises anxiety which is converted into physical symptoms.	e. Schizophreni f. Drug abuse g. Delusion disorders
iv.— The patient has an impaired ego functioning reality testing and judgement is affected.	h. Suicidal
v.— The patient has conflict between Id and superego where ego is not able to meditate effectively.	i. Conversion reaction.
vi.— The patient is fixated at the anal stage of psychosexual development. Defenses used are regression, isolation undoing and reaction formation.	j. Hypochondrias. k. Phobias
vii.— The patient feels guilty and develops a self-punishing attitude, even attempts to commit suicide.	

viii.—The patient has difficulty in having relationship with family members. He is regressed and fixated at the oral stage of psychosexual development.

ix.— The patient has dependency for love and affection. Develops ambivalent feelings towards parents.

6. Fill in the blanks from the words given below:
Mental Retardation, Substance abuse, Organic mental disorders, Anxiety, Excitement, Somatoform disorders.

(i) In....................physiological changes are increased.
(ii) In....................characteristic symptoms are increased, motor activity, elated mood and increased thought.
(iii) In.....................the patient has repeated presentation of physical symptoms with a persistent request for medical investigation.
(iv) In.......................there is arrested and incomplete development of the mind which is especially characterized by impairment of skill and is manifested during development period.
(v) In........................there is impairment of brain tissue functions due to such factors as head injurym toxic conditions or encephalitis.

7. List the Nursing Diagnoses of the Patient with Anxiety.

8. List the Nursing Diagnoses of the Patient with Delusional Disorders.

KEY

Comprehensive Test of Chapter VIII

1. (i) Assessment and identification of needs.
   (ii) Plan of action.
   (iii) Implementation of plan
   (iv) Evaluation

2. (i) Data collection
   (ii) Analysis of data
   (iii) Nursing diagnosis or identification of nursing problems.

3. (i) Determining priorities
   (ii) Setting goals
   (iii) Selecting nursing actions
   (iv) Developing/writing nursing care plan

4. (i) Independent nursing actions
   (ii) Dependent nursing actions;

5.

1.	g	4.	e	7.	c
2.	h	5.	a	8.	f
3.	i	6.	b	9.	d

6. (i) Anxiety
   (ii) Excitement
   (iii) Somatoform Disorders
   (iv) Mental Retardation
   (v) Organic Brain Disorders

7. * Exaggerated fear
   * Impaired communication
   * Lowered self-esteem
   * Disturbed sleep pattern
   * Increased activity
   * Self-care deficit.
   * Changed psychological status
   * Decreased orientation
   * Altered socialization
   * Disturbed eating pattern
   * Dehydration

8. * Suicidal ideation and attempts
   * Increased weight loss
   * Loss of interest
   * Impaired communication
   * Reduced self-esteem and self-concept
   * Decreased appetite
   * Decreased activity
   * Altered affect, apathy, ambivalence
   * Reduced attention and concentration
   * Increased ideas of worthlessness
   * Decreased sleep
   * Self-care deficits.

CHAPTER IX

OTHER ASPECTS OF PSYCHIATRIC NURSING

UNIT XXIV
COMMUNITY MENTAL HEALTH NURSING

UNIT OUTLINE

* Concept of the National Mental Health Programme for India.
* Objectives of the programme.
* Approaches to the National Mental Health Programme.
* Definition of community mental health nursing.
* Factors leading to mental health problems/ disorders.
* Approaches to community mental health
  - Primary prevention.
  - Secondary prevention, Crisis intervention.
  - Tertiary prevention.

Community Facilities
  - Day Hospital/Centre
  - Half-way Houses
  - Group homes
  - Foster homes
  - Sheltered workshops
  - Mental health emergency care; Hot line, walk-in-clinics and home visits
  - Self-help groups
* Application to Nursings.
* Better Study Section.

INTENDED LEARNING BEHAVIOUR

After reading this unit you will be able to:
* Explain the National Mental Health Programme for India.
* List the objectives of the National Mental Health Programme.
* Apply the knowledge of approaches to be used in community mental health.
* Define community mental health nursing.
* Identify the factors leading to mental health problems.
* Explain the role of the nurse at:
  - The primary prevention level.
  - Secondary prevention and crisis intervention.
  - The tertiary prevention level.
* Describe the role of the nurse in community support.

COMMUNITY MENTAL HEALTH NURSING

CONTENT

INTRODUCTION

Community mental health services include all those activities in the community connected with mental health other than the institutional or hospitalized setting. The community approach focuses on the total population of a defined geographical area rather than an individual patient. Emphasis is mainly on preventive service, provision of a continuous, comprehensive system of services designed to meet all mental health-related needs in the community. Mental health care is provided through education, consultation, brief psychotherapy, crisis intervention and follow-up care.

CONCEPT OF NATIONAL MENTAL HEALTH PROGRAMME

India is a signatory State to the Alma Ata Declaration which envisages health for all by the year 2000 as the goal and primary health care or an approach. Health has been defined not as merely absence of diseases but as a state of positive well-being—physical, mental and social. Mental health, therefore, forms an essential part of total health and as such must form an integral part of the national health policy.

The National Mental Health Programme Policy (1982) has been formulated with the following objectives:

OBJECTIVES

a) To ensure availability and accessibility of minimum mental health care for all in the foreseeable future, particularly to the most vulnerable and under-priveleged sections of the population.

b) To encourage the population on mental health knowledge of general health care in social development.

c) To promote community participation in mental health services development and to stimulate efforts towards self-help in the community.

APPROACHES TO NATIONAL MENTAL HEALTH PROGRAMME

To achieve the objectives the following approaches were formed:

I) DIFFUSION OF MENTAL HEALTH SKILLS

Instead of centralising mental health skills and expertise in an urbanized community it should reach periphery (i.e. the primary health care structure at the community level like Primary Health Centre, Subcentre and Village level workers). Mental health care must start at the grassroot level.

II) APPROPRIATE APPOINTMENT OF TASKS IN MENTAL HEALTH CARE

The tasks to be performed at each level (village workers, subcentre, primary health centre, district hospital, regional hospital) will be specified and a referral system set up so that the total system works in an integrated fashion.

III) EQUITABLE AND BALANCED TERRITORIAL DISTRIBUTION OF RESOURCES

Every effort will be made to introduce or strengthen mental health first in those regions which are at present deprived of it or where it is seriously deficient.

IV) INTEGRATION OF BASIC MENTAL HEALTH CARE INTO GENERAL HEALTH SERVICES

This will facilitate in dealing with patients without gross psychiatric disturbances. It will enable the health worker to identify psychosocial problems. Psychiatric mental health workers will be able to identify and relate psychosocial factors contributing to ill-health.

V) LINKAGE TO COMMUNITY DEVELOPMENT

Involvement of state, district and block leadership in the implementation of the mental health programme to ensure community involvement in preventive efforts directed at psycho-social problems like alcohol, drug abuse, behaviour of childhood and adolescence, delinquency and other avoidable problems.

VI) MENTAL HEALTH CARE

It should include

A) TREATMENT:

1. Primary health care at the village and subcentre levels.
2. Primary health centre
3. District hospital
4. Mental hospitals and teaching psychiatric units.

B) REHABILITATION SUB-PROGRAMME (PREPARATION OF PERSONNEL)

C) PREVENTION SUB-PROGRAMME. (PREPARATION OF PERSONNEL)

VII) MENTAL HEALTH TRAINING

VIII) MENTAL RETARDATION AND DRUG DEPENDENCE

Though these are not mental illnesses still the health workers should be able to counsel the parents, provide public education and know-how to refer such children to social welfare agencies for rehabilitation. The National Mental Health Policy indicates clearly the role of community mental health workers, including the Mental Health Nurse.

DEFINITION

Community Mental Health Nursing is the application of knowledge of psychiatric nursing in preventing, promoting and maintaining mental health of the people, to help in early diagnosis and care and to rehabilitate the clients after mental illness.

In community living, the individual may go through stressful situations. He/she may be able to cope with stress, and adjustment takes place. Sometimes this stress leads to mental illness.

FACTORS LEADING TO PROBLEMS

Mental health/illnesses have natural histories of the same kind as physical diseases despite many unknown factors of agents, host and environment.

I. **AGENT FACTORS** : May be Biological, Psychosocial, and Socio cultural.

II. **HOST FACTORS ARE MAINLY INTRINSIC** : These may be:
   (i) Demograhic characteristics such as age, sex, ethnicity prone to mental illness.
   (ii) Biological characteristics such as genetic factors, biochemical levels as in schizophrenic disorders.
   (iii) Social and Economic Factors such as neurotic and schizophrenic disorders, personality disorders.
   (iv) Life Style factors such as personality traits, type of physique, type of personality, use of alcohol or drugs.

III. **ENVIRONMENTAL FACTORS (EXTRINSIC)** : Inadequate parent education, lack of proper community integration leading to drug and alcohol abuse and social insecurity are some of the examples.

APPROACHES TO COMMUNITY MENTAL HEALTH

Community mental health can be attained through:

* Use of a multidisciplinary approach, including all the mental health team workers.
* The following concepts should be kept in mind by all the team members:
  i) Primary prevention of mental illness.
  ii) Secondary prevention of mental illness.
  iii) Tertiary prevention.

PRIMARY PREVENTION

Primary prevention means lowering the rate of new cases of mental disorders in a population by counteracting forces which may produce illness, like providing health education to vulnerable groups of teenagers, homeless families.

The emphasis in primary prevention is mainly on health devleopment and effective coping abilities of an individual.

The community mental health nurse has a significant role in primary prevention. The factors which a community mental psychiatric nurse should emphasize are:

I) BIOLOGICAL AND PHYSICAL FACTORS.
II) PSYCHOSOCIAL FACTORS.
III) SOCIOCULTURAL FACTORS.

BIOLOGICAL AND PHYSICAL FACTORS

BIOLOGICAL FACTORS :— The community health nurse has a significant role specially in prenatal and postnatal care. It will help in reduction of mental retardation and organic mental disorders. Special follow-up during antenatal on nutrition, vaccination, avoidance of the use of drugs and alcohol, repeated x-rays, prevention of repeated abortions, genetic counselling to the couple with a high risk of chromosomal abnormalities like mongolism, family history of mental retardation, AIDS with associated mental disorders. Encourage abortion of a defective foetus, if diagnosed in utero.

PHYSICAL FACTORS :— For the growth of a child minimum facilities such as food, shelter and clothing are required. Parents need to be prepared for thc acceptance of a new child in the family.

A childless couple should be guided for the investigation. Encourage the couple to go for adoption for their mental health. The names of agencies can be given to the parents in this connection.

PSYCHOSOCIAL FACTORS

The individual needs to learn all those competencies by which he/she can cope with a crisis situation such as *(i) opportunities for learning needed competencies.*

A. PHYSICAL COMPETENCIES :— For example, coordination of muscles, protecting oneself from injuries. A child may not learn these competencies because of overprotection by parents. He is not given any opportunity to learn.

B. INTELLECTUAL COMPETENCIES :— A child/individual is not exposed to such type of stimulation. For example, exposure to the use of a computer.

C. EMOTIONAL COMPETENCIES :— In a stressful situation, a solution is provided by the parents. So the child does not learn to cope with his emotional problem. It is not his/her fault. Use of drugs by the son is not treated because of a social stigma unless hospitalization is required. The child needs to be given an opportunity to face emotional stress. For example, coping alone at home in the absence of mother for four to five hours will enable the child to develop confidence.

D. SOCIAL COMPETENCIES :— (i) *Opportunities need to be provided* for group interaction, socialization with guests and friends, so that the child learns to accept his strengths and weakness. He/she makes an effort to improve on his weakness.

If opportunities to learn basic competencies are not provided to the child/individual, he may find it difficult to cope with stressful situations and may have maladjustment in difficult situations.

(ii) Fostering of Clear Values — A conflict in values of what an individual learns and what he sees leads to maladjustment and mental disorders. For example, a child has learnt copying during an examination. This is bad. She finds all the children in the class are copying and the teacher is not able to find out. However, this child does not copy. As a result, others get very high scores and an area of their choice in higher education, whereas this child who was not copying does not get the area of his choice due to a comparatively low score. This causes a conflict in values of the child.

(iii) Preparation of an individual to cope with changes such as adolescence, marriage, pregnancy, childbirth, family planning, marriage of children, old age.

At each life situation preparation is required due to different demands. The client may look for support from within the family or from the health professional.

SOCIOCULTURAL FACTORS

To help people cope with stress, mental health education is necessary, specially public education about causes leading to mental disorders by putting up exhibitions, T.V. plays, radio talks and use of mass media.

For reducing social isolation, a social support system should be developed. For example, a drug-addict-to-drug-addict programme, anticipatory guidance for the risk groups, widows, adolescents, primi mothers, death of spouse, divorce, group disaster like earthquakes or bomb explosions. *PRIMARY PREVENTION* includes mental health education through exhibitions on "How to live mentally healthy", "Mental health is part of physical health," "Prevention of mental illness" are few of the examples of the theme for health education. School talks on problems of children and where to go for help. Education to teachers and parents on maintaining a healthy environment at school and home. Mass media stage plays in schools and colleges, street plays are some of the other methods which can be adopted to educate the community to prevent maladaptive behaviour or mental disorders.

TO RECALL

- Concept of the National Mental Health Programme (India)
- Objectives and approaches.
- Definition of community mental health nursing.
- Mental illness/disorders are also caused-like physical disorders by interaction of agent, host and environment.
- Approaches to community mental health nursing are:
  - — Primary Prevention
  - — Secondary Prevention
  - — Tertiary Prevention

PRIMARY PREVENTION means lowering the rate of new cases of mental disorders in a population. Factors for Primary Prevention

- — Biological and Physical Factors
- — Psychosocial factors
- — Sociocultural Factors

SECONDARY PREVENTION

Secondary prevention of mental disorders aims at early detection and prompt treatment of maladaptive behaviour in an individual's family and community setting. *The emphasis is on minimizing the duration of illness.*

The approach of the community mental health nursing in secondary prevention should be early detection and prompt intervention of high–risk individual such as recently divorced or widowed, high school dropouts, retirement. In these crisis situations, intervention helps the individual to recover fast, otherwise precipitation of crisis leads to anxiety, fear, guilt, shame and helplessness.

CRISIS AND BALANCING FACTORS

Crisis is an initial disturbance that results from a stressful event or a perceived threat to self. Crisis is self-limiting, that means within four to six weeks the individual is able to cope with the crisis situation.

In crisis a person is at a turning point. He/she faces a problem that he can't easily solve by using his/her usual coping mechanisms. As a result, there is increased tension and anxiety and the individual is less able to find a solution. The individual feels helpless and emotionally upset.

Crisis can be *Maturational;* demands for various stages of development which an individual needs to cope with, for example, adolescence, adult, old age.

Situational such as loss of employment, severe suicidal ideation, marital dispute, change from a rural to urban setting, technological changes.

Adventitious crisis: Accidental, uncommon or unexpected crisis. For example, both the parents die and the child is left alone.

Though the crisis is self-limiting, sometimes intervention is required.

Crisis intervention is the process by which an individual is helped to cope with a crisis in his/her life situation, so as to bring his/her level of functioning to that of the precrisis level.

The community mental health nurse needs to identify the available outpatient and inpatient treatment within the community. Partial/short-term hospitalization like day-care cantres can be utilized.

Hot Lines Service Link — It is a telephone service link through which help can be extended. *Walk-in-clinics,* where the patient can walk in any time of the day or night to get professional help. The community needs to be oriented for the available service and its utilization.

Efforts should be made to minimize the duration of sickness. If a client requires drugs, or physical therapy (ECT), the psychiatrist should be consulted immediatly. Follow-up should be done to ensure the improvement or deterioration of the client's mental and physical health. Crisis intervention must be considered a very significant aspect of secondary prevention. Crisis assessment and effect of balancing factors in stress are presented in the figure no. 32 at page no. 431

TERTIARY PREVENTION

Tertiary prevention means reducing the rate of recurrence of illness. Even with a primary prevention approach and crisis intervention at the secondary level, some persons would require hospitalization for emotional and mental disorders.

The goal of tertiary prevention is to reduce the prevalence of long-term disabilities and problems due to mental disorders.

Tertiary prevention includes prompt and intensive inpatient care, rehabilitation, after-care and resocialization.

Intensive inpatient care for emotional disorders will prevent it from becoming chronic. It will also enable the individual to return to his home or society as early as possible. Through the community mental health approach the following therapeutic services can be provided by the nurse:

A) TREATMENT AND FOLLOW-UP

The community mental health nurse needs to ensure the type of psychotropic drugs the patient is taking. She also needs to ensure maintenance of dose, supervision of safe intake of drugs, observation of side-effects, educating family members to observe for side-effects and report.

B) INDIVIDUAL AND FAMILY THERAPY

The patient has to go back to his family. So it is very essential that the family is helped to meet the stress. Family support needs to be identified in helping the patient.

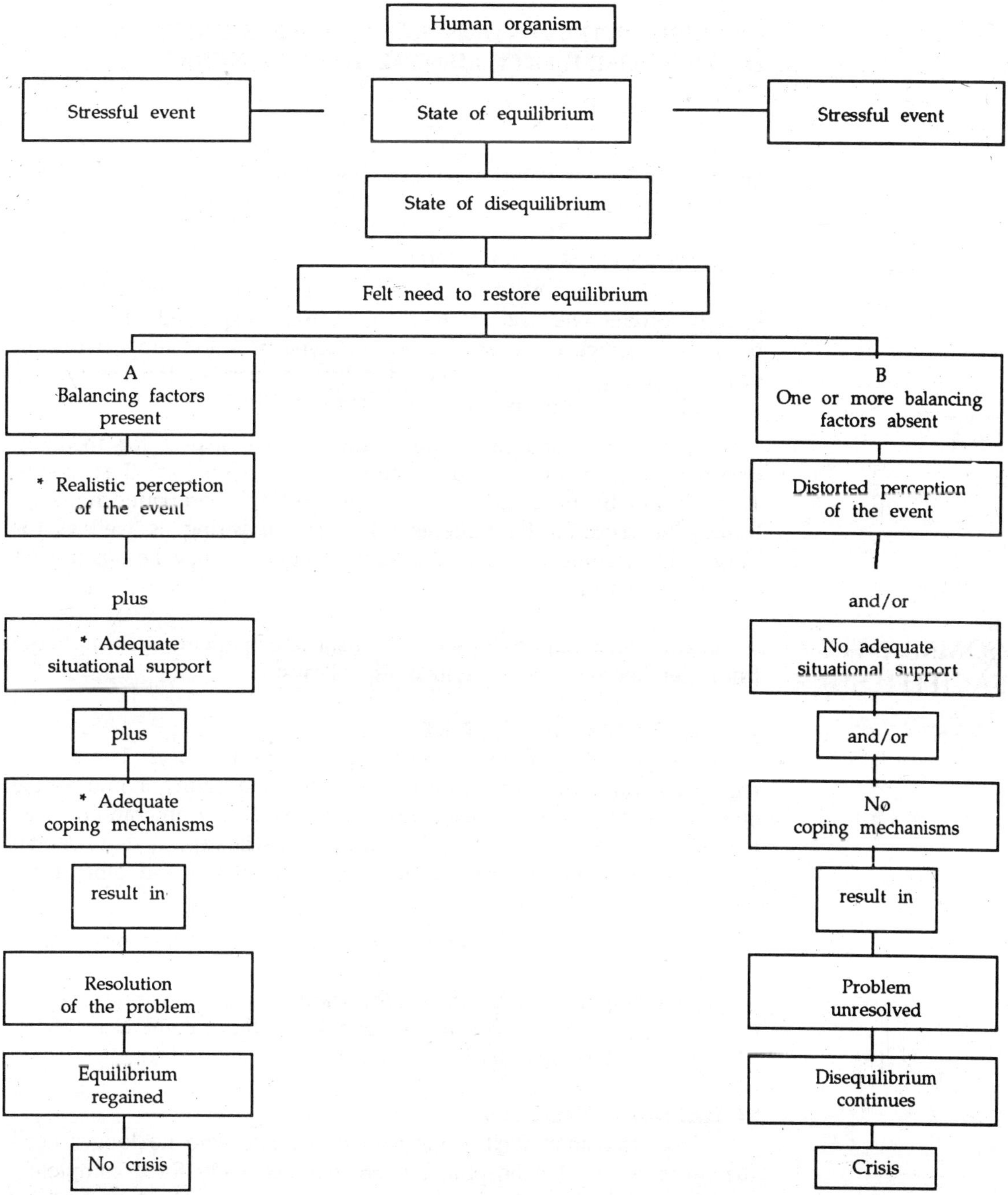

* Balancing factors.

Fig. 32 : Crisis Assessment Paradigm: Effect of balancing factors in a stressful event.

Source: From Aguilera D.C., & Messick J.H. (1982) Crisis Intervention— Theory & Methodology, 4th edition. St. Louis, The C.V. Mosby Co., p. 65

C) CRISIS INTERVENTION IS ANOTHER SIGNIFICANT ROLE OF THE COMMUNITY MENTAL HEALTH NURSE.

D) INTERACTIONAL SKILLS TRAINING

Social skill training can be given to develop effective interaction and communication abilities. For example, 'drug addict group', Alcoholic Anonymous Groups.

E) OCCUPATIONAL TRAINING

The patient needs to be rehabilitated and helped to become socially productive. His interest area can be exploited and he can be helped to pick up a job. He would come back for support during stress. This support can be provided by members of the family and the community and mental health team.

Rehabilitation and after-care is an essential aspect for mentally disordered patients. They need to readjust themselves outside the hospital. They should be provided with *'safe and human'* therapeutic housing. It may be required for patients who are recovering as well as for those with chronic diseases. Therapeutic housing may be supervised or unsupervised.

COMMUNITY FACILITIES

Community facilities for mentally disordered patients after discharge from the hospital are described as follows:

1. DAY HOSPITAL/ CENTRES

A hospital programme organized on a day-time basis. The patient receives a full range of treatment, services and return home at the end of the day. The concept, introduced by D.E. Cameran in 1946, is now being used in rehabilitation and psychiatric care. A day hospital is staffed by a trained psychiatric nurse, psychitarist and other team members.

In India, day hospitals/centres are available, though less for mentally ill but comparatively better for mentally retarded.

The family feels relief for a few hours in a day and develops coping energy for the rest of the time when the patient is at home. The patient develops discipline and routine.

2) HALF-WAY HOUSES

It is a transition facility for mental patients who no longer need the full services of a hospital but are not yet ready for a completely independent living. They need supervision for medication and for carrying on domestic activities. If they are still in job, they will leave for the job and come back to this half-way house. Medical facilities are regularly provided.

3) GROUP HOMES

These homes may belong to a hospital or rented by 15 to 20 mentally ill recovering patients. These ex-patients stay together, meet their financial commitments and live in a society like other members. They try to provide moral, emotional and social support to each other. If one of the members is leading towards relapse, they try to help him by providing support.

4) FOSTER HOMES

It is a home in which a patient recovering from a mental disorder is placed in a voluntary family by a social agency for family care. The family is paid by the agency. Placement may be temporary or permanent. The patient gets a home-like environment.

5) SHELTERED WORKSHOP

The patient may find it difficult to compete for employment. He should be encouraged to attend a sheltered workshop, which is a work-oriented rehabilitation facility with a controlled working environment to fulfil the individual's vocational goals. In these workshops ex-long-term mentally ill patients can utilize their experience and abilities by relearning. This will help them make progress towards a normal living and economic independence.

6) MENTAL HEALTH EMERGENCY CARE

Hot Line — A telephone line maintained by trained personnel for the purpose of providing crisis intervention. There are voluntary organizations in India providing such services.

Walk-in-clinic— It is a 24-hour psychiatric emergency room in which diagnostic or therapeutic service is available without an appointment.

Home Visit by the community health team/individual during a crisis situation.

7) SELF-HELP GROUPS

Self-help groups in the community will help the individual as well as members of the family. Alcoholic anonymous groups, drug addiction groups, groups of patients with mental retardation are few of the examples.

Community mental health nursing aims at providing comprehensive, continuous care to the people. The aim is to reduce the number of mentally ill patients through primary prevention; early diagnosis and limiting the disability; through secondary prevention and rehabilitation through use of community facilities by tertiary prevention.

The community mental health nurse applies her knowledge of the nursing process in assessment, planning, implementation intervention and evaluation to provide comprehensive care to patients.

TO RECALL

a. Secondary Prevention aims at early detection and prompt treatment of maladaptive behaviour in an individual, family and community.

* Crisis can be maturational, situational and adventitious.

b. Tertiary Prevention aims at reducing the recurrence of disease.

* Services given by nurse
  * Treatment and follow-up
  * Individual and family therapy
  * Crisis intervention
  * Interactional skills training
  * Occupational training

c. Community Facilities
  * Day hospital/centres
  * Half-way homes
  * Group homes
  * Foster homes
  * Sheltered workshops
  * Mental health emergency care, hot line, walk-in-clinic, home visit.
  * Self-help groups.

APPLICATION TO NURSING

Reading of this unit on Community Mental Health Nursing will enable the reader to develop a concept about the National Mental Health Programme in India. The learner will be able to identify her/his role in primary, secondary and tertiary levels of prevention. Reading of this unit will enable the nurse to mobilise community facilities for helping the psychiatric patients.

BETTER STUDY SECTION OF UNIT XXIV

1. VOCABULARY (Use Dictionary)

Anticipatory	Integration
Approach	Intrinsic
Competencies	Maladaptive
Conflict	Prevalence
Coping	Postnatal
Detection	Precipitation
Envisages	Prenatal
Extrinsic	Vulnerable
Fostering	Voluntary

2. ASSIGNMENTS

* Make notes on the 'Alcoholic Anonymous Group'.

* Prepare a plan of activities for school children to promote their mental health.
* Write notes on approaches to the national mental health programme (Refer to Report on the National Mental Health Programme).

3. STUDY QUESTIONS

(a) List three objectives of the National Mental Health Policy.

(b) Define the following terms:
   * Primary Prevention
   * Secondary Prevention
   * Tertiary Prevention

(c) List the role of the nurse in Primary Prevention of Mental Disorders.

(d) List four community facilities for mentally ill patients after discharge from hospital.

4. READING REFERENCE

1. Coleman J.C. *Abnormal Psychology and Modern Life.* (Fifth edition) Scott, Foresman and Company, Illinois (1976).

2. Director-General of Health Services— *Report on the National Mental Health Programme for India (1987).*

3. Mitchel R.G. *Essential Psychiatric Nursing.* Churchill Livingstone (1986).

4. Park J.E. & Park K. *Textbook of Preventive and Social Medicine,* Thirteenth edition, Banarsi Dass Bhanot, Jabalpur (1991)

5. Shives L.R. *Basic Concepts of Psychiatric Mental Health Nursing. (Second edition).* J.B. Lippincott Company, Philadelphia (1990).

6. Wilson H.S. Kneisl, C.R. *Psychiatric Nursing.* Addision Wesley Publishing Company, California (1979).

UNIT XXV
PSYCHIATRIC MENTAL HEALTH NURSE AND MENTAL HEALTH TEAM, SCOPE AND LEGAL ISSUES

UNIT OUTLINE

Introduction of the Mental Health Team.

A. Members of the Mental Health Team.

B. Scope of the Psychiatric Mental Health Nurse.
   — Changing roles of the Nurse.
   — Role of the Nurse in various settings.
   — Basic skills for psychiatric nursing
   — Career opportunities for the Psychiatric Nurse.

C. Legal Aspects of Psychiatric Nursing
   * Overview of the Indian Mental Act 1987.
   * Admission of the Mentally ill patient.
   * Discharge of the Mentally ill patient.
   * Leave of absence.
   * Protection of human rights.
   * Role of the Nurse in Legal Psychiatry.
   * Standards of Psychiatric Mental Health Nursing Practice.

Application to Nursing.

Better Study Section.

INTENDED LEARNIG BEHAVIOUR

After reading this unit, you will be able to:

a) Discuss the role of various team members.

b) Describe the role of the Psychiatric Mental Health Nurse.

c) Explain the career opportunities for the psychiatric Nurse.

d) Describe the Indian Mental Health Act 1987.

e) Identify the procedure of admission, discharge and leave of absence of patients.

f) Test the standards of Psychiatric Mental Health Nursing Practice.

A MENTAL HEALTH TEAM

INTRODUCTION

Team work is significant in any setting more so in a mental health setting. The milieu needed to care for the patient depends upon the qualification, experience, skilful handling of the situation by all members of the team with a similar approach. For promotion of a therapeutic environment members of various disciplines coordinate their activities.

MEMBERS OF MENTAL HEALTH TEAM

Members of the mental health team are:

— Psychiatric Nurse Clinical Specialist
— Registered Nurse working in a Psychiatric Unit/Hospital
— Psychiatrist
— Clinical Psychologist
— Psychiatric Social Worker
— Psychiatric Para-Professionals
— Psychiatric Aids, ECT Technician
— Occupational Therapist
— Recreational Therapist
— Diversional/Play Therapist
— Creative Art Therapist
— Clergyman

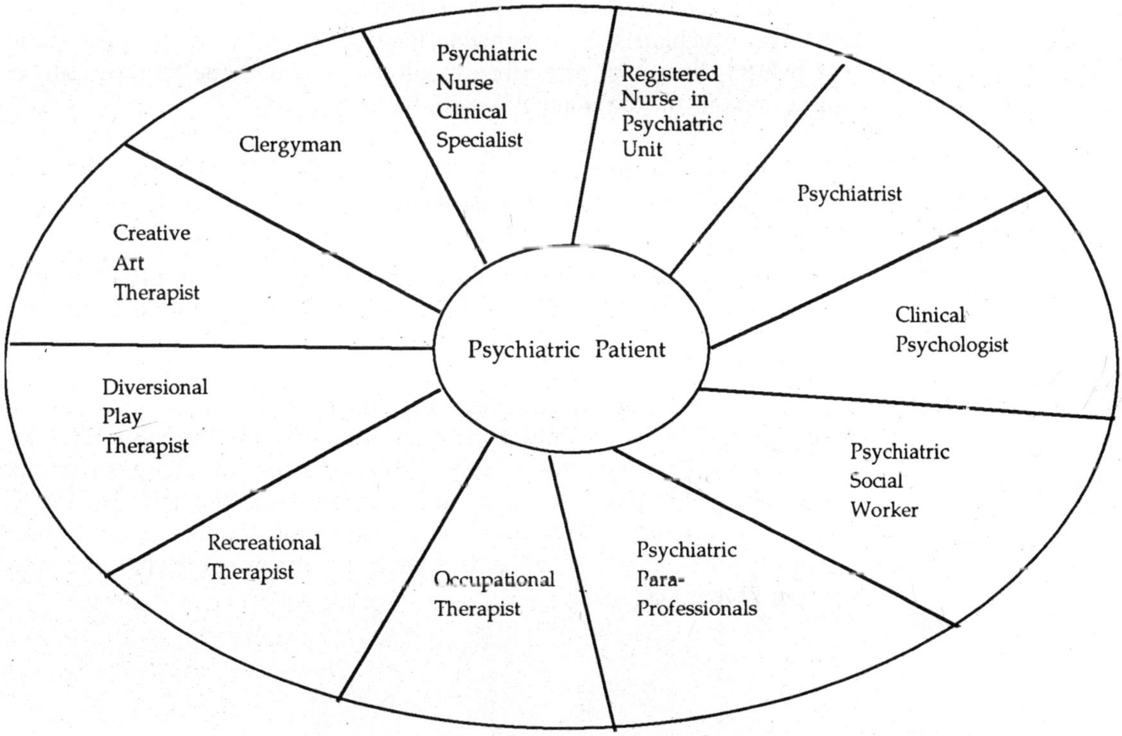

Fig. 33 : Psychiatric Mental Health Team

PSYCHIATRIC NURSE CLINICAL SPECIALIST

Psychiatric Nurse Clinical Specialist should have a Master's Degree in Nursing, preferably with post-graduate research work. She provides individual, group and family psychotherapy in a hospital and community setting. Participates actively in primary, secondary and tertiary prevention of mental disorders. Takes up resposibility of teaching, administration and research, besides publishing work in a mental health/illness setting. Works as a leader, can practise independently.

REGISTERED NURSE IN PSYCHIATRIC UNIT/HOSPITAL

Registered Nurse goes through a General Nursing and Midwifery Programme or B.Sc. Nursing, Post-basic B.Sc. Nursing Programme, Diploma in Nursing Education and Administration with an elective course in Psychiatric Nursing. She/he develops skill in caring for mental patients, in hospital settings, works with the clinical nurse specialist in a community mental health setting. Gives holistic nursing care by assessing patients' mental, social, physical, psychological and spiritual needs.

Opportunities are available to update knowledge through continuing education, inservice edcuation, workshops and courses conducted by open universities.

PSYCHIATRIST

Doctor with post-graduation in Psychiatry should have at least two to three years of residence training.

The psychiatrist is responsible for diagnosis, treatment, prevention of mental disorders, prescribes medicines and somatic therapy, serves as a leader of the mental health team.

CLINICAL PSYCHOLOGIST

Clinical psychologist needs to have a doctoral degree in clinical psychology and should be registered with the Clinical Psychologists' Association.

Performs the role of diagnostic tests, deals with interpretation and evaluation of findings of tests. Implements a programme of behaviour modification.

PSYCHIATRIC SOCIAL WORKER

She/he is a graduate in social work and a post-graduate in psychiatric social work. Plays a significant role in assessing the individual, family and community adaptive and support system. Helps in discharge planning, counselling for job placement and follow-up on the job. She/he is aware of the state laws and legal rights of her/his patients and protects these rights. She/he is skilled iin interview techniques and group dynamics.

PSYCHIATRIC PARA-PROFESSIONALS

PSYCHIATRIC NURSING AIDS/ATTENDANTS

High School educational level. They are given training on the job. They assist in maintaining the therapeutic environment and provide care under supervision.

ECT TECHNICIANS

These technicians go through a training period of six to nine months. Their role is to prepare the ECT machine and other articles and give ECT under the supervision of a psychiatrist or anesthetist.

AUXILLARY PESONNEL

Are volunteer housekeepers or clerical staff who come in contact with the patient. They should be given inservice education to interact with the patient therapeutically.

OCCUPATIONAL THERAPIST (O.T.)

Occupational Therapist (O.T.) goes through specialized training. He/she has a pivtol role to play by using manual and creative techniques to assess the interpersonal responses of the patient. Patients are helped to develop skill in the area of their choice and become economically independent. They are helped to work in a sheltered workshop.

In a hospital setting , the patient may think that doing jobs like gardening, cleaning the locker are belittling him and he avoids going for OT.

If O.T. is planned in a meaningful manner it is very significant in treatment and early recovery of the patient. The therapist focuses on vocational skills and activities of daily living (ADL) to raise the self-concept of the patient.

RECREATIONAL THERAPIST

Recreational therapist plans activities to stimulate the patient's muscles coordination, interpersonal relationship and socialization. Recreational and occupational therapies are always need-based. No single approach can be used ***(Refer to Nursing Care Plans in Chapter—VIII).***

DIVERSIONAL PLAY THERAPIST

Makes observation of a child/patient during his play. The behaviour of the child while playing, the types of toys and his reaction toward the doll, beating, calling or throwing are the focus of attention. The therapist explores the behaviour of the child and relates to conditions like phobia, child abuse, separation or any other condition.

CREATIVE ART THERAPIST

An arts graduate, he/she encourages the patient to express his work freely with colours. The therapist analyses the use of bright colours leading to light, faded colours which have a meaning, live figures drawn by the patient. A boat sinking in the river. An accident. Analysis will help in bringing the repressed feelings of the patient to a conscious level.

CLERGY MAN

Religious persons from different religions may be asked to come to the hospital unit once a week so that the patient can have a spiritual discussion or make a confession if he/she desires.

TO RECALL

Members of the Mental Health Team
Psychiatric Nurse Clinical Specialist
Psychiatrist Registered Nurse working in a Psychiatric Unit
Clinical Psychologist
Psychiatric Social Worker
Psychiatric Para-Professional
Psychiatric Nursing Aides
ECT Technician
Auxillary Personnel
Occupational Therapist
Recreational Therapist
Diversional/play Therapist
Creative Art Therapist
Clergy Man

B. SCOPE OF PSYCHIATRIC MENTAL HEALTH NURSE

INTRODUCTION

Advances in the past few decades in the fields of psychiatry and nursing have re-emphasized the role of psychiatric nursing in various settings. The role of a psychiatric nurse is changing from giving custodial care to the dynamic approach in giving care for recovery of the patient. Every nurse who performs a simple nursing procedure is giving psychiatric nursing care to the patient. For example, how she communicates a message to the patient, allows the patient to talk and have mental catharsis. The nurse gives holistic care to the patient with emphasis on the psychological component which is a core component of human needs.

CHANGING ROLE

The role of a psychiatric mental health nurse is changing due to various factors, such as:

(1) Increased awareness of the consumer that is patient, as an individual and as a member of the family and other groups.
(2) Awareness of the community in early detection and treatment of mental disorders and utilization of psychiartic hospitals and dispensaries.
(3) Awareness of the value of continuity of care throughout the patient's illness, involving a variety of community facilities.
(4) The multidisciplinary team approach to psychiatric practice, and increasing therapeutic responsibility of each member, including the nurse.
(5) Reorganization of the physical structure of the hospital in care of mentally ill patients eg. open doors, disappearance of physical restraints, therapeutic milieu, legal restrictions.
(6) Increasing effort to rehabilitate patients, both in and out of hospital, to prevent their physical, mental and social deterioration.
(7) Expansion of the psychiatric services within general hospitals.
(8) Emphasis of mental health services in the national health policy.

ROLE OF NURSE IN VARIOUS SETTINGS

The role of a psychiatric mental health nurse can be in various settings:

i) The psychiatric institutional setting. ii) The general hospital setting. iii) The extramural health services (Those services which are existing beyond hospital or walled settings).

Essential skills required for giving effective care are:

(i) Skill of Basic Nursing— It is a professional preparation of the nurse with general nursing and midwifery or B.Sc. in Nursing (ii) Technical Nursing is the advanced qualification that is M.Sc. in Psychiatric Mental Health Nursing, Diploma in Psychiatric Nursing. (iii) Occupational Nursing Skills. (iv) Recreational Nursing Skills, (v) Interpresonal Nursing Skills, (vi) Observational and (vii) Skills of communication.

INPUT

OUTPUT

PROCESS

NURSE EDUCATOR

NURSE ADMINISTRATOR

NURSE RESEARCHER

CAREER OPPORTUNITIES IN VARIOUS SETTINGS

BASIC SKILLS (Input)

* Basic Nursing.
* Technical Nursing.
* Observational.
* Interpersonal.
* Communication.
* Organizational.
* Occupational.
* Recreational.

PSYCHIATRIC INSTITUTION

* O.P.D.
* Wards.
* Therapies
  — ECT.
  — Psychotherapy.
* Day Hospital/Centres.
* Family Care Units.
* Child Guidance Clinics.
* Mental Retardation Clinics.
* Psychiatric Nursing Homes.
* Community Mental Health Centres.
* Rehabilitation Centres.
* Halfway Houses.

GENERAL HOSPITAL

* Psychiatric Unit.
* Casualty & Emergency.
* Paediatric & Well baby Clinic.
* Obstetrical Nursing.
* Cardiac Nurshing.
* Geiratric Nursing.
* Pre-post Surgery Unit.
* School Health Nursing.
* Occupational Health Nursing.

EXTRA MURAL SERVICE

* Health Education Programme in Community.
* Programme for
  — School teacher.
  — School children.
  — Adolescents.
  — Parents.
  — Pregnant women.
  — Elderly people.
  — Physically handicaped.
  — Follow-up care.
* Collaboration with related agencies
  — Social wel fare agency.
  — Employment agencies.
* Individual & Group Consultation.
* Drug deaddict.
* Alcoholic addict.
* Suicide prevention team.
* Team member for protection of women from Bettery.

TEACHING INSTITUTION

* Teaching in university nursing programme.
* Schools of Nursing Programmes.
* M.P.H.W. Programme.
* Distant education teaching.

OUTPUT

* Promotion of Mental Health.
* Prevention of Mental Illness.
* Care and Rehabilitation on Mentally Ill.

Fig. 34 : Table describing the Preparation of Psychiatric Nurse, her role in Various Settings and its outcome.

The role of the nurse in all the settings is of an educator, administrator and researcher. It will definitely depend on the nurse's educational preparation to take up these roles.

So the role of the nurse will vary according to:
(a) the setting in which she is working.
(b) her position in the team and the type of nursing preparation i.e. advanced or basic.
(c) essential basic skills or competencies expected by the nurse.
(d) flexibility ability of the nurse in various settings e.g. listener, health educator, administrator etc.
(e) ability to recognize and ultilize the therapeutic potential/abilities of an individual patient in a particular situation.
(f) coordination, communication and decision-making abilities within the team.
(g) responsibility for health promotion, preventive action and case finding, nursing care and treatment, continuity of care and participation in community-need programmes.
(h) ability to take up teaching roles in educational programmes/conduct inservice education programmes.
(i) ability to do research work and use findings for improvement of patient care.

Role of the nurse in psychiatric institutions and extramural services has been discussed throughout the text of this book. Few examples from her role in a general setting are described below:

SETTING	INTERVENTIONS
EMERGENCY/ CASUALTY NURSING	Crisis intervention for the relatives during stress. Unexpected sickness of a family member causes anxiety. Burns 40% , accident of a child, sudden pain in the chest are crisis situations for an individual and the family which will need intervention.
OUTPATIENT DEPARTMENT	Diagnosed with a disease. For example, cancer, diabetes, tuberculosis. All this leads to a level of anxiety. The patient and his/her relatives are confused, distressed and need help in this crisis situation.
OBSTETRICAL NURSING	Helping mother in labour. She is in great stress and anxiety. Prenatal counselling for the sex of the child. Postnatal counselling if the child is male or female and not of what the couple desired to have. Support to primi mother. Provide support to parents with a still-born child or born with congenital deformities.

SETTING	INTERVENTIONS
CARDIAC NURSING	Encourage the relatives and the patient to talk out their anxiety. Red signal feeling in the patient and relatives in educating the intensity of sickness. Caring for the patient and his/her relatives.
CANCER/ ONCOLOGIC NURSING	Providing support to a family member. Helping the patient to learn to tolerate pain. Helping terminally ill to die peacefully.
SCHOOL HEALTH NURSING	Helping the child to cope with his/her physical handicap. Handling the behaviour problem. Identifying maladaptive behaviour Education to parents.
INDUSTRIAL/ OCCUPATIONAL HEALTH NURSING	Crisis intervention during occupational hazards. Teaching stress management. Helping during an anxiety attack, specially during the stress of production. Helping employers during the stress.

Fig. 35 : Table describing the sample of Career Opportunities for Psychiatric Nurse other than the Psychiatric Setting.

TO RECALL

* Changing role of the Nurse due to
  — Awareness of the consumers.
  — Awareness of the community in early detection of diseases.
  — Awareness of the value of continuity of care.
  — Multidisciplinary team approach
  — Reorganization of the physical set-up of a mental hospital.
  — Rehabilitation of mentally ill patients.
  — Extended mental health services approach.
  — Emphasis on mental health in the national health policy.
* Role of the Nurse in Various Settings
  The nurse works as an educator, administrator and researcher with essential basic skills to promote mental health, prevent mental illness and care for chronically ill patients.
* Career Opprtunities for the Psychatric Mental Health Nurse.

C. LEGAL ASPECTS OF PSYCHIATRIC NURSING

INTRODUCTION

The Psychiatric Mental Health Nurse should be sufficiently aware of the legal aspects of psychiatry. This will help her to protect the patients' right and avoid in giving poor advice or innocentaly involving herself in legal issues.

OVERVIEW OF INDIAN MENTAL ACT 1987

The Indian Mental Act, 1987, is an amendment of the Indian Lunacy Act, 1912. The present Act recognizes the crucial role of treatment and care of mentally ill persons. It also incorporates the latest knowledge and recent concepts in the field of mental health. The emphasis in the new Act is on discarding custodial care, segregating mental patients from the community and incorporating better provisions relating to treatment and care. Judicial safeguards for patients' rights have been provided for the first time to prevent any indignity or cruelty to the mentally ill. It introduces humanitarian considerations. There is an explicit protection of their human rights.

ADMISSION OF MENTALLY ILL PATIENT

The psychiatric patient can be admitted by the Medical Officer Incharge of the hospital on request even without the application made by the patient. Similarly, the person who is admitted can be discharged within 24 hours. Psychiatric patients can be admitted like the physically ill patients. Admission of mentally ill patients can be on:

i. Voluntary basis.
ii. Under special circumstances.
iii. Admission by the Police officer or Magistrate.

(I) ADMISSION ON VOLUNTARY BASIS

Any person (except a minor) who considers himself to be a mentally ill person and desires to be admitted to any psychiatric hospital or psychiatric nursing home for treatment, may request the Medical Officer Incharge for being admitted on a voluntary basis.

A minor voluntary patient can be admitted at the request of his/her guardian.

The patient is admitted for 24 hours. Then a board, consisting of two Medical Officers, will decide whether such a voluntary patient needs further treatment or should be discharged. In that case the treatment is continued for a period of not exceeding 90 days at a time.

(II) ADMISSION UNDER SPECIAL CIRCUMSTANCES

Any mentally ill person who does not, or is unable to, express his willingness for admission as a voluntary patient, may be admitted or kept as an inpatient in a psychiatric hospital or psychiatric nursing home on an application made by his/her relative or friend. If the Medical Officer Incharge is satisfied that in the interest of the mentally ill person it is necessary to keep him/her under treatment, he/she is kept as an inpatient in the hospital.

Application on a prescribed form shall be accompanied by two medical certificates from two medical officers, one of whom should be in Government Service. They should explain the condition of the mentally ill patient, such that he should be treated as an inpatient in a psychiatric hospital.

(III) ADMISSION BY THE POLICE OFFICER & MAGISTRATE

A police officer, under Section 23 of the Indian Mental Health Act, 1987, may take into protection any person found wandering within the limits of his station. The officer should have reason to believe that the person is mentally ill and is incapable of taking care of himself. He can be dangerous by reason of his mental illness.

Such a patient is produced before a nearby magistrate within 24 hours of detention.

The magistrate shall:

(a) examine the person to assess his capacity to understand.
(b) cause him to be examined by a medical officer, and
(c) make such inquiries about the person as he may deem necessary.

If the medical officer certifies and the magistrate is satisfied that the person is mentally ill, he is treated as an inpatient in the psychiatric hospital. This is in the interest of the patient's health and personal security.

DISCHARGE OF MENTALLY ILL PATIENT

The Medical Officer Incharge of a psychiatric hospital or psychiatric nursing home may on the recommendation of two medical practitioners, one of whom shall preferably be a psychiatrist, by order in writing, direct the discharge of any person, other than a volunatry patient detained or undergoing treatment as an inpatient. Such a patient should thereupon be discharged from the psychiatric hospital or physchiatric nursing home, provided there is no order from any other authority like the Superintendent of Prison.

LEAVE OF ABSENCE

Any application for leave or absence on behalf of a mentally ill person (not being a mentally ill prisoner) undergoing treatment as an inpatient in any psychiatric hospital or psychiatric nursing home may be made to the Medical Officer Incharge.

The application should be submitted duly signed by the relatives who had admitted the patient. It should be accompanied by a bond specifying.

(i) to take proper care of the mentally ill person.
(ii) to prevent the mentally ill person from causing injury to himself or to others, and
(iii) to bring back the mentally ill to the psychiatric hospital on the expiry of the leave period.
(iv) in case the patient is not brought back after the expiry of the leave period the magistrate needs to be informed.

MCNAUGHTON'S CASE AND RULES

CRIMINAL LIABILITY

The prisoner McNaughton was indicted for the murder of Edward Drummond in 1843. McNaughton wanted to kill British Prime Minister Sir Robert Peel (1843) under the influence of his delusions, but by mistake he shot his secretary Edward Drummond on the back. He was tried and was found "not guilty on the ground of insanity." The case created a great sensation and the House of Lords invited learned judges for their reasons and opinions. Tindel, Chief Justice, answered several questions. The answers have now come to be known as Mc Naughton's Rule (s) all over the world. In India, Section 84 of the Indian Penal Code (Act 45 of 1860) states that "nothing is an offence which is done by a person, who at the time of doing it by reason of unsoundness of mind is incapable of knowing the nature of the act or that he is doing what is either wrong or contrary to law." The policy of the Criminal Law is to control not only the sane but also the insane person as far as possible. Hence, an insane person is not *IPSO FACTO* protected. He must bring himself within the exception of Section 84 of the Indian Penal Code to escape liability.

MARRIAGE

Marriage of a lunatic who is so found by inquisition is void, even if it was celebrated during a lucid interval (Lucid interval is when an insane shows that the mind was sufficiently recovered to enable him understand the nature of the act and that any delusion which he still suffers does not affect the act. The acts of a person during a lucid interval possess the same validity and involve him in the same responsibility as the acts of a sane man). If the fact of mental illness or treatment has been kept from the knowledge of the other party, it would also amount to fraud.

Under Section 12 of the Hindu Marriage Act of 1955 a marriage with a person who was an idiot or a lunatic can be declared null. Section 5 (ii), introduced by Act 68 (1976), states that at the time of marriage neither party:

a) is incapable of giving a valid consent.......(due to)........unsoundness of mind; or

b) though capable of giving consent, has been suffering from mental disorders of such a kind or to such an extent as to be unfit for marriage and the procreation of children; or

c) has been subject to recurrent attacks of insanity or epilepsy.

Either party to a marriage may present an application for judicial separation,where the other party has been continuously of unsound mind for a period not less than two years immediately preceding the presentation of the petition (Section 10) as he or she may apply for divorce if the other party has been incurablity of unsound mind for a continuous period of not less than three years before the petition (Section 13)

ADOPTION

A Hindu Male 'who is of sound mind', is not a minor can adopt a child, with the consent of his wife unless '....she has been declared by a court to be of unsound mind.' (Act 78, 1965, Section 7)

A Hindu Female 'who is of sound mind, is not a minor' and is not married can adopt a child. It she is married and her husband........has been declared by court to be of unsound mind (Act, 78, 1956, S.8)

RIGHT TO VOTE

Under Act 326 of the Constitution of India, no person declared to be of unsound mind can vote.

WITNESS

Under the Indian Evidence Act (Section 5, 118) a lunatic is not incompetent to testify in the court as a witness unless he is prevented from understanding the questions put to him and giving rational answers to them.

TESTAMENTARY DISPOSITION

Testamentary capacity is regulated by the Indian Succession Act 39 (1925). It includes the following points:

1) A will must be in writing.
2) A will need not be registered.
3) It must be signed by testator in the presence of two witnesses.
4) A legatee cannot attest the will.
5) An executor (s) is usually appointed under the will by the testator, and will carry out terms after his/her death
6) The will may be revoked or modified anytime before the death of the testator.
7) A will takes effect only after the death of the testator, it is said to be 'ambulatory' and to speak from the grave.
8) The applicable to wills is contained in the Indian Succession Act. Under Section 59 of that Act, "Every person of sound mind not being minor may dispose of his property by will."
   Explanation 4 of Section 59 states that "no person can make a

will while he is in such a state of mind, whether arising from intoxication or from illnesses or from anyother cause. That he does not know what he is doing."

TRANSFER OF PROPERTY

The Transfer of Property Act relates to transfer of immovable property. Section 7 declares "that only persons competent to contract and entitled to transferable property are authorised to do so (that is transfer). Such property of some other person like a guardian or trustee" can effect a valid transfer.

CONTRACT

A contract begins with an offer and its acceptance. An offer is defined under the Indian Contract Act (1872 S. 11) where one person signifies to another his willingness to do or to abstain from doing anything with a view to obtaining the assent of that other to such act or, forebearance he is said to make a proposal.' A person is said to be of 'Sound Mind' for the purpose of a contract, if at the time of making a contract he is capable of understanding it and of forming a rational judgement as to effect upon his interests.'

THE NARCOTIC DRUGS AND PSYCHOTROPIC BSTANCES ACT (NDPSA), 1985

In India the Opium Act of 1857 was revised first in 1878. The Dangerous Drug Act of 1930 included, among the other drugs, opium and its alkaloids and cocaine. In 1950, the Opium Act of 1878 was revised as The Opium and Revenue Laws Act 1950.

On 16th September 1985, the above mentioned Acts were repealed and NDPSA Act 61 of 1985 was enforced. The Act includes:

a) Narcotic Drugs (cannabis, cocaine, coca leaf, opium, poppy straw and all manufactured, 'drugs').
b) Psychotropic Substances (76 drugs and their derivatives are, for example diazepam, pentazocine, phenobarbital).

If any person produces, possesses, transports, imports, exports drugs or Psychotropic Substance except 'ganja' he shall be punishable with:
(i) RI (Rigorous imprisonment) for not less than ten years which may extend to 20 years and
(ii) and a fine of not less than one lach rupees which may extend to two lakh rupees.
(iii) Punishment for repeat offence is RI for not less than 15 years which may extend to 30 years. And a fine of not less than 1.5 lakh rupees which may extend to 3 lakh rupees.

However, if a person is carrying small quantities e.g. 250 gms of heroin, 5 gms of charas, 5 gms of opium, 125 gms of cocaine, then the punishment is simple imprisonment which may extend to one year or a fine (unspecified) or both. For less than 500 gms of ganja imprisonment is five years.

If a person is found to be trafficking more than or equal to 1 kg of pure heroin, punishment is death penalty.

PROTECTION OF HUMAN RIGHTS OF MENTALLY ILL PERSONS

Under Section 81 of the Indian Mental Health Act, 1987:

(1) No mentally ill person shall be subjected during treatment to any indignity (physical or mental) or cruelty.

(2) No mentally ill person under treatment shall be used for purposes of research, unless:

(i) such research is of direct benefit to him for purposes of diagnosis or treatment, and

(ii) such a patient being a voluntary patient, has given consent in writing or where such a person (whether or not a voluntary patient) is incompetent by reason of minority or otherwise to give a valid consent, the guardian or any other person who can give consent on his behalf has given consent in writing.

ROLE OF NURSE IN LEGAL PSYCHIATRY

* The nurse needs to be aware of the Indian Mental Health Act, 1987.
* She should be qualified to work in a psychiatric ward/ or go through a continuing education programme.
* She should be aware of the procedure of admission and discharge.
* If the patient does not report after the expiry of the leave period, she needs to immediately inform the concerned psychiatrist.
* She should be aware of the rights of a patient to protect him from undergoing treatment/research which may not benefit him.
* Should obtain informed consent for treatment and procedures, such as:
  - (i) explanation about the procedure to the patient (if he can follow) otherwise relatives should be explained.
  - (ii) advantages of therapy.
  - (iii) risks associated with the therapy.
  - (iv) answer to any question which relatives need to clarify.
  - (v) answer any alternative therapies and their effectiveness.
  - (vi) written consent.
  - (vii) the patient and his/her relatives have the right to refuse treatment and withdraw consent specially for physical treatment such as ECT.
* Maintenance of confidentiality of records. The records and correspondance should not be made available to the patient, relatives or any third party, as records can be misused by anyone for humiliating the patient and his/her family or taking away the property.
* Maintain the standards of nursing care. Nursing standards are maintained according to preparation of the nurse and the supervisory help she is getting.

The American Nurses' Association has laid down Psychiatric Mental Health Nursing Practice Standards as follows:

STANDARDS

i. Data are collected through pertinent clinical observations based on knowledge of the Arts and Science, with particular emphasis on psychosocial and biophysical science.
—Data collection is done through various sources.

ii. Clients are involved in the assessment, planning, implementation and evaluation of their nursing care programme to the fullest extent of their capabilities.
— Based on the client's capabilities.

iii. The problem-solving approach is utilized in developing nursing care plans.

iv. Individuals, families and community groups are assisted achieving satisfying and productive patterns of living throu health teaching.
— appropriate techniques are used for health teaching.

v. The activities of daily living (ADL) are utilized in a goal-direct way in work with clients.
— Activities are planned based on the patient's need, strengt and levels of functioning.

vi. Knowledge of somatic therapies and related clinical skills is utilize in working with clients.
— Observation and effects of each therapy are recorded and discussed with the client and his/her family.

vii. The environment is structured to establish and maintain a therapeutic milieu.
— Effects of the environment on the individual are observed, analysed and interpreted.
The environment is modified according to the client's needs.

viii. The nurse participates, with interdisciplinary teams, in assessing, planning, implementing and evaluating programmes and other mental health activities.
— She plays a pivtol role in the care of the patient.

ix. Psychotherapeutic interventions are used to assist clients to achieve maximum development.

x. The practice of individual, group or family psychotherapy requires appropriate preparation and recognition of accountability for the practice.
— Preparation of the nurse to function as a primary therapist.

xi. The nurse participates, with other members of the community, in planning and implementing mental health services that include the broad continum of promotion of mental health, prevention of mental illness, treatment and rehabilitation.
— participates in community mental health care.

xii. Learning experiences are provided for other nursing care personnel through leadership, supervision and teaching.
— Accepts leadership roles and responsibilities.

xiii. Responsibility is assumed for continuing educational and professional development and contributions are made to the professional growth of others.
— updates self-knowledge and other professionals.

xiv. Contribution to nursing and the mental health field are through innovation in theory and practice and participation in research.
— Conducts research studies, implements the findings.

When the nurse fails to meet a standard of care, it is referred to as negligence.

* The nurse should intelligently avoid getting involved in questions such as whether the patient should make a will about his/her property.
* The nurse should avoid giving wrong information. She must confirm with the psychiatrist in case of doubt.
* Maintain an accurate record of observation as they can be used as legal documents any time, especially medicine record, mental status examination record, the nurse's notes.
* Protection of the patient from physical or sexual assault or any.

INTENTIONAL TORTS

Intentional torts are when others interfere in an individual's privacy, mobility, property or personal interests. These rights of the individual should be protected. Some of the examples of intentional torts are:

Battery — The intentional touching of another without the consent of the client.

Assault — An intentional act which places another in fear that an immediate battery (violent beating) is about to be committed on him.

False Imprisonment — An intentional act which prevents an individual from moving about and wherever he wants to be.

Defamation — Publication of a false statement about an individual made either verbally or in some other form to the third person. This damages his reputation.

Violation of Privacy — Revealing personal information about an individual which may belittle him or interfere in his personal private life.

Intentional Infliction of Emotional Distress — Intentional infliction of an individual with severe emotional unrest.

* Constant observation of the patient with suicidal ideation.
* Providing therapeutic milieu for the recovery of the patient.

It is essential for the psychiatric mental health nurse to be aware of legal aspects of psychiatry because ignorance is no bliss.

TO RECALL

Overview of the Indian Mental Act, 1987
Admission of the mentally ill patient
- **Admission on a voluntary Basis**
- **Admission under special circumstnces**
- **Admission by the Police Officer and the Magistrate**

Discharge of the mentally ill patient
Leave of Absence
Protection of Human Rights
Role of the Nurse in Legal Psychiatry
- **Standards of Nursing**
- **Intentional Torts**
  1. **Battery**
  2. **Assault**
  3. **False imprisonment**
  4. **Defamation**
  5. **Violation of Privacy**
  6. **Infliction of Emotional Distress**

APPLICATION TO NURSING

Reading of this unit on the legal aspects of psychiatric nursing will help the student nurse to identify her significant role in protecting the rights of the patient. She would be able to develop skills in caring for the patient according to nursing standards. She will also identify her pivtol role in a mental health team.

BETTER STUDY SECTION OF UNIT XXV

1. VOCABULARY (use dictionary)

Belittling	Holistic
Capabilities	Humanitarian
Catharsis	Intensity
Coordinate	Interaction
Crucial	Judicial
Custodial	Pivotal
Detention	Somatic
Deterioration	Violation
Dynamic	

2. ASSIGNMENT
   Make notes of the Indian Mental Health Act, 1987.

3. STUDY QUESTIONS
   a. List the members of the Mental Health Team.
   b. List career opportunities for the psychiatric mental health nurse in an institutional, psychiatric institution, general hospital and extramural setting.

c. Explain the standard for psychiatric mental health nursing practice.
d. Write the procedure for admission and discharge of the patient in a psychiatric ward.

4. READING REFERENCE

The American Nurses' Association: ***Standards Psychiatric Mental Health Nursing Practices,*** American Nursing Association,2420 Pershing Road, Kansas City, Missouri 64108 (1973).

John A., Riberira M.O., Buckle D., ***The Nurse in Mental Health Practice.*** Report on the Technical Conference, the World Health Organization, Geneva (1963).

Kalkman, M.E., Davis A.J. ***New Dimensions in Mental Health Psychiatric Nursing,*** McGraw Hill Book Company (1974).

Lego S. ***The American Handbook of Psychiatric Nursing.*** J.B. Lippincott Company, Philadelphia (1984).

Matheny, R.V., Topalis M. ***Psychiatric Nursing.*** **Sixth** edition. The C.V. Mosby Company (1974)

Mearness D.F. & Taylor C.M. ***Essentials of Psychiatric Nursing*** (Ninth edition) The C.V. Mosby Company, Saint Louis (1974).

Murthy B.V. ***Forensic Psychiatry,*** Bangalore (1957).

Report of the Joint Committee, ***The Mental Health Bill,*** Lok Sabha Secretariate, New Delhi (1978)

Gupta N. ***A Short Text Book of Psychiartry,*** New Delhi (19-

Sharma , Shridhar. ***Mental Hospitals in India.*** Directorate-General of Health Services, New Delhi (1990).

Shives L.R. ***Basic Concepts of Psychiatric Mental Health Nursing.*** Second edition J.B. Lippincott Company, Philadelphia (1990).

Wison, S.H.& Kneisl C.R. ***Psychiatric Nursing*** **Addison**-Wesley Publishing Company, California (1979).

UNIT XXVII

EMERGING TREADS IN PSYCHIARTRIC MENTAL HEALTH NURSING

UNIT OUTLINE

Introduction

* Challenges for the Nurse
* Demographic changes
* Social changes
* Economic changes
* Technological Changes
* Gap in mental and physical health care

Issues and Trends

* Preparation of the Nurse
* Standards for Psychiatric Mental Health Nursing
* Development for a Code of Ethics
* Participation in legal issues
* Changing role of the psychiatric Mental Health Nurse
* Cost of effective nursing care
* Focus of care
* Role of the Mental Health Nurse in Research

Application to Nursing
Better Study Section.

INTENDED LEARNING BEHAVIOUR

After reading this unit, you will be able to:

a) Identify the challenges Psychiatric Mental Health Nurse has to face in terms of:
   - Demographic changes
   - Social changes
   - Economic changes
   - Technological changes
   - Gap in mental and physical health care

b) Identify the Issues and emerging trends in psychiatric mental health nursing in terms of:
   - Upgrading qualification of nursing education.
   - Setting standards
   - Participation in legal aspects
   - Changing role of the psychiatric mental health nurse.
   - Cost-effective nursing care
   - Focus of care
   - Role of the mental health nurse in research.

CONTENT

INTRODUCTION

During the period of rapid change, a nurse needs to make wise decisions on several nursing issues, such as making a list of nursing diagnosis, participating in decision-making concerning national mental health care issues, deciding on alternatives to hospital care. The psychiatric nurse faces various challenges because of changes in the patient care approach.

CHALLENGES FOR THE NURSE

There are various challenges which a psychiatric mental health nurse faces due to demographic changes, social changes, economic changes, technological changes and the gap in mental and physical health care.

1. DEMOGRAPHIC CHANGES

a) Type of Family :— With the nuclear family system the disturbed behaviour of the child or family member gets immediate attention. Hence, the family approaches the community nurse, health centre or hospital from where the patient may be referred for psychiatric help. The nuclear family leads to other types of difficulties such as anxiety of working parents for leaving children in a crech.

The nurse needs to be prepared in counselling parents and families. She also needs to update her knowledge in the field of psychiatric mental nursing.

b) Stress of Urbanization:— Staying in an urban community with lack of resources and ambitious goals, competitive spirit in the people is increasing. Urbanization leads to various other types of stresses such as housing, transport, lack of supplies etc. The individual may or may not be able to cope with the stresses.

The Mental Health Nurse needs to help these individuals to identify the incongruence of goals with the means they have.

c) Increasing Number of Elderly Groups :— Sudden change in the family system has also brought changes in the life style of the old people. Decreased economic status due to retirement and neglect by members of the family bring unique challenges for a Psychiatric Mental Health Nurse. She needs to help in two major fields: *Psychogeriatrics* and *Geropsychiatry.*

Psychogeriatrics is special psychiatric care for patients who are elderly. *Geropsychiatry* is care of aging psychiatric patients.

The nurse needs to develop knowledge and skill in caring for elderly patients.

2. SOCIAL CHANGES

The individual in society is becoming more and more aware of his socical rights. Efforts are made to maintain intergroup and interagroup

loyalties. Otherwise, the individual feels isolated.
Peer Group Pressures specially on adolescent groups lead to various types of maladative behaviour like delinquency, dropouts from school or drug abuse.

The Psychiatric Mental Health nurse needs to conduct programmes in school health such as counselling sessions for adolescent groups, awareness programmes for teachers and parents on drug abuse, AIDS or behaviour problem.

3. ECONOMIC CHANGES

With the fast growing industrialization in India people are under stress to maintain standards of living. They take up certain bad habits like alcoholism and excessive smoking which lead to health problems

The Psychiatric Mental Health Nurse needs to identify various areas in which help can be extended to an individual, the family and the community.

4. TECHNOLOGICAL CHANGES

Mass media, television, other electronic systems and computers have brought a lot of changes in the people. The impact of education is vivid and strong in the people when they watch or hear something.

Mental Health Nursing personnel should take a leading role in educating the public through these mass media on issues like: developmental tasks of the child, adolescents, adults, needs of the elderly people, factors leading to drug abuse and alcoholism, its prevention and cure.

5. GAP IN MENTAL AND PHYSICAL HEALTH CARE

Health is defined with all physical, social, spiritual, emotional and mental components. Priority is given to physical care. There are only 45 mental hospitals in India (1987). These hospitals need to be staffed with trained psychiatric personnel, whereas there is practically no dearth of such experts in general hospitals.

ISSUES AND TRENDS

These challenges raise the following issues:

* Are the nurses educationally prepared to take up these challenges ?
* Are there any standards of psychiatric mental health nursing to maintain quality care ?
* Are there codes of ethics for nursing personnel ?
* Are the nurses participating in legal aspects of psychiatric mental health care ?
* Are the nurses prepared to take up roles in various psychiatric settings listed below:
  — Clinical health worker/Staff Nurse

— Clinical nurse specialist
— Nurse psychotherapist
— Psychiatric nurse educators
— Psychiatric nurse leader.

* Are the psychiatric mental health nurses able to give cost-effective care ?
* Are they able to attend to the target groups

— Children	— Mentally retarded
— Women	— Follow-up of chornic
— Youth	— mental illness
— Elderly	

* Are the nurses doing research in the area of psychiatric mental health nursing ?

1. PREPARATION OF NURSE

The existing educational programme for nursing in India includes:
— Doctorate in Nursing
— M.Phil. in Nursing
— M. Sc. in Nursing
— General Nursing and Midwifery
— Diploma in Psychiatric Nursing

General Nursing and Midwifery (GNM) programme has 30 hours of psychiatric nursing and four weeks of clinical experience. It is an orientation programme in psychiatric nursing. B.Sc. Nursing prepares a student to take up the role of first-level-care providers in a psychiatric mental health nursing setting. M.Sc. in Psychiatric Mental Health Nursing produces nurse clinicians but their number is not more than 20-30. M. Phil and Doctorate in Nursing are getting prepared to take up research in the field of Psychiatric Nursing.

A beginning is made with nursing personnel developing an insight into updating their knowledge in psychiatric mental health nursing, through bridge courses like Diploma in Psychiatric Nursing. The trend of open university will provide an opportunity for these bridge courses.

2. STANDARDS FOR PSYCHIATRIC MENTAL HEALTH NURSING

Standards need to be developed in psychiatric mental health nursing. The American Nurses' Association has developed standards of nursing. Quality of nursing can be ensured if there are laid—down standards of psychiatric mental health nursing.

3. DEVELOPMENT OF CODE OF ETHICS

A code of ethics provides protection to a practising nurse in clinical and community health nursing settings. This is very important for the psychiatric mental health nurse because of her taking up independent roles like psychotherapy, conducting group talks, maintaining patients' confidentiality and protecting their rights. A clearly developed and defined code of ethics will strengthen the efficiency of the psychiatric mental health nurse.

4. PARTICIPATION IN LEGAL ISSUES

Protection of the patient for his human and legal rights *(Described in Unit XXV under Legal Aspects of Psychaitric Mental Health Nursing).* The client's right to refuse a particular treatment or care, protection from confinement, restrictions, and intentional torts. Informed consent for therapies. These are a few of the legal issues in which the nurse has to participate with knowledge of the rights of the patient and her role.

5. CHANGES IN ROLE OF PSYCHIATRIC MENTAL HEALTH NURSE

(a) Staff Nurse — In the preceding chapters of this book the role of the staff nurse has been identified as multidimensional. Peplau stated that psychiatric nurses did not need to bring the patient to the therapy or the therapy to the patient because 'nurses are the therapy'. The nurses are therapy in psychiatric inpatient mileu, group therapy, individual therapy and family therapy.

The change in the staff nurse's role is significant. Nursing care plans described in Chapter VIII emphasize the role of the nurse in making nursing diagnosis, setting goals, planning of care, implementation and evaluation of nursing care. The staff nurse needs to update her knowledge to give holistic care to patients.

(b) Clinical Nurse Specialist — In India, the number of clinical nurse specialists in the field of psychiatric mental health nursing is very few. Their role is in an educational therapeutic and consultative setting. In the clinical setting, they should provide consultative services to nursing personnel and demonstrate practising of therapies. She should conduct inservice education programmes for various psychiatric mental health workers. Take up research studies to improve patient care, initiate and participate in curriculum revision/changes. More and more psychiatric clinical nurse specialists need to be prepared.

(c) Nurse Psychotherapist A clinical nurse specialist in the field of psychiatric mental health nursing develops competency to give individual, group and family psychotherapy.

Psychotherapy skill with knowledge update is an important issue. The patient finds the nurse psychotherapist available in the hospital, at the subcentre, in the community and even during home visits. Availability of a competent nurse in the field of psychiatric mental health nursing provides confidence to the clients. On the other hand, going to psychotherapist clients may take time in decision making and the crisis situation by then may become difficult to handle.

The nurse needs to take up psychotherapy roles like individual therapy, group therapy, interpersonal relationship, skill communication techniques,helping clients to socialize. Conduct inservice education for various workers in a clinical and community setting, identify the areas of research and implement the findings of research.

(d) Psychiatric Nurse Educators — Psychiatric nursing has been taught mainly by psychiatrists. They are able to impart knowledge about the basis of diseases and psychodynamics but it is the nurse educator who needs to teach the nursing component/care of the patient with various symptoms.

The number of nurses in the teaching field of psychiatric mental health nursing needs to enhanced. This is a big challenge for nursing curriculum planners.

A psychiatric mental health nurse needs to take up teaching of psychiatric nursing at the graduate, postgraduate and doctoral levels. She should be able to give expert guidance to research scholars.

Psychiatric mental health nurses are taking up these roles, but very few prepared nurse educators are available. The number needs to be enhanced.

(e) Psychiatric Nurse Leader — The other significant issue for the psychiatric mental health nurse is to take up the role of a nurse leader. She should participate in legal issues, national mental health acts, rights of patients and other significant issues.

6. COST-EFFECTIVE NURSING CARE

Quality nursing care will reduce the cost of patient care. Studies need to be conducted to find out the cost in preparation of the nurse and her quality of giving nursing care.

7. FOCUS OF CARE

The challenge confronting the psychiatric mental health nurse is to focus care on significant groups: children, women, youth, elderly people, mentally retarded and chronic mentally ill patients. To prevent maladjustment and maladaptive behaviour, these target groups need to be helped.

8. ROLE OF NURSE IN PSYCHIATRIC MENTAL HEALTH & RESEARCH

The nurse has an important role in research activities for improving the care of the patient. She/he is in constant contact with the patient. Observations made by the nurse contribute to the patient's diagnosis and treatment.

She participates in research done by various professionals. She conducts research in the area of therapies used for the patient. The skills, techniques and methods needto be developed in order to practise nursing effectively. A psychiatric mental health nurse can develop various teaching modules and put them to test. For example, a training module can be developed to impart training to mentally retarded persons. Research studies can be carried out for compliance of treatment and recovery of the patient. Family support and recovery of the patient can be done by the nursing personnel.

The emerging trends in nursing are more towards independent and collaborative roles. Mental health nursing needs to develop a list of nursing diagnoses.

TO RECALL

Challenges for the Nurse
* Demographic changes
* Stress or urbanization
* Social changes
* Economic changes
* Technological changes
* Gap in mental and physical health care

Issues and Trends
* Preparation of the nurse in the psychiatric mental health field
* Standards for psychiatric mental health nursing
* Development of a code of ethics
* Participation in legal issues

Changing Role of Psychiatric Mental Health Nurse as

a) Staff Nurse
b) Clinical Nurse Specialist
c) Clinical Psychotherapist
d) Psychiatric Nurse Educator
e) Psychiatric Nurse Leader.

* Cost-effective nursing care
* Focus of care target groups like children, adolescents, women, youth, elderly groups, mentally retarded, chronic mentally ill patients.
* Role of the nurse in psychiatric mental health research.

APPLICATION TO NURSING

Reading of this unit on emerging trends in nursing will enable the learner to identify the challenges in nursing. She will be able to identify the need of updating her knowledge by going through the postgraduate courses.

BETTER STUDY SECTION OF UNIT XXVI

1. **VOCABULARY** (Use dictionary)

Challenges	Incongruence
Collaborative	Intragroup
Competitive	Intergroup
Compliance	Issues
Contributes	Restrains
Enhanced	Revision
Emphasize	Significant
	Stress
	Trends

2. **ASSIGNMENT**

   Make a list of the issues and emerging trends with the role of the psychiatric mental health nurse.

3. **STUDY QUESTIONS**

   Identify and list the challenges for the psychiatric mental health nurse at levels of:
   — Staff Nurse
   — Ward Sister
   — Nurse Teacher
   — Assistant Nursing Superintendent
   — Nursing Superintendent

4. **READING REFERENCES**

World Health Organization. ***Organization of Mental Health Services in Developing Countries.*** WHO Technical Report Series No. 564, 31-36 (1975).

Johnson B.S. ***Adaptation and Growth of Psychiatric Mental Health Nursing.*** 2nd ed. J.B. Lippincott Company, Philadelphia (1989).

Beek, Rawlins and Williams. ***Mental Health Psychiatric Nursing. A Holistic Life Cycle Approach.*** 2nd ed. The C.V. Mosby Company, Toronto (1988).

COMPREHENSIVE TEST ON CHAPTER IX

1. List approaches to the National Mental Health Programme:
   i.
   ii.
   iii.
   iv.
   v.
   vi.
   vii.
   viii.

2. List three obejectives of the National Mental Health Programme Policy (1982)
   i.
   ii.
   iii.

3. Place an appropriate term from Column B in the space given along with the statement in Column A.

	COLUMN 'A'	COLUMN 'B'
i.	It means lowering the rate of new cases of mental disorders.	A. Secondary Prevention
ii.	When others interfere in the individual's privacy, mobility, property or personal interest.	B. Indian Lunacy Act, 1912
iii.	It is a transition facility for mental patients who no longer need the full services of hospital but not ready to live independently.	C. Indian Mental Health Act, 1987
iv.	It aims at early detection and prompt treatment.	D. Intentional torts.
v.	No mentally ill person shall be subjected during treatment to any indignity (whether physical or mental) or cruelty.	E. Foster Homes
		F. Primary prevention
		G. Half-way houses.

4. Fill in the blank space with the words provided in parenthesis.
   Clinical Nurse Specialist, Registered Nurse, Assault, Battery, the Indian Lunatic Act, 1912 the Indian Mental Health Act, 1987, Walk-in Clinic, Crisis Intervention, Day Centre.

i .... is self limiting within four to six weeks.
ii .... is 24 hours psychiatric emergency room for diagnostic or therapeutic services.
iii. .... is an amendment of ....
iv .... is the intentional touching of another person without the consent of the client.
v. ....should take up the role of a researcher also.

KEY

Comprehensive Test of Chapter IX

1. (i) Diffusion of mental health skills to the periphery of the health service system.
   (ii) Appropriate appointment of tasks in mental health care.
   (iii) Equitable and balanced territorial distribution of resources.
   (iv) Integration of basic mental health care into general health services.
   (v) Linkage to community development.
   (vi) Various aspects of mental health care.
   (vii) Mental health training.
   (viii) Mental retardation and drug dependence.

2. (i), To ensure availability and accessibility of minimum mental health care for all.
   (ii) To encourage the population on mental health knowledge of general health care in social development.
   (iii) To promote community participation in mental health service development.

3 (i) F
   (ii) D
   (iii) G
   (iv) A
   (v) C

4. (i) Crisis
   (ii) Walk-in Clinic
   (iii) (a) Indian Mental Health Act, 1987
   (b) Indian Lunacy Act, 1912
   (iv) Battery
   (v) Clinical Nurse Specialist.

APPENDIX

ICD-10 CLASSIFICATION OF MENTAL AND BEHAVIOURAL DISORDERS

LIST OF CATEGORIES

FOO—FO9
ORGANIC, INCLUDING SYMPTOMATIC, MENTAL DISORDERS

FOO DEMENTIA IN ALZHEIMER'S DISEASE

- F00.0 Dementia in Alzheimer's disease with early onset
- F00.1 Dementia in Alzheimer's disease with late onset
- F00.2 Dementia in Alzheimer's disease, atypical or mixed type
- F00.9 Dementia in Alzheimer's disease, unspecified

FO1 VASCULAR DEMENTIA

- F01.0 Vascular dementia of acute onset
- F01.1 Multi-infarct dementia
- F01.2 Subcortical vascular dementia
- F01.3 Mixed cortical and subcortical vascular dementia
- F01.8 Other vascular dementia
- F01.9 Vascular dementia, unspecified

F02 DEMENTIA IN OTHER DISEASES CLASSIFIED ELSEWHERE

- F02.0 Dementia in Pick's disease
- F02.1 Dementia in Creutzfeldt-Jakob disease
- F02.2 Dementia in Hutington's disease
- F02.3 Dementia in Parkinson's disease
- F02.4 Dementia in human immunodeficiency virus [HIV] disease
- F02.8 Dementia in other specified diseases classified elsewhere

F03 UNSPECIFIED DEMENTIA

A fifthe character may be added to specify dementia in F00-F03, as follows:

.x0 Without additional symptoms

.x1 Other symptoms, predominantly delusional
.x2 Other symptoms, predominantly hallucinatory
.x3 Other symptoms, predominantly depressive
.x4 Other mixed symptoms

F04 ORGANIC AMNESIC SYNDROME, NOT INCLUDED BY ALCOHOL AND OTHER PSYCHOACTIVE SUBSTANCES

F05 DELIRIUM, NOT INCLUDED BY ALCOHOL AND OTHER PSYCHOACTIVE AND TO PHYSICAL DISEASE

F05.0 Delirium, not superimposed on dementia, so described
F05.1 Delirium, superimposed on dementia
F05.8 Other delirium
F05.9 Delirium, unspecified

F06 OTHER MENTAL DISORDERS DUE TO BRAIN DAMAGE AND DYSFUNCTION AND TO PHYSICAL DISEASE

F06.0 Organic hallucinosis'
F06.1 Organic catatonic disorder
F06.2 Organic delusional [schizophrenia-like] disorder
F06.3 Organic mood [affective] disorders
.30 Oranic manic disorder
.31 Organic bipolar disorder
.32 Organic dperessive disorder
.33 Organic mixed affective disorder
F06.4 Organic anxiety disorder
F06.5 Organic dissociative disorder
F06.6 Organic emotionally liable [asthenic] disorder
F06.7 Mild cognitive disorder
F06.8 Other specified mental disorders due to brain damage and dysfunction and to physical disease
F06.9 Unspecified mental disorder due to brain damage and dysfunction and to physical disease

F07 PERSONALITY AND BEHAVIOURAL DISORDERS DUE TO BRAIN DISEASE, DAMAGE AND DYSFUNCTION

F07.0 Organic personality disorder
F07.1 Postencephalitic syndrome
F07.2 Postconcussional syndrome
F07.8 Other organic personality and behavioural disorders due to brain disease, damage and dysfunction
F07.9 Unspecified organic personality and behavioural disorder due to brain disease, damage and dysfunction

F09 UNSPECIFIED ORGANIC OR SYMPTOMATIC MENTAL DISORDER

F10-F19 MENTAL AND BEHAVIOURAL DISORDERS DUE TO PSYCHOACTIVE SUBSTANCE USE

F10.- Mental and behavioural disorders due to use of alchol
F11.- Mental and behavioural disorders due to use of opioids
F12.- Mental and behavioural disorders due to use of cannabinoids
F13.- Mental and behavioural disorders due to use of sedatives or hypnotics
F14.- Mental and behavioural disorders due to use of cocaine
F15.- Mental and behavioural disorders due to use of other stimulants, including caffeine
F16.- Mental and behavioural disorders due to use of hallucinogens
F17.- Mental and behavioural disorders due to use of tobacco
F18.- Mental and behavioural disorders due to use of volatile solvents
F19.- Mental and behavioural disorders due to multiple drug use and use of other psychoactive substances

Four- and five-character may be used to specify the clinical conditions, as follows :

Flx.0 Acute intoxication
- .00 Uncomplicated
- .01 With trauma or other bodily injury
- .02 With other medical complications
- .03 With delirium
- .04 With perceptual distortions
- .05 With coma
- .06 With convulsions
- .07 Pathological intoxication

Flx.1 Harmful use

Flx.2 Dependence syndrome
- .20 Currently abstinent
- .21 Currently abstinent, but in a protected environment
- .22 Currently on a clinically supervised maintenance or replacement, regime [controlled dependence]
- .23 Currently abstinent, but receiving treatment with aversice or blocking drugs
- .24 Currently using the substance [active dependence]
- .25 Continuous use
- .26 Episodic use [dipsomania]

Flx.3 Withdrawal state
- .30 Uncomplicated
- .31 Convulsions

Flx.4 Withdrawal state with delirium
- .40 Without convulsions

.41 With convulsions

Flx.5 Psychotic disorders
- .50 Schizophrenia like
- .51 Predominantly delusional
- .52 Predominantly hallucinatory
- .53 Predominantly polymorphic
- .54 Predominantly depressive symptoms
- .55 Predominantly manic symptoms
- .56 Mixed

Flx.6 Amnesic syndrome

Flx.7 Residual and late-onset psychotic disorder
- .70 Flashbacks
- .71 Personality or behaviour disorder
- .72 Residual affective disorder
- .73 Dementia
- .74 Other persisting cognitive impairment
- .75 Late-onset psychotic disorders

Flx.8 Other mental and behavioural disorders

Flx.9 Unspecified mental and behavioural disorder

F20-F29 SCHIZOPHRENIA, SCHIZOTYPAL AND DELUSIONAL DISORDERS

F20 SCHIZOPHRENIA

- F20.0 Paranoid schizophrenia
- F20.1 Hebephrenic schizophrenia
- F20.2 Catatonic schizophrenia
- F20.3 Undifferentiated schizophrenia
- F20.4 Post-schizophrenic depression
- F20.5 Residual schizophrenia
- F20.6 Simple schizophrenia
- F20.8 Other schizophrenia
- F20.9 Schizophrenia, unspecified

A fifth character may be used to classify course :
- .x0 Continuous
- .x1 Episodic with progressive deficit
- .x2 Episodic with stable deficit
- .x3 Episodic remittent
- .x4 Incomplete remission

.x5 Complete remission
.x8 Other
.x9 Period of observation less than one year

F21 SCHIZOTYPAL DISORDER

F22 PERSISTENT DELUSIONAL DISORDERS
F22.0 Delusional disorder
F22.8 Other persistent delusional disorders
F22.9 Persistent delusional disorder, unspecified

F23 ACUTE AND TRANSIENT PSYCHOTIC DISORDERS
F23.0 Acute polymorphic psychotic disorder without symptoms of schizophrenia
F23.1 Acute polmorphic psychotic disorder with symptoms of schizophrenia
F23.2 Acute schizophrenia-like psychotic disorder
F23.3 Other acute predominantly delusional psychiotic disorders
F23.8 Other acute and transient psychotic disorders
F23.9 Acute and transient psychotic disorders unspecified

A fifth character may be used to identfy the presence or absence of associated acute stress:
.x0 Without associated acute stress
.x1 With associated acute stress

F24 INDUCED DELUSIONAL DISORDER

F25 SCHIZOAFFECTIVE DISORDERS
F25.0 Schizoaffective disorder, manic type
F25.1 Schizoaffective disorder, depressive type
F25.2 Schizoaffective disorder, mixed type
F25.8 Other schizoaffective disorders
F25.9 Schizoaffective disorder, unspecified

F28 OTHER NONORGANIC PSYCHOTIC DISORDERS

F29 UNSPECIFIED NONORGANIC PSYCHOSIS

F30-F39
MOOD [AFFECTIVE] DISORDERS

F30 MANIC EPISODE
F30.0 hypomania
F30.1 Mania without psychotic symptoms
F30.2 Mania with psychotic symptoms
F30.8 Other manic episodes
F30.9 Manic episode, unspecified

F31 BIPOLAR AFFECTIVE DISORDER

F31.0 Bipolar affective disorder, current episode hypomanic
F31.1 Bipolar affective disorder, current episode manic without psychotic symptoms
F31.2 Bipolar affective disorder, current episode manic with psychotic symptoms
F31.3 Bipolar affective disorder, current episode mild or moderate depression
.30 Without somatic symptoms
.31 With somatic symptoms
F31.4 Bipolar affective disorder, current episode severe depression without psychotic symptoms
F31.5 Bipolar affective disorder, current episode severe depression with psychotic symptoms
F31.6 Bipolar affective disorder, current episode mixed
F31.7 Bipolar affective disorder, currently in remission
F31.8 Other bipolar affective disorders
F31.9 Bipolar affective disorder, unspecified

F32 DEPRESSIVE EPISODE

F32.0 Mild depressive episode
.00 Without somatic symptoms
.01 With somatic symptoms
F32.1 Moderate depressive episode
.10 Without somatic symptoms
.11 With somatic symptoms
F32.2 Severe depressive episode without psychotic symptoms
F32.3 Severe depressive episode with spsychotic symptoms
F32.8 Other depressive episodes
F32.9 Depressive episode, unspecified

F33 RECURRENT DEPRESSIVE DISORDER

F33.0 Recurrent depressive disorder, current episode mild
.00 without somatic symptoms
.01 With somatic symptoms
F33.1 Recurrent depressive disorder, current episode moderate
.10 Without somatic symptoms
.11 With somatic symptoms
F33.2 Recurrent depressive disorder, current episode severe without psychotic symptoms
F33.3 Recurrent depressive disorder, current episode severe with psychotic symptoms
F33.4 Recurrent depressive disorder, currently in remission
F33.8 Other recurrent depressive disorders
F33.9 Recurrent depressive disorder, unspecified

F34 PERSISTENT MOOD [AFFECTIVE] DISORDER

F34.0 Cyclothymia
F34.1 Dysthymia
F34.8 Other persistent mood [affective] disorders
F34.9 Persistent mood [affective] disorder, unspecified

F38 OTHER MOOD [AFFECTIVE] DISORDERS
F38.0 Other single mood [affective] disorders
.00 Mixed affective episode
F38.1 Other recurrent mood [affective] disorders
.10 Recurrent brief depressive disorder
F38.8 Other specified mood [affective] disorder

F39 UNSPECIFIED MOOD [AFFECTIVE] DISORDER

F40—F48
NEUROTIC, STRESS-RELATED AND SOMATOFORM DISORDERS

F40 PHOBIC ANXIETY DISORDERS
F40.0 Agoraphobia
.00 Without panic disorder
.01 With panic disorder
F40.1 Social phobias
F40.2 Specific (isolated) phobias
F40.8 Other phobic anxiety disorders
F40.9 Phobic anxiety disorder, unspecified

F41 OTHER ANXIETY DISORDER
F41.0 Panic disorder [episodic paroxysmal anxiety]
F41.1 Generalized anxiety disorder
F41.2 Mixed anxiety and depressive disorder
F41.3 Other mixed anxiety disorders
F41.8 Other specified anxiety disorders
F41.9 Anxiety disorder, unspecified

F42 OBSESSIVE—COMPULSIVE DISORDER
F42.0 Predominantly obsessional thoughts or ruminations
F42.1 Predominantly compulsive acts [obsessional rituals]
F42.2 Mixed obsessional thoughts and acts
F42.8 Other obsessive-compulsive disorders
F42.9 Obsessive-compulsive disorder, unspecified

F43 REACTION TO SEVERE STRESS, AND ADJUSTMENT DISORDERS
F43.0 Acute stress reaction
F43.1 Post-traumatic stress disorder
F43.2 Adustment disorders
.20 Brief depressive reaction
.21 Prolonged depressive reaction
.22 Mixed anxiety and depressive reaction
.23 With predominant disturbance of other emotions
.24 With predominant disturbace of conduct

.25 With mixed disturbance of emotions and conduct
.28 With other specified precdominant symptoms
F43.8 Other reactions to severe stress
F43.9 Reaction to severe stress, unspecified

F44 DISSOCIATIVRE {CONVERSION} DISORDERS
F44.0 Dissociative amnesia
F44.1 Dissociative fugue
F44.2 Dissociative stupor
F44.3 Trance and possession disorders
F44.4 Dissociative motor disorders
F44.5 Dissociative convulsions
F44.6 Dissociative anaesthesia and sensory loss
F44.7 Mixed dissociative {conversion} disorders
F44.8 Other dissociative {conversion} disorders
.80 Ganser's syndrome
.81 Multiple personality disorder
.82 Transient dissociate {conversion} disorders occurring in childhood and adolescence
.88 Other specified dissociative {conversion} disorders
F44.9 Dissociative {conversion} disorder, unspecified

F45 SOMATOFORM DISORDERS
F45.0 Somatization disorder
F45.1 Undifferentiated somatoform disorder
F45.2 Hypochondriacal disorder
F45.3 Somatoform autonomic dysfunction
.30 Heart and cardiovascular system
.31 Upper gastrointestinal tract
.32 Lower gastrointestinal tract
.33 Respiratory system
.34 Genitourinary system
.38 Other organ or system
F45.4 Persistent somatoform pain disorder
F45.8 Other somatoform disorders
F45.9 Somatoform disorder, unspecified

F48 OTHER NEUROTIC DISORDERS
F48.0 Neurasthenia
F48.1 Depersonalization-derealization syndrome
F48.8 Other specified neurotic disorders
F48.9 Neurotic disorder, unspecified

F50-F59
BEHAVIOURAL SYNDROMES ASSOCIATED WITH PHYSIOLOGICAL DISTURBANCES AND PHYSICAL FACTORS

F50 EATING DISORDERS
- F50.0 Anorexia nervosa
- F50.1 Atypical anorexia nervosa
- F50.2 Bulimia nervosa
- F50.3 Atypical bulimia nervosa
- F50.4 Overeating assocaited with other psychological distubances
- F50.5 Vomiting associated with other pshchological disturbances
- F50.8 Other eating disorders
- F50.9 Eating disorder, unspecified

F51 Nonorganic sleep disorders
- F51.0 nonorganic insomnia
- F51.1 Nonorganic hypersomnia
- F51.2 Nonorganic disorder of the sleep-wake schedule
- F51.3 Sleepwalking {somnambulism}
- F51.4 Sleep terrors {night terrors}
- F51.5 Nightmares
- F51.8 Other nonorganic sleep disorders
- F51.9 Nonorganic sleep disorder, unspecified

F52 SEXUAL DYSFUCTION, NOT CAUSED BY ORGANIC DISORDER OR OR DISEASE
- F52.0 lack or loss of sexual desire
- F52.1 Sexual aversion and lack of sexual enjoyment
  - .10 Sexual aversion
  - .11 lack of sexual enjoyment
- F52.2 Failure of genital response
- F52.3 Orgasmic dysfunction
- F52.4 Premature ejaculation
- F52.5 Nonorganic vaginismus
- F52.6 Nonorganic dyspareunia
- F52.7 Excessive sexual drive
- F52.8 Other sexual dysfunction, not caused by organic disorders or disease
- F52.9 Unspecified sexual dysfunction, not caused by organic disorder or disease

F53 MENTAL AND BEHAVIOURAL DISORDERS ASSOCIATED WITH THE PUERPERIUM, NOT ELSEWHERE CLASSIFIED

- F53.0 Mild mental and behavioural disorders associated with the puerperium, not elsewhere classified
- F53.1 Severe mental and behavioural disorders associated with the puerperium, not

elsewhere classified

F53.8 Other mental and behavioural disorders associated with the puerperium, not elsewhere classified

F53.9 Puerperal mental disorder, unspecified

F54 PYSCHOLOGICAL AND BEHAVIOURAL FACTORS ASSOCIATED WITH DISORDERS OR DISEASES CLASSIFIED ELSEWHERE

F55 ABUSE OF NON-DEPENDENCE-PRODUCING SUBSTANCES

F55.0 Antidepressants
F55.1 Laxatives
F55.2 Analgesices
F55.3 Antacids
F55.4 Vitamins
F55.5 Steroids or hormones
F55.6 Specific herbal or folk remedies
F55.8 Other substances that do not produce dependence
F55.9 Unspecified

F59 UNSPECIFIED BEHAVIOURAL SYNDROMES ASSOCIATED WITH PHYSIOLOGICAL DISTURBANCES AND PHYSICAL FACTORS

F60-F69
DISORDERS OF ADULT PERSONALITY AND BEHAVIOUR

F60 SPECIFIC PERSONALITY DOSORDERS

F60.0 paranoid personality disorder
F60.1 Schizoid personality disorder
F60.2 Dissocial personality disorder
F60.3 Emotionally unstable personality disorder
.30 Impulsive type
.31 Borderline type
F60.4 Histrionic personality disorder
F60.5 Anankasitic personalily disorder
F60.6 Anxious {avoidant} personality disorder
F60.7 Dependent personality disorders
F60.8 Other specific personality disorders
F60.9 Personality disorder, unspecified

F61 MIXED AND OTHER PERSONALITY DISORDERS

F61.0 Mixed personality disorders
F61.1 Troublesome personality changes

F62 ENDURING PERSONALITY CHANGES, NOT ATTRIBUTABLE TO BRAIN DAMAGE AND DISEASE

F62.0 Enduring personality change after catastrophic experience
F62.1 Enduring personality change after psychiatric illness
F62.8 Other enduring personality changes
F62.9 Enduring personality change, unspecified

F63 HABIT AND IMPULSE DISORDERS
F63.0 pathological gambling
F63.1 pathological fire-setting {pyromania}
F63.2 Pathological stealing {kleptomania}
F63.3 Trichotillomania
F63.8 Other habit and impulse disorders
F63.9 Habit and impulse disorder, unspecified

F64 GENDER IDENTITY DISORDERS
F64.0 Transsexualism
F64.1 Dual-role transvestism
F64.2 Gender identity dosorder of childhood
F64.8 Other gender identity disorders
F64.9 Gender identity disorder, unspecified

F65 DISORDERS OF SEXUAL PREFERENCE
F65.0 Fetishism
F65.1 Fetishistic transverstism
F65.2 Exhibitionism
F65.3 Voyeurism
F65.4 Paedophilia
F65.5 Sadomasochism
F65.6 Multiple disorders of sexual preference
F65.8 Other disorders of sexual preference
F65.9 Disorder of sexual preference, unspecified

F66 PSYCHOLOGICAL AND BEHAVOURAL DISORDERS ASSOCIATED WITH SEXUAL DEVELOPMENT AND ORIENTATION
F66.0 Sexual maturation disorder
F66.1 Egodystonic sexual orientation
F66.2 Sexual relationship disorder
F66.8 Other psychosexual development disorders, unspecified
F66.9 Psychosexual development disorder, unspecified

A fifth character may be used to indicate association with:
.xo Heterosexuality
.x1 homosexuality
.x2 Besexuality
.x8 Other, including prepubertal

F68 OTHER DISORDDERS OF ADULT PERSONALITY AND BEHAVIOUR

F68.0 Elaboration of physical symptoms for pshchological reasons
F68.1 Intentional production or feigning of symptoms or disabilities, either physical or psychological {factitious disorder}
F68.8 Other specified disorder of adult personality and behaviour

F69 UNSPECIFIED DISORDER OF ADULT PERSONALITY AND BEHAVIOUR

F70-F79
MENTAL RETARDATION

F70 Mild mental retardation

F71 Moderate mental retardation

F72 Severe mental retardation

F73 Profound mental retardation

F78 Other mental retardation

F79 Unspecified mental retardation

A fourth character may be used to specify the extent of associated behavioural impairment:

F7x.0 No, or minimal, impairment of behaviour
F7 x.8 Other impairments of behaviour
F7x.9 Without mention of impairment of behaviour

R80-F89
DISORDERS OF PSYCHOLOGICAL DEVELOPMENT

F80 SPECIFIC DEVELOPMENTAL DISORDERSA OF SPEECH AND LANGUAGE

F80.0 Specific speech articulation disorder
F80.1 Experssive language disorder
F80.2 Receptive language disorder
F80.3 Acquired aphasia with epilepsy {landau-kleffner syndrome}
F80.8 Other developmental disorders of speech and language
F80.9 Developmental disorder of speech and language, unspecified

F81 SPECIFIC DEVELOPMENTAL DISORDERS OF SCHOLASTIC SKILLS

F81.0 Specific reading disorder
F81.1 Specific spelling disorder
F81.2 Specific disorder of arithmetical skills
F81.3 Mixed disorder of scholastic skills

F81.8 Other developmental disorders of scholastic skills
F81.9 Developmental disorder of scholastic skills, unspecified

F82 SPECIFIC DEVELOPMENTAL DISORDER OF MOTOR FUNCTION

F83 MIXED SPECIFIC DEVELOPMENTAL DISORDERS

F84 PERVASIVE DEVELOPMENTAL DISORDERS
F84.0 Childhood autism
F84.1 A typical autism
F84.2 Rett's syndrome
F84.3 Other childhood disintegrative disorder
F84.4 Overactive disorder associated with mental retardation and stereotyped movements
F84.5 Asperger's syndrome
F84.9 pervasive developmental disorder, unspecified

F88 OTHER DISORDERS OF PSYCHOLOGICAL DEVELOPMENT

F89 UNSPECIFIED DISORDER OF PSYCHOLOGICAL DEVELOPMENT

F90-F98
BEHAVIOURAL AND EMOTIONAL DISORDERS WITH ONSET USUALLY OCCURRING IN CHILDHOOD AND ADOLESCENCE

F90 HYPERKINETIC DISORDERS
F90.0 Disturbance of activity and attention
F90.1 Hyperkinetic conduct disorder
F90.8 Other hyperkinetic disorders
F90.9 Hyperkinetic disorder, unspecified

F91 CONDUCT DISORDERS
F91.0 Conduct disorder confined to the family context
F91.1 Unsocialized conduct disorder
F91.2 Socialized conduct disorder
F91.3 Oppositional defiant disorder
F91.8 Other conduct disorders
F91.9 Conduct disorder, unspecified

F92 MIXED DISORDERS OF CONDUCT AND EMOTIONS
F92.0 Depressive conduct disorder
F92.8 Other mixed disorders of conduct and emotions
F92.9 Mixed disorder of conduct and emotions, unspecified

F93 EMOTIONAL DISORDERS WITH ONSET SPECIFIC TO CHILDHOOD
F93.0 Separation anxiety disorder of childhood

F93.1 Phobic anxiety disorder of childhood
F93.2 Social anxiety disorder of childhood
F93.3 Sibling revalry disorder
F93.8 Other childhood emotional disorders
F93.9 Childhood emotional disorder, unspecified

F94 DISORDERS OF SOCIAL FUCTIONING WITH ONSET SPECIFIC TO CHILDHOOD AND ADOLESCENCE

F94.0 Elective mutism
F94.1 Reactive attachment disorder of childhood
F94.2 Disinhibited attachment disorder of childhood
F94.8 Other childhood disorders of social fuctioning
F94.9 Childhood disorders of social functioning, unspecified

F95 TIC DISORDERS

F95.0 Transient tic disorder
F95.1 Chronic motor or vocal tic disorder
F95.2 Combined vocal and multiple motor tic disorder {de la Tourette's syndrome}
F95.8 Other tic disorders
F95.9 Tic disorder, unspecified

F98 OTHER BEHAVIOURAL AND EMOTIONAL DISORDERS WITH ONSET USUALLY OCCURRING IN CHILDHOOD AND ADOLESCENCE

F98,0 Nonorganic enuresis
F98.1 Nonorganic encopresis
F98.2 Feeding disorder of infancy and childhood
F98.3 Pica of infancy and childhood
F98.4 Stereoyped movement disorders
F98.5 Stuttering {stammering}
F98.6 Cluttering
F98.8 Other specified behavioural and emotional disorders with onset usually occurring in childhood and adolescence
F98.9 Unspecified behavioural and emotional disorders with onset usually occurring in childhood and adolescence

F99
UNSPECIFIED MENTAL DISORDER

F99 MENTAL DISORDER, NOT OTHERWISE SPECIFIED

Reproduced by Permission from :-
The ICD-10 Classification of Mental and Behavioural Disorders. Clinical Descriptions and diagnostic Guidlines. Geneva, World Health Organization, 1992 (PP 22-40)

GLOSSARY

AFFECTIVE DISORDERS — Illness in which mood changes is the primary and dominant symptom.

AFFECTIVE TONALITY — Changes which occur in affect or mood of the patient.

AIDS — Acquired Immuno-Deficiency Syndrome.

AKATHISIA — It is E. P. S., Characterise with difficulties in sitting still or strong urge to move about.

ALCOHOLIC ANONNYMOUS GROUPS — It is a group of recovering alcoholics and the attitude of each member towards the addict is tolerant and constructive.

ALCOHOLISM — It is a chronic dependence characterized by compulsive drinking of alcohol to such a degree that it produces mental disturbance, interfers with social and economic functioning.

ALZHEMIER'S DISEASE — It is a type of presenile dementia occuring between 40 to 50 years of age.

ANTI-PARKINSONIAN AGENT — The specific drug to treat extrapyremidal side effects of antipsychotic agent.

ANTI-PSYCHOTIC AGENT — Also known as a Neuroptic Drug has major clinical use in the treatment of psychosis.

ANXIETY — It is a pervasive feeling of dread, apprehension and impending disaster.

ASSESSMENT — It is the systematic and purposeful collection of data on the health status of the patient.

BABINSKI SIGN — The toes extends upward when the sole is gentally stimulated due to less of function of the upper motor neuron.

BINGE EATING — Repeated taking of a large quantity of food and drink in a short time It is also known as Buliamia Nervosa.

BULIMIA NERVOSA — See Binge eating.

CONVERSION DISORDER — There are somatoform disorders in which repressed inner conflicts are unconsciously converted or transformed into physical symptoms that have no organic basis.

CRISIS — It is an initial disturbance that results from a stressful event or a percieved threat to self.

CRISIS INTERVENTION — It is the process by which an individual is helped to cope with a stressful situation.

DAY HOSPITAL/CENTRE — A hospital programme organized on a day time basis.

DELIRIUM — It is a state of clouded consciousness in which attention cannot be sustained, the environment is wrongly percieved and disturbances of thinking are present.

DEMENTIA — It is a disease of brain, usually a chronic or progressive in nature with disturbances of multiple higher cortical functions. Produces decline in intellectual functioning. It can be senile and presenile.

DEPERSONALIZATION — It is a state of mind in which self of the individual appears to him as unreal.

DOUBLE — Bound Communication — The child is not able to discriminate the sort of message being conveyed.

DRUG ABUSE — It is a pathological use of drug or alcohol with impairment in social and occupational functioning.

DRUG DEPENDENCE — A state psychic, sometimes also physical resulting from taking a drug.

ENCOPRESIS — It is repeated voluntary or involntary passage of feaces in day or night time in one's clothing after the age of 4 years.

EPILEPSY — It is a group of disorders associated with disturbances in the electrical discharges of brain cells. Grand mal epilepsy, status epilepticus, petti mal epilepsy psychomotor seizures, epileptic psychosis.

EXTRAPYRAMIDAL SYMPTOMS — These symptoms include motor restlessness, parkinsonism, akathisia, dystonia, tardive dyskinesia and neuroleptic malignant syndrome.

FOSTER HOMES — A home in which patient recovering from a mental disorder stays with a family.

GAS — General adaptation syndrome.

GENETIC COUNSELLING — Providing information and guidance regarding relevant facts about inherited pathology.

GROUP HOMES — The ex-patients stay together.

HALF-WAY HOUSES — It is a transition facility for mental patients who no longer need the full services of a hospital but are not yet ready for a completely independent living.

HOMEOSTASIS — It is defined as the maintenance of a normal steady state in the body.

HOT-LINE SERVICES — It is a telephone link services through which professional help can be extended.

HUNTIGTON'S CHOREA — Characterized by a chronic, progressive chorea occurs between the ages of 30 to 50 years.

INTENTIONAL TORTS — When others interfere in an individual's privacy, property or personal interests.

INVOLUTIONAL MELANCHOLIA — It is a mental disorder occuring in a late middle life or during the menopausal period.

KORSAKOFF SYNDROME — The type of dementia develops from a delirium tremens which does not completely recover due to thiamine deficiency.

LETHALITY — Capable of causing death.

LIMBIC SYSTEM — The part of brain that includes portions of cerebral cortex, the thalamus and certain subcortical structures.

LTG — Long Term Goal.

LUPUS ERYTHEMATOUS — A collagen (or connective tissues) disease of unknown origin.

MALADAPTIVE LEARNING — When an individual is not able to learn the correct or adaptive techniques to solve the problems of life.

MONGOLISM — A chromosomal disorder characterised by an extra chromosome, mongloid features, a round flat face, eyes seems to slant, mildly or severely retarded.

MR — Mental Retardation is a disorder characterized by significant subaverage intellectual functioning, an I. Q. of 70 or below.

MSE — Mental Status Examination.

MULTIPLE PERSONALITY— Two or more personalities exist in one individual. One personality at a time is dominant and works at a conscious level at one time.

NEGLIGENCE — When nurse fails to meet a standard of care.

NMS — Neuroleptic Malignant Syndrome; a complication of antipyschotic agents.

NEURASTHENIA It is a neurotic condition marked by fatigue, insomnia, aches, pains, irritability depression and difficulty in concentration.

NEUROSIS — It is mild to moderately servere illness of the personality in which ego function of reality testing is not affected intensively and maladjustment to life is limited.

NURSING DIAGNOSIS — It is a statement of patient's actual and potential problems.

NURSE-PATIENT-RELATIONSHIP — It is an interaction process in which the nurse fulfills her role by using her professional knowledge and skill to help the patient.

NURSING PROCESS — It is an organized, systematic method of giving individualized nursing care to the patient.

OCN —Obsessive Compulsive Neurosis in which obsessions or compulsion are the significant source of distress and interfere with the individual's ability to function.

OCULOGYRIC CRISIS — Occurs in dystonia which is EPS, eyes look upward, head is turned to one side.

ORGANIC MENTAL DISORDER — Involve impairment of brain tissue functions.

PARKINSON'S DISEASE — Occurs before the age of 30 years. Majority of the cases are reported between 50 and 70 years of age. L. Dopa is the drug which brings improvement.

PARKINSONISM — Patient hows motor retardation, mask like face, rigidity of muscles, tremors of hands and shuffling gaits (EPS).

PHOBIA — It is an exaggerated pathological fear of a specific type of stimulus or situation.

PICA — Persistent Craving for unnatural, non-nutritive substances such as hair, paint, chalk found in pregnant women and children.

PICK'S DISEASE — It is degenerative disorder of the nervous system. Usually occurs in 45 to 50 years of age.

POSTNATAL CARE — The care following child birth.

PRENATAL CARE — The care during the period between conception and birth.

PRESENILE DEMENTIA — See dementia.

PREVENTION — means lowering the rate of new cases of mental disorders in a population.

PSYCHALGIA — Patient complains of severe prolonged pain without any organic pathology.

PSYCHIC DEPENDENCE — Psychic dependence occurs when the drug is central to a person's thoughts, emotions and activities.

PSYCHIATRIC EMERGENCY — It is a sudden onset of unusual disordered or socially inappropriate behaviour caused by an emotional or physiological situation.

PSYCHOGENIC FAGUE — It is an amnesic dissociated state in which the individual flees or runs away from home, forgets his entire past but not the basic skills.

PSYCHOPATIC PERSONALITY — It is also described as antisocial reaction starts before the age of 15 years with such behaviour as lying, stealing, trauncy atc.

PSYCHOPYSIOLOGICAL DISORDERS — represent a group of ailment in which emotional stress is contributing factor to physical problems.

PSYCHOSIS — It is a very serious illness of the personality which involves impairment of ego functions. Reality testing is markedly impaired. There are signs of grave maladjustment to life.

PSYCHOSOMATIC DISORDERS — See Psychophysiological disorders.

RAPPORT — It is a relationship of mutual sympathy and understanding especially between patient and therepist.

RUMINATION — The act of persistently pondering about a problem.

SCHIZOPHRENIC DISORDERS —Characterized in general by distortion of thinking, perception and inappropriate or blunted affect. Delusion and hallucination are present.

SECONDARY PREVENTION — It aims at early detection and prompt treatment.

SELF HELP GROUP — Members of the group help themselves and group members.

SHELTERED WORKSHOP — Ex-long-term mentally ill patients work under supervision.

SOMATOFORM DISORDERS — The patient has repeated presentation of physical symptoms with a persistent request for medical investigation inspite of negative findings and reassurance by the doctor.

SOMNAMBULISM — It is a disorder in which patient walks and does all the acitivities during sleep.

STG — Short Term Goal.

STRESS — A state of physical or psychological strain which imposes demands for adjustment upon the individual.

SUICIDE — It is an act or instance or taking one's own life voluntarily.

TARDIVE DYSKINESIA — It is characterized by involuntary rhythemic, stereotyped movements, protrusion of tongue, puffing of cheeks, chewing movements involuntary movements of extremities and truck occurs due to abrupt termination of antipsychotic drugs.

TERTIARY PREVENTION — Aims at reducing the reoccurance of disease.

TIC DISORDERS — It is repeated involuntary contraction of a small group of muscles.

TOURETT'S DISORDER — A sterotyped movement disorder characterized by repeated, involuntary rapid movements of various muscle. Groups involving vocal tics such as grunts, barks,sniffs etc.

TRUANCY — Absence from school without permission.

VANDALISM — Willful defacement or destruction of property.

VEGITATIVE LEVEL — State of deterioration in which the patient is immobile, out of contact with the environment, unresponsive to questioning and ultimately has to be fed and toileted.

WALK IN CLINICS — Patient/client can walk in any time of the day or night for professional help.

WITHDRAWAL SYMPTOM — It is an organic mental disorder following stopping or reduction in theintake of a substance such as alcohol, opioids etc.

WITHDRAWN BEHAVIOUR — It is an attempt in which the patient tries to avoid social interaction.

LIST OF REFERENCES

Augilera D.C., & Messick J.H. *Crisis Intervention Theory and Methodology*. (Fourth Edition). St. Louis : The C.V. Mosby Co: (1982, p.65).

Almedia E.M., & Chapman, *The Interpersonal Basis of Psychiatric Nursing*. G.P. Putnam's Sons, New York (1972).

Beck, Rawlins and Williams. *Mental Health Psychiatric Nursing — A Holistic Life Cycle Approach*. (Second Edition), The C.V. Mosby Company, Toronto (1988).

Berlo, D.K. *The Process of Communication*. Holt, Rinehart and Winston, New York (1963).

Bimla Kapoor. *A Textbook of Psychiatic Nursing,* Vol. I Kumar Publishing House, Delhi, (1992).

Calvin S. Hall. *A Primer of Freudian Psychology*. New American Library, New York, Ontario (1979).

Cavener, J. & Brodie H.K. *Signs and Symptoms in Psychiatry* J.B. Lippincott, Philadelphia.

Coleman James C. *Abnormal Psychology and Modern Life* (Fifth Edition), Scott, Foresman and Company, Glenview, Illinois (1976).

Goldenson, R.M. *Longman Dictionary of Psychology and Psychiatry*. New York (1984).

Haderson and Gillespie's. *Textbook of Psychiatry for Students and Practioners* (Tenth Edition), Oxford, University Press, London (1974).

John A.; Reberira, Buckle D. *The Nurse in Mental Health Practice*. Report on Technical Conference, WHO, Geneva (1963).

Johnson Barbara Schoen. *Adaptation and Growth : Psychiatric Mental Health Nursing*. J.B. Lippincott Company, Philadelphia (1989).

Kalkman M.E. & Davis A.J. *New Dimensions in Mental Health Psychiatric Nursing* (Fourth Edition). McGraw Hill Book Company, New York (1974).

Karnosh L.J. and Mereness, R.V. *Essentials of Psychiatric Nursing* (Sixth Fdition), English Language Book Society (1985).

Kaplan H.L., Sadock B.J. *Comprehensive Textbook of Psychiatry* (Fifth Edition), Vol. I &II, Williams and Wilkins, Baltimore (1989).

Keys. J. and Hoffling C.K. *Basic Psychiatric concepts in Nursing*. (Fourth Edition), J.B. Lippincott Company (1980).

Kolb L.C. and Brodie H.K.M. *Modern Clinical Psychiatry* (Tenth Edition), W.B. Saunders

Company. Philadephia (1982).

Lego Suzanne. ***The American Handbook of Psychiatric Nursing.*** J.B. Lippincott Company, Philadephia (1984).

Mitchell R.G. ***Essential Psychiatric Nursing.*** Churchil Living Stone, New York (1986).

Park, J.E. and Park, K. ***Textbook of Preventive and Social Medicine,*** (Thirteenth Edition), J.B. Lippincott Company, Philadelphia (1990).

Sharma, S. ***Mental Hospitals in India,*** DGHS, New Delhi (1990).

Shives, L.R. ***Basic Concepts of Psychiatric Mental Health Nursing.*** (Second Edition) J.B. Lippincott Company, Philadelphia (1990).

Soloman P. & Patch V. ***Handbook of Psychiatry.*** J.B. Lippincott Company, philadelphia (1985).

Symposium on Suicide- Medico pastrol Association-Pottery Road, Moorthy Press, Bangalore, India.

Taylor C. M. ***Essentials of Psychiatric Nursing.*** (Eleventh Edition), The C.V. Mosby Company, London (1982).

The American Nruse's Association. ***Standards, Psychiatric Mental Health Practices.*** ANA, 2420 Pershing Road, Kansas City, Missouri 64108 (1973).

Topalis M. and Matheny R. ***Psychitric Nursing*** (Fifth Edition). The C.V. Mosby Company (1970).

Travelbee Joyce. ***Intervention in Psychiatric Nursing Process in the One-to-one Relationship*** (Ninth Edition), F.A. Davis Company, Philadelphia (1976).

Tripathi K.D. ***Essentials of Medical Pharmacology.*** Jaypee Brothers House, Delhi (1990).

Walker, J.J. ***Essentials of Clinical Psychiatry.*** J.B. Lippincott Company, London (1985).

Wilson H.S., Kneisl C.S. ***Psychiatric Nursing*** (Second Edition), Addison Wesley Publishing Company, Nursing Division, California (1983).

World Health Organization. ***Organization of Mental Health Services in Developing Countries.*** WHO Technical Report Series No. 564, 31-36 (1975).

World Health Organization. ***The ICD-10 Classification of Mental and Behavioural Disorders. Clinical Descriptionand Diagnostic Guidelines,*** Geneva, WHO (1992).

INDEX

F

G

H

I

READER'S OPINION

1. Did you have any difficulty in understanding the language?

   Yes ....

   No ....

   If yes, mention the page and paragraph numbers where you had difficulty

   Page No. ....

   Para No. ....

2. Did the material in the study guide help you in achiving the objective mentioned in the begining of each unit?

   ....

   ....

3. Did you try the better study section questions?

   a) If yes, give your suggestions

   ....

   (i) What it easy?

   (ii) Was it difficult?

4. Did you take the assignment?

   Yes ....

   No ....

   a) Was the assignment helpful?

   b) Mention the assignment which was helpful ....

5. Did the chapter test help you in doing review?

   Give your comments.

   ....

   ....

6. Would you like to add anything in the chapter to learn the subject better.

   ....

   ....

Students are advised to fill up the above mentioned form and send it at the following address :

Dr. Bimla Kapoor

(Director and Professor)

School of Health Science IGNOU

Maidan Garhi, New Delhi.